Acupuncture in Clinical Practice

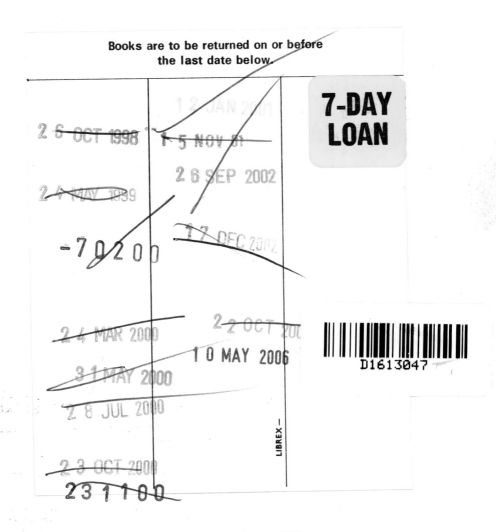

Acupuncture in Clinical Practice

A practical guide to the use of acupuncture and related therapies

Bai Xinghua MD
Lecturer in Acupuncture, Beijing College of Acupuncture and Moxibustion,
Beijing, People's Republic of China

English Consultant

RB Baron

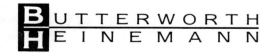

Butterworth-Heinemann
Linacre House, Jordan Hill, Oxford OX2 8DP
A division of Reed Educational & Professional Publishing Ltd

A member of the Reed Elsevier plc group

OXFORD   BOSTON   JOHANNESBURG
MELBOURNE   NEW DELHI   SINGAPORE

First published 1996

© Reed Educational & Professional Publishing Ltd 1996

British Library Cataloguing in Publication Data
A catalogue record for this book is available from the British Library.

Library of Congress Cataloguing in Publication Data
A catalogue record for this book is available from the Library of Congress.

ISBN 0 7506 2670 4

Composition by Genesis Typesetting, Rochester
Printed and bound in Great Britain by The Bath Press, Somerset

Contents

Acknowledgements		viii
Preface		ix
About the authors		x
Introduction		xi
Treatment of diseases and disorders		1
1	Abnormal fetal position	3
2	Acne vulgaris	3
3	Acute gastroenteritis	5
4	Acute intestinal obstruction	6
5	Acute mastitis	8
6	Acute soft tissue injury	10
7	Acute tonsillitis	11
8	Alcohol withdrawal	13
9	Allergic rhinitis	14
10	Alopecia areata	16
11	Amenorrhoea	17
12	Angina pectoris	19
13	Appendicitis	20
14	Arrhythmia	22
15	Bacillary dysentery	24
16	*Bi* syndrome	25
17	Brandy nose	29
18	Bronchial asthma	29
19	Calcaneodynia	32
20	Cardiac neurosis	33
21	Central retinitis	35
22	Cervical spondylopathy	36
23	Childhood anorexia	38
24	Childhood hyperkinetic syndrome	40
25	Chloasma	41
26	Cholecystitis	41
27	Cholelithiasis	43
28	Chronic bronchitis	45
29	Chronic diarrhoea	48
30	Chronic pelvic inflammatory disease	49
31	Chronic pharyngitis	51
32	Competition syndrome	52
33	Constipation	53
34	Costal chondritis	55
35	Cutaneous pruritus	56
36	Cystic hyperplasia of the breast	58
37	Cystitis	59
38	Developmental disability	61
39	Diabetes mellitus	62
40	*Dian* and *kuang* syndromes	64
41	Drug withdrawal	66
42	Dysfunction of the temporomandibular joint	68
43	Dysfunctional uterine bleeding	68
44	Dysmenorrhoea	70
45	Eczema	72
46	Epidemic keratoconjunctivitis	74
47	Epididymitis	75
48	Epilepsy	77
49	Epistaxis	80
50	Erythromelalgia	82
51	External humeral epicondylitis	83
52	Facial spasm	84
53	Female infertility	86
54	Flat wart	88
55	Furunculosis	89
56	Gastritis	90
57	Gastrointestinal neurosis	93

58	Gastroptosis	95
59	Habitual miscarriage	96
60	Headache	97
61	Haemorrhoids	100
62	Herpes zoster	102
63	Hiccups	103
64	High fever	105
65	Hypertension	106
66	Hyperthyroidism	108
67	Hysteria	110
68	Impotence	112
69	Influenza	114
70	Insufficient lactation	115
71	Intercostal neuralgia	116
72	*Jue* syndrome	117
73	Leukorrhagia	120
74	Lochiorrhagia	122
75	Lumbar muscle strain	123
76	Malaria	124
77	Male infertility	126
78	Meniere's disease	128
79	Menopausal syndrome	130
80	Morning sickness	132
81	Motion sickness	133
82	Mumps	134
83	Myocarditis	135
84	Myopia	137
85	Neurodermatitis	139
86	Neurosism	141
87	Nocturnal enuresis	143
88	Obesity	144
89	Otitis media suppurativa	146
90	Pancreatitis	147
91	Paralytic strabismus	149
92	Parkinson's disease	150
93	Peptic ulcer	152

94	Peripheral facial paralysis	154
95	Phantom limb pain	156
96	Pharyngeal paraesthesia	157
97	Postconcussional syndrome	158
98	Postpartum uterine contractions	159
99	Premenstrual syndrome	160
100	Prolapse of the uterus	162
101	Prostatitis	164
102	Ptosis	165
103	Raynaud's disease	166
104	Recurrent ulcer of the mouth	167
105	Retention of placenta	169
106	Retention of urine	170
107	Scapulohumeral periarthritis	172
108	Sciatica	174
109	Seborrhoeic dermatitis	176
110	Seminal emission	177
111	Sequelae of cerebrovascular accident	179
112	Simple glaucoma	182
113	Stiff neck	183
114	Stye	184
115	Suppurative nasal sinusitis	185
116	Thecal cyst	187
117	Thromboangiitis obliterans	188
118	Tinnitus and hearing loss	190
119	Tobacco withdrawal	192
120	Toothache	193
121	Trigeminal neuralgia	194
122	Urinary stones	196
123	Urticaria	199
124	Vomiting	200
125	*Wei* syndrome	202

Appendices: Details of therapies and techniques   207

Appendix 1 The 14 meridians and their acupuncture points   209

Appendix 2 Extraordinary acupuncture
              points   219
Appendix 3 Auricular therapy   227
Appendix 4 Blood-letting puncturing   242
Appendix 5 Chiropractic   244
Appendix 6 Cupping   245
Appendix 7 Electroacupuncture   248
Appendix 8 Hot salt compress therapy   250
Appendix 9 Point implantation therapy   251

Appendix 10 Point injection therapy   253
Appendix 11 Scalp acupuncture   255

Glossary   260

Bibliography   263

Useful addresses   264

Index   267

Acknowledgements

I am very grateful to my English language consultant, RB Baron of Albion, California, USA, who provided unfailing support and encouragement, as well as revising, editing, and computerizing the entire manuscript.

I am also grateful to have received the very professional support and advice of Mary Seager and Claire Hutchins of Butterworth-Heinemann, Oxford, UK.

My thanks to Liu Xiaoyan, who revised the transliterated spelling of the Chinese acupuncture points; and to Li Nan, who drew the exquisite illustrations for the book.

RB and I would also like to thank Cynthia J. Huang, Jim Wilcox and Allison Wolfe for their professional and moral support during the preparation of the manuscript.

Finally, my grateful thanks to my wife, Cheng Xiaoli. Without her loving support and dedication, it would have been impossible to publish this book.

Preface

Acupuncture has a long history in China. Its influence is felt in the lives of all Chinese people. I remember when I was a little boy I saw my mother punctured with many needles. This seemed so cruel and ruthless that it made a very deep impression on me. Now I know that acupuncture is a miracle of medical history, ranking alongside the four great inventions of ancient China: gunpowder, the compass, paper making, and printing.

The question that often occurs to me now is how this invasive therapeutic method arose so naturally in ancient times that there is no definitive record of its origins. It is as if its principles and applications sprang forth full blown from nature. An answer to this mystery may be found in a popular Chinese legend.

It is said that during the Wudi period (the earliest recorded Chinese civilization, around 2600–2200 B.C.), severe flooding spread over the country and brought great disaster to the people. Emperor Yao appointed his minister Gun to harness the river and control the flood. Gun's attempts to obstruct the flood by erecting dykes and dams failed. Gun's son, Yu, was appointed by the next emperor, Shun, to continue his father's work. Drawing a lesson from his father's failure, Yu dredged canals according to the physical features of the terrain to lead the water to the sea. After thirteen years of hard work, the floods subsided. Up until the present, Yu is still praised for his contributions and the excellence of his moral character.

It is reasonable to deduce that the ancient Chinese invented acupuncture based on the correspondence between the microcosm (the human body) and the macrocosm (the universe). They compared the meridians of the human body to the earth's rivers, and the *qi* and blood flowing through the meridians to the rivers' waters. They then activated the meridians by puncturing with needles to remove obstructions and promote the flow of *qi* and blood, just as they dredged the rivers to manage the flood.

I offer this book as a compass, in the hope that it may guide you in your navigation of the rivers and seas of the body during your practice of acupuncture and related therapies.

Bai Xinghua
Lecturer of Acupuncture and Moxibustion
Beijing College of Acupuncture and Moxibustion

About the Authors

Bai Xinghua was born in a small village in North East China in 1964. He completed his Bachelor's degree in Medicine in 1986 and his Master's degree in Acupuncture (at the Beijing College of Traditional Chinese Medicine) in 1989. He has been working as a lecturer and acupuncturist since 1989. He is a member of the Chinese Association of Acupuncture and Moxibustion and he has published numerous articles and books on the subject of Traditional Chinese Medicine, the most recent of which is 'Chinese Auricular Therapy and Practical Auricular Point and Area Map' (Scientific and Technical Documents Publishing House, Beijing 1994).

R.B. Baron, of Albion, California, USA, received her Bachelor's degree in Modern Chinese History from the University of California-Santa Cruz in 1991. She has been living in Shanghai and Beijing since 1991, where she has translated a range of scientific and literary materials. She first collaborated with Dr. Bai on his recent book, *Chinese Auricular Therapy and Practical Auricular Point and Area Map.*

Introduction

Although the development of science and technology has brought great progress in diagnostic techniques, modern medicine still provides no effective treatment for many diseases and disorders. More importantly, many modern drugs have been found to have severe iatrogenic side effects. As a result, traditional Chinese medicine (TCM), with a history stretching over 5000 years, is gaining an increasing international recognition and welcome. The wide indications, effectiveness, safety, simplicity and economy of acupuncture and other traditional drugless therapies such as moxibustion, cupping and auricular therapy offer ideal treatment for a wide range of diseases and disorders.

Acupuncture in Clinical Practice is a practical handbook for practitioners of acupuncture and related traditional Chinese therapies, including auricular therapy, blood-letting puncturing, chiropractic, cupping, electroacupuncture, hot salt compress therapy, moxibustion, point implantation therapy, point injection therapy and scalp acupuncture. The core of the book is an alphabetical guide to the treatment of 125 diseases and disorders of internal and surgical medicine, gynaecology, paediatrics, dermatology and the sensory organs as well as miscellaneous problems. For each condition the guide discusses the aetiology, differentiation and treatment using the various therapies. Technical details of the therapies are given in the 11 appendices which follow and the book concludes with a glossary of major terms, a bibliography and a list of contact addresses for those wishing to further their interest and involvement in the practice of acupuncture and related therapies.

In the treatment guide, for each disease and disorder, prominence is given to the three factors which most directly influence therapeutic results, i.e. **correct differentiation of syndromes**, **accurate selection of points** and **selection of appropriate therapies**. Syndromes are differentiated on the basis of thorough diagnosis according to the principles of traditional Chinese medicine. Points are selected according to differentiation of syndromes, and appropriate therapies are then chosen according to syndrome or condition. When this process is followed, the arrow of treatment will unerringly strike the target of disease or disorder.

Differentiation of syndromes

Syndrome (*zheng* in Chinese) is a special term used in traditional Chinese medicine. Syndromes are determined by analysing the symptoms and signs of a disease or disorder at various stages of its course in accordance with the meridian, *zangfu* and Eight Principles theories of TCM. Correct differentiation of syndromes can determine the position, nature, development and prognosis of the condition at each of its stages, and is essential for effective treatment.

It is well known that patients with the same disease, or even a patient during different stages of the course of a disease, may present different syndromes due to differences in age, sex, constitution, season, etc. For instance, the common cold is classified into wind-cold and wind-heat types; wind-cold type is further classified into excessive and deficient syndromes. A person who has a cold may present Taiyang, Shaoyang and Yangming syndromes at different stages of its course. In this situation, *different syndromes of the same disease* should be treated using different and appropriate methods, based on the patient's particular circumstances. For example, for a common cold of the wind-cold type, wind-cold is expelled; for a common cold of the wind-heat type, wind is expelled and heat dispelled. For a common cold of the deficient type, antipathogenic *qi* is strengthened; for a common cold of the excessive type, exogenous pathogens are eliminated.

On the other hand, patients with different diseases may present the same syndrome. For instance, hyperactivity of the liver *yang* is a common syndrome of various diseases including glaucoma, hypertension, and Meniere's disease. When treating *different diseases with the same syndrome*, an accurate diagnosis should first be established according to differences in aetiology and pathology. The syndrome should then be differentiated according to the theories of traditional Chinese medicine.

Accurate differentiation of syndromes is one of the most difficult skills for practitioners of TCM to master. However, syndromes are relatively consistent despite the complexity of a disease's manifestations. Standardization of syndromes will be very helpful to students of TCM. This guidebook standardizes the syndromes of 125 diseases and disorders according to the author's experience, as well as that of other practitioners, in order to allow students more easily to master differentiation of the syndromes and build a strong foundation for accurate diagnosis and effective treatment.

Selection of appropriate points

Acupuncture points are like herbs. Each has its own properties. Selecting acupuncture points is similar to prescribing herbal medicine; good results in acupuncture and other traditional drugless therapies are dependent on choosing the proper points to be treated.

A typical acupuncture prescription usually includes three different kinds of points: local, distal and points that are clinically effective for treating specific symptoms. The three types of points may be used singly or in combination.

Any local point can be used to treat local problems. For instance, Yingxiang (LI20) is used for treating nasal problems; Xiyan (Ex20) is used for problems of the knee.

Distal points are selected according to meridian theory. The meridians, which connect the upper to the lower and the inside with the outside, unify the human body into an organic whole. Therefore, points on the lower part of the body can be used to treat problems of the upper part. This is especially true for points below the elbows and knees. For instance, the Large Intestine meridian connects with the teeth, so Hegu (LI4), the *yuan* (source) point of the Large Intestine meridian, is an important distal point for treating toothache. The Stomach meridian connects internally with the stomach, so Zusanli (S36), the *he* (sea) and lower *he* (confluent) point of the Stomach meridian, is the most important distal point for treating stomach problems.

Many points have been proven through clinical experience to be effective for treating specific symptoms. For example, Dazhui (Du14), the meeting point of the Du meridian and the Hand and Foot Yang meridians, functions to dispel heat and expel exogenous pathogens, so it is one of the most important points for treating high fever and the common cold. Fenglong (S40), the *luo* (collateral) point of the Stomach meridian, functions to strengthen the spleen and stomach and eliminate phlegm, so it is widely used for treatment of diseases caused by accumulation of pathogenic phlegm, such as *dian* and *kuang* syndromes and epilepsy.

Selection of appropriate therapies

It is said that necessity is the mother of invention. Numerous traditional therapies have been developed according to local requirements over the course of TCM's 5000 year history. It is recorded in *The Classic of Medicine* that various therapies evolved regionally, since people living in different areas usually suffer from different kinds of diseases and disorders according to varying climate, diet, and living conditions. For instance, people in eastern China, who live near the sea, eat a lot of seafood and salt, which may produce heat in the interior and consume the blood. Accordingly, puncturing using stone needles (*bianshi*, a cuneiform needle which originated in the Neolithic Age), an ideal method for discharging pus and blood to cure carbuncles and furuncles, was developed in this area. The nomadic people of the north, where it is very cold, are constantly moving in search of new pastures and drink a lot of milk, so they are susceptible to invasion of exogenous wind and abdominal distension. Therefore moxibustion, which functions to expel cold and warm the body, was developed in this area.

Each therapy presented in this guide has certain advantages. It is very important to select the appropriate therapy in each case in order to attain the best therapeutic results. In some cases, it is suggested that several methods be used either consecutively or in combination, according to the characteristics of the therapies and the condition of the disease or disorder.

Clinically, the primary difference between modern pharmacotherapy and traditional drugless therapies, especially acupuncture, lies in the method of treatment. In modern medicine, the doctor prescribes medicine and the patient takes it. This limited interaction is not sufficient in acupuncture, in which practitioners not only prescribe points but also puncture and stimulate them throughout the course of treatment. Therefore, in addition to correct differentiation of syndromes, accurate selection of points and selection of appropriate therapies, the following aspects should also be emphasized when using acupuncture.

Accurate location of points

When disease or disorder is present in the body, there will usually be positive signs such as tenderness, eminence, scleroma, or angiectasis present on or near points corresponding or related to the area of the problem. The positive signs may be found precisely on acupuncture points determined according to proportional measurement or anatomical landmarks; however, in many cases location may vary slightly. For example, Yanglingquan (G34), the *he* (sea) and lower *he* (confluent) point of the Gallbladder meridian, is an important point for treating gallbladder problems. However, the tender point in cases of gallbladder problems such as cholecystitis and cholelithiasis is usually found about 0.8–1.2 *cun* below the theoretical position of Yanglingquan (G34).

It is therefore necessary to detect positive signs by means of palpation and inspection in order to determine the exact location of points corresponding to the problem being treated. *Neijing, the Classic of Medicine*, recommends first pressing the point and only puncturing it if the patient feels sensations of tenderness or relief. This is especially important when puncturing specific body points such as back-*shu* points, *he* points and auricular points.

Concentration of the mind

Acupuncture is not a purely physical therapy. Acupuncture consists of the application of needles to stimulate and balance the meridian *qi* in order to treat diseases and disorders. The power of the will, unique to human beings, is essential to this process. In *qigong*, the practice of the mental control of *qi*, *qi* can be directed along the meridians by will alone. Acupuncture also makes use of the mind's ability to control the flow of *qi*. *The Classic of Medicine* states that the key to

acupuncture is first to regulate the mind. The practitioner should visualize holding the needle as if it were a tiger or dragon, while deeply experiencing the flow of *qi* and carefully observing the patient's reactions. The patient should cultivate positive belief and confidence in the efficacy of the treatment, while concentrating the mind on the needling sensation in the affected area. A quiet and comfortable environment will help both patient and practitioner better to concentrate their minds.

Individual differences

Acupuncture stimulates the flow of *qi* and a needling sensation in affected areas of the body in order to dispel pathogens and rebalance the normal functions. Because each person responds differently to acupuncture, the human factor plays an important role in this process. For instance, it is well known that people have differing levels of sensitivity to the transmission of *qi*. People who are sensitive will have much better therapeutic results than those who are not. Additionally, the needling sensation one person experiences may vary when the same point is punctured by another practitioner. This not only reflects differences in the practitioners' skill, but also indicates that the transmission of *qi* experienced by the patient is related to innate qualities of the individual practitioner. An article in *The Classic of Medicine* called 'Appoint Occupations According to Ability' states that people selected for training in acupuncture and moxibustion should be soft-spoken, contained, skilful and attentive.

Precautions

Of course, the practitioner must be reponsible for strictly sterilizing needles between patients to prevent the possible transmission of blood-borne diseases such as hepatitis or AIDS. Patients should also take responsibility for protecting their own health by verifying with the practitioner prior to treatment that the needles have been sterilized.

Treatment of diseases and disorders

1 Abnormal fetal position

Abnormal fetal position refers to all fetal positions other than normal occipitoanterior position, including occipitotransverse and occipitoposterior positions and breech, footling and compound presentation. It is a primary cause of difficult labour. Various factors may result in abnormal fetal position, including deformity of the pelvis or uterus, fetal abnormality, placenta previa and flaccidity of the abdominal muscles.

Aetiology and differentiation of syndromes

Traditional Chinese medicine classifies abnormal fetal position as difficult labour, and considers it to be caused either by deficiency or stagnation of the *qi* and blood. There are usually no additional symptoms accompanying abnormal fetal position.

Treatment

Moxibustion

Acupuncture point:

Zhiyin   (B67)

Both the uterus and the urinary bladder are located in the lower abdomen and connect either directly or indirectly with the Chong and Ren meridians. Zhiyin (B67), the *jing* (well) point of the Urinary Bladder meridian, is the meeting point of the Urinary Bladder and Kidney meri-

dians. The classical literature of traditional Chinese medicine cites numerous cases of successful treatment of difficult labour due to abnormal fetal position by the application of moxibustion to Zhiyin (B67). Many modern reports also indicate that this method is a very safe and effective method of correcting abnormal fetal position to facilitate delivery.

Treatment with moxibustion should be started during the seventh or eighth month of pregnancy. The recipient should empty the bladder, loosen clothing and sit with the feet on a low stool. Apply moxa roll moxibustion to bilateral Zhiyin (B67) for 10–15 minutes, once a day. Four treatments constitute one course.

Reexamine 24 hours after each treatment and every day for three days following correction of abnormal fetal position, then once a week until delivery. Start a new course of treatment in the event of relapse.

Remarks

- Moxibustion is very effective for correcting abnormal fetal position. In many cases, two or three treatments are sufficient.
- Moxibustion is not suitable for correcting abnormal fetal position due to uterine deformity, fetal abnormality, or narrow pelvis.
- This method may not be applied in cases of habitual premature labour or toxaemia of pregnancy.

2 Acne vulgaris

Acne vulgaris is a common problem of adolescence. It is caused by hypersteatosis combined with proliferation and hyperkeratosis of the epithelia of the follicular orifices, leading to accumulation of sebum cutaneum and subsequent bacterial infection. Primarily affected are the face and chest. Skin lesions include pimples, pustules, scleroma and cysts.

Aetiology and differentiation of syndromes

According to traditional Chinese medicine, acne vulgaris is caused either by exogenous wind-heat invading the lungs or by overindulgence in spicy or greasy food, resulting in accumulation of heat in the stomach and intestines. There are usually no general symptoms accompanying localized manifestations.

Treatment

Body acupuncture

Main acupuncture points:

Quchi	(LI11)
Hegu	(LI4)
Zusanli	(S36)
Xuehai	(Sp10)
Sanyinjiao	(Sp6)
Feishu	(B13)

Quchi (LI11) and Hegu (LI4), the *he* (sea) and *yuan* (source) points respectively of the Large Intestine meridian, are punctured to regulate the stomach and intestines and dispel heat. Zusanli (S36), the *he* (sea) and lower *he* (confluent) point of the Stomach meridian, functions to activate the meridians and regulate the stomach and intestines. Xuehai (Sp10) (Sea of Blood in Chinese) is one of the most important points for treating skin conditions. Sanyinjiao (Sp6), the meeting point of the three Foot Yin meridians, functions to strengthen the liver and spleen. The lungs function to nourish the skin, so Feishu (B13), the back-*shu* point of the lungs, is punctured to regulate the lungs and expel wind-heat. This point is usually pricked with a three-edged needle and then cupped for 15–20 minutes to draw blood.

Auxiliary points are chosen according to meridian theory:

- For skin lesions of the face, Sibai (S2), Xiaguan (S7), Jiache (S6), and Zanzhu (B2) are added.
- For skin lesions of the chest, Danzhong (Ren17) and Jianjing (G21) are added.
- For skin lesions of the back, Dazhui (Du14), Fengchi (G20), and Fengmen (B12) are added.

All points are punctured using the reducing method, once a day or once every other day. Ten treatments constitute one course.

Electroacupuncture

Points used are the same as for body acupuncture. Select one or two pairs of points each time. Puncture until a needling sensation is achieved; then connect the needles to an electrical stimulator. Apply continuous wave stimulation of the highest bearable intensity for 20–30 minutes, once a day or once every other day. Ten treatments constitute one course.

Blood-letting puncturing

Acupuncture points:

Dazhui	(Du14)
Feishu	(B13)
Geshu	(B17)
Dachangshu	(B25)
Weizhong	(B40)

Select one or two points each time. Prick with a three-edged needle, then cup for 10–15 minutes to draw blood. Treat once every other day. This method is usually used in conjunction with other therapies to increase stimulation.

Auricular therapy

Main auricular points:

Areas corresponding to the affected regions: tap with a plum blossom needle to cause bleeding.

Lung: expels wind.

Stomach, Large Intestine: dispel heat from the stomach and intestines.

Endocrine, Midpoint of Rim, Adrenal Gland: regulate endocrine function to relieve inflammation.

Apex of Ear: blood-letting puncturing of this point with a three-edged needle dispels heat.

Auxiliary auricular points:

For itching, Heart, Ear Shenmen and Centre of Ear are added.

Use auricular taping with strong manipulation and blood-letting puncturing where indicated, twice a week. Five treatments constitute one course.

Remarks

- ☯ Traditional therapies are effective for treating acne vulgaris; two or more therapies are usually combined to increase stimulation.
- ☯ The patient should eat less fatty and oily foods and more fruit and vegetables to regulate the bowel function.
- ☯ The patient should wash the skin with soft soap or sulphur soap to cleanse cutaneous sebum.

3 Acute gastroenteritis

Acute gastroenteritis is an acute inflammation of the intestines caused by overindulgence in food or alcohol or consumption of contaminated food, occurring mainly in the summer and autumn. It is characterized by sudden onset of abdominal pain, diarrhoea and vomiting. Dilute or watery stool may be passed ten or more times each day. In cases with severe vomiting, disturbance of the electrolyte balance with subsequent lowered blood pressure or muscle spasms may occur.

Aetiology

Traditional Chinese medicine classifies acute gastroenteritis as diarrhoea. It is considered to be caused primarily by either invasion of the intestines by damp-heat, overindulgence in food or alcohol, or consumption of contaminated food, resulting in dysfunction of the stomach and intestines so that liquid and solid cannot be separated and diarrhoea occurs.

Differentiation of syndromes

- Acute gastroenteritis due to attack on the stomach and intestines by pathogenic cold.
  Characterized by sudden onset of nausea, vomiting, abdominal pain, and diarrhoea; accompanied by chills, headache, feeling of cold in the hands and feet, greasy whitish tongue coating and tense pulse
- Acute gastroenteritis due to invasion of the stomach and intestines by pathogenic damp-heat.
  Characterized by fetid vomiting, abdominal pain, foul smelling diarrhoea, burning sensation in the anus, fever, thirst, scanty yellowish urine, greasy yellowish tongue coating and rapid slippery pulse.
- Acute gastroenteritis due to damage of the stomach and intestines by improper diet.
  Characterized by abdominal pain alleviated following defecation, eructation with fetid odour, nausea, vomiting, sulphurous smelling diarrhoea, thick greasy tongue coating and slippery pulse.

Treatment

Body acupuncture

Main acupuncture points:

Tianshu	(S25)
Shangjuxu	(S37)
Zusanli	(S36)

Tianshu (S25) and Shangjuxu (S37), the front-*mu* point of the large intestine and lower *he* (confluent) point of the Large Intestine meridian respectively, are treated in combination to strengthen the large intestine's function of transportation. These points are used for treating all problems of the large intestine. Zusanli (S36), the *he* (sea) and lower *he* (confluent) point of the Stomach meridian, functions to regulate both the stomach and intestines.

Auxiliary points and appropriate methods of manipulation are selected according to differentiation of syndromes.

- For acute gastroenteritis due to attack on the stomach and intestines by pathogenic cold, moxibustion is added on Tianshu (S25) and Shenque (Ren8) to warm the meridians and expel cold.
- For acute gastroenteritis due to invasion of the stomach and intestines by pathogenic damp-heat, Chize (L5) and Weizhong (B40) are added and pricked with a three-edged needle, then cupped for 10–15 minutes to dispel damp-heat.
- For acute gastroenteritis due to damage of the stomach and intestines by improper diet, Neiguan (P6) and Gongsun (Sp4) are added and punctured using the reducing method to strengthen the stomach and spleen.
- For cases with severe vomiting, Neiguan (P6) is added and punctured using the reducing method to subdue rebellious rising of the stomach *qi* and stop vomiting.

Treat once or twice a day. Five treatments constitute one course.

Auricular therapy

Auricular points:

Stomach, Large Intestine, Abdomen: correspond to the affected areas of the body; regulate the functions of the stomach and large and small intestines.

Spleen: the spleen governs transportation and transformation of water and dampness, so Spleen is treated to strengthen the spleen and eliminate dampness.

Sympathesis: alleviates spasm of the smooth muscles to relieve pain.

Ear Shenmen, Occiput: tranquillize the mind and relieve pain.

Apex of Ear: blood-letting puncturing of this point with a three-edged needle relieves inflammation and pain.

Use auricular taping and blood-letting puncturing where indicated, once a day or once every other day. Five treatments constitute one course.

Remarks

☯ Both body acupuncture and auricular therapy are very effective for treating acute gastroenteritis; in most cases there will be great improvement in such symptoms as diarrhoea, abdominal pain and vomiting after only one or two treatments.
☯ In cases with severe disturbance of the water/electrolyte balance, concurrent emergency measures should be undertaken.

4 Acute intestinal obstruction

Acute intestinal obstruction, or acute ileus, is a commonly seen acute abdominal condition. It is classified into the following types:

● Mechanical intestinal obstruction, due to organic diseases such as internal or external hernia, intestinal adhesion, cancer of the intestinal wall, twisted bowel, intussusception or congenital malformation of the intestines. These conditions can create stricture of the intestines which affects transportation of material in the intestines.
● Dynamic intestinal obstruction, subclassified into two types:
  – Paralytic intestinal obstruction, due to abdominal surgery, peritonitis, spinal cord injury, retroperitoneal haematoma or inflammation, or colicky abdominal pain, leading to temporary loss of peristalsis which affects transportation of material in the intestines.
  – Spastic intestinal obstruction, due to foreign objects in the intestines, irritating food or lead poisoning, with resulting enterospasm which affects transportation of material in the intestines.
● Angiomesenteric intestinal obstruction, caused by mesenteric embolism or thrombosis, with resulting disturbance of blood circulation to the intestines which affects transportation of mate-

rial in the intestines. Acute ileus is marked by pain and distension in the abdomen, vomiting and lack of defecation with flatus. Additional physical signs include borborygmi, visible intestinal peristalsis and peristaltic wave.

Aetiology

Traditional Chinese medicine classifies acute intestinal obstruction as *guange* (obstruction and rejection in Chinese). Primarily affected is the large intestine. According to the *The Classic of Medicine*, the large intestine is one of the six hollow *fu* organs and controls the transportation of waste materials out of the body following digestion. Dysfunction may result from obstruction by foreign bodies, depletion of bodily fluid, stagnation of *qi* and blood, or toxic pathogens.

Differentiation of syndromes

● Acute intestinal obstruction of the excessive heat type.
  Characterized by paroxysmal abdominal colic, nausea, fetid vomit, abdominal distension and lack of defecation with flatus; accompanied by fever, dry mouth, desire for cold drinks, scanty

yellowish urine, dark red tongue with thick coating and slippery wiry or full rapid pulse.
- Acute intestinal obstruction due to contraction of the intestines by pathogenic cold.
  Characterized by abdominal pain and distension with paroxysmal exacerbation, aggravated by cold and alleviated by warmth; watery vomit, lack of defecation with flatus; accompanied by aversion to cold, feeling of cold in the abdomen and extremities, thick whitish tongue coating and tense wiry pulse.
- Acute intestinal obstruction due to stagnation of *qi*.
  Characterized by severe abdominal distension with intermittent and unfixed pain aggravated by pressure; vomiting, lack of defecation with flatus; accompanied by feeling of fullness in the chest, greasy whitish tongue coating and wiry pulse.
- Acute intestinal obstruction due to stagnation of blood.
  Characterized by persistent severe stabbing pain in the abdomen aggravated by pressure; possible mass, vomiting; scanty stool resembling coffee grounds or lack of defecation with flatus; dark red or purple-spotted tongue and uneven pulse.
- Acute intestinal obstruction due to deficiency of *qi*.
  Characterized by severe distension of the entire abdomen; vomiting, lack of defecation with flatus; accompanied by pale complexion, shortness of breath, lassitude, profuse perspiration, pale tongue with whitish coating and weak pulse.
- Acute intestinal obstruction due to depletion of the bodily fluid.
  Characterized by abdominal distension and pain; nausea, vomiting and lack of defecation with flatus; accompanied by dizziness, blurred vision, dry mouth, dry whitish or yellowish tongue coating and soft pulse.

Treatment

Body acupuncture

Main acupuncture points:

Tianshu	(S25)
Dachangshu	(B25)
Shangjuxu	(S37)
Zusanli	(S36)
Daheng	(Sp15)
Neiguan	(P6)

The main pathogenesis of acute intestinal obstruction is blockage of the large intestine. Tianshu (S25) and Dachangshu (B25), the front-*mu* and back-*shu* points respectively of the large intestine and Shangjuxu (S37), the lower *he* (confluent) point of the Large Intestine meridian, are treated in combination to promote peristalsis and remove obstruction. Zusanli (S36), the *he* (sea) and lower *he* (confluence) point of the Stomach meridian, is the most important point for treating gastrointestinal problems. Daheng (Sp15), located on the bilateral sides of the abdomen, is a local point for treating intestinal obstruction. Neiguan (P6), the *luo* (collateral) point of the Pericardium meridian and one of the eight confluence points connecting with the Yinwei meridian, functions to subdue rebellious rising of the stomach *qi* and arrest vomiting.

Auxiliary points and appropriate methods of manipulation are chosen according to differentiation of syndromes.

- For acute intestinal obstruction of the excessive heat type, heat is expelled by adding and puncturing Hegu (LI4), Dazhui (Du14) and Zhigou (SJ6) using the reducing method, or pricking Dazhui (Du14) with a three-edged needle and then cupping for 10–15 minutes to draw blood.
- For acute intestinal obstruction due to contraction of the intestines by pathogenic cold, the intestines are warmed and cold expelled by adding and puncturing Guanyuan (Ren4) and main points using heat-producing manipulation, and applying moxibustion as needed. Shenque (Ren8) is added but not punctured; only moxibustion is applied.
- For acute intestinal obstruction due to stagnation of *qi*, Zhongwan (Ren12) is added and punctured using the reducing method to promote the flow of *qi* and relieve distension.
- For acute intestinal obstruction due to stagnation of blood, Hegu (LI4), Taichong (Liv3) and Sanyinjiao (Sp6) are added and punctured using the reducing method to promote circulation of blood and relieve pain.
- For acute intestinal obstruction due to deficiency of *qi*, the intestines are strengthened to remove obstruction by adding and puncturing Guanyuan (Ren4), Qihai (Ren6) and Zhongwan (Ren12) using the reinforcing method, or adding moxibustion as needed.
- For acute intestinal obstruction due to depletion of the bodily fluid, Zhigou (SJ6), Sanyinjiao

(Sp6) and Taixi (K3) are added and punctured using the reinforcing method to increase the bodily fluid and moisten the bowels.

Treat twice a day. Ten treatments constitute one course.

Electroacupuncture

Points used are the same as for body acupuncture. Select two or three pairs of points each time. Puncture the points until a needling sensation is achieved, then connect the needles to an electrical stimulator. Apply intermittent wave stimulation of the strongest bearable intensity for 30 minutes. Treat once a day or once every other day. Ten treatments constitute one course.

Moxibustion

Acupuncture points:

Tianshu	(S25)
Daheng	(Sp15)
Guanyuan	(Ren4)
Qihai	(Ren6)
Shenque	(Ren8)
Zhongwan	(Ren12)
Dachangshu	(B25)

Apply either moxa roll moxibustion for 15–20 minutes, five to seven medium sized moxa cones, or hot salt compress for 30–60 minutes. Treat three to four points, twice a day. Ten treatments constitute one course.

Moxibustion functions to expel cold, promote the flow of *qi* and blood, and strengthen the functions of the organs. It is therefore suitable for treating acute intestinal obstruction due to contraction of the intestines by pathogenic cold, stagnation of the *qi* or blood, or deficiency of *qi* or bodily fluid.

Remarks

- The causes of acute intestinal obstruction are complex. A diagnosis must first be established in each case, so that proper and timely treatment may be chosen.
- Traditional therapies regulate intestinal peristalsis, increase intestinal secretion and absorption and promote the circulation of blood to the intestines and are therefore beneficial for removing intestinal obstruction.
- Changes in symptoms and signs should be closely observed during treatment with traditional therapies. If after two or three days there is no improvement or the condition worsens, additional measures should be undertaken.
- Traditional therapies should be applied as soon as possible following abdominal surgery in order to promote peristalsis and prevent intestinal adhesions.

5 Acute mastitis

Acute mastitis is an acute suppurative inflammation of the breast caused by the *Staphylococcus aureus* bacterium. It occurs primarily in primiparae women during the breast-feeding period, with onset generally occurring three to four weeks following delivery. There is often a history of cracked or inverted nipple or galactostasis prior to onset. In the initial stage, the breast is red and swollen with localized hard and tender regions; after several days the hard inflamed mass softens and an abscess forms. General symptoms may include high fever, chills, headache, nausea, poor appetite and even septicaemia.

Aetiology

According to traditional Chinese medicine, primarily affected in acute mastitis are the liver and stomach. The liver dominates the flow of *qi* and the Liver meridian passes through the nipples. Mental injury which damages the liver may result in stagnation of the liver *qi*, affecting milk secretion and causing accumulation of milk in the breasts, leading to mastitis. The Stomach meridian, which also distributes through the breasts, is rich in both *qi* and blood; improper diet such as overindulgence in spicy or greasy foods may result in accumulation of heat in the Stomach meridian which combines with milk to cause redness, swelling and pain in the breasts. Acute mastitis may also be caused by invasion of the breasts by exogenous heat and toxins through cracked nipples.

Differentiation of syndromes

- Acute mastitis due to stagnation of the liver *qi*.
  Characterized by distension, pain and swelling of the breast which may occur prior to delivery; accompanied by distension in the chest and hypochondriac region, frequent sighing, depression or irritability, poor appetite, whitish tongue coating and wiry pulse.
- Acute mastitis due to hyperactivity of the stomach-fire.
  Characterized by sudden onset of distension, pain and swelling of the breast following delivery; usually accompanied by high fever, chills, headache, thirst and preference for cold drinks, poor appetite, red tongue with yellowish coating and rapid slippery pulse.
- Acute mastitis due to deficiency of the spleen and stomach.
  Characterized by long-standing diabrotic abscess secreting milk or pus; accompanied by lassitude, pale complexion, poor appetite, abdominal distension, pale tongue with whitish coating and weak pulse.

Treatment

Body acupuncture

Main acupuncture points:

Jianjing	(G21)
Neiguan	(P6)
Danzhong	(Ren17)
Rugen	(S18)

Jianjing (G21), the meeting point of the Gallbladder meridian and the San Jiao, Stomach and Yangwei meridians, is punctured obliquely forward for 0.5–0.8 *cun* to dredge the meridians and relieve pain and swelling. Neiguan (P6), the *luo* (collateral) point of the Pericardium meridian and one of the eight confluence points connecting with the Yinwei meridian, is punctured to promote the flow of *qi*. Danzhong (Ren17) and Rugen (S18) are local points for treating mastitis.

Auxiliary points and appropriate manipulation are chosen according to differentiation of syndromes.

- For acute mastitis due to stagnation of the liver *qi*, Taichong (Liv3) and Sanyinjiao (Sp6) are added and punctured using the reducing method to promote the flow of the liver *qi*.
- For acute mastitis due to hyperactivity of the stomach fire, Neiting (S44), Shaoze (SI1) and Dazhui (Du14) are pricked with a three-edged needle to draw several drops of blood and clear away heat and toxins.
- For acute mastitis due to deficiency of the spleen and stomach, the spleen and stomach are strengthened by adding and puncturing Zusanli (S36), Sanyinjiao (Sp6) and Qihai (Ren6) using the reinforcing method, or applying moxibustion as needed.

Blood-letting puncturing and cupping therapy

Points chosen are the same as for body acupuncture, or Huatuojiaji (Ex 46 T2-T8) may be substituted. Prick with a three-edged needle or tap with a plum blossom needle to cause mild bleeding, then cup for 15 minutes to draw blood and clear away heat and toxins.

Treat two to three points each time, once every other day. Three treatments constitute one course. This method is most suitable for treating mastitis due to hyperactivity of the stomach-fire.

Auricular therapy

Auricular points:

Chest, Thoracic Vertebrae: correspond to the affected areas of the body. Locate positive points; tape both frontal and dorsal surfaces to increase stimulation. Auricular points corresponding to the breast are located between Chest and Thoracic Vertebrae and between Thoracic Vertebrae and the scaphoid fossa.

Stomach: the Stomach meridian distributes through the breasts, so Stomach is taped to activate the meridian and dispel heat and toxins.

Liver: regulates the flow of *qi*.

Endocrine, Adrenal Gland: main anti-inflammation points.

Subcortex: regulates the nervous and endocrine functions.

Ear Shenmen: main point for relieving pain.

Apex of Ear: blood-letting puncturing of this point with a three-edged needle dispels heat and toxins, alleviates swelling and relieves pain.

Use auricular taping with strong manipulation and blood-letting puncturing where indicated, twice a week. Five treatments constitute one course.

Remarks

☙ Extensive clinical findings indicate that acupuncture is very effective for treating acute mastitis in the initial stage. There will often be great improvement in signs and symptoms, or even a complete cure, after one to three treatments.
☙ In cases of abscess or diabrotic mastitis, acupuncture is usually combined with moxibustion to promote natural diabrosis and completely discharge pus to improve healing.
☙ For cases complicated by septicaemia, additional emergency methods should be undertaken concurrent with traditional therapies.

6 Acute soft tissue injury

Acute soft tissue injury refers to sprain or contusion of the soft tissues, including the muscles, tendons, ligaments or joint capsules. It usually occurs on the shoulder, elbow, wrist, fingers, lumbus, hip, knee or ankle. Manifestations include swelling, pain and impaired joint movement.

Aetiology

According to traditional Chinese medicine, acute soft tissue injury is caused by external trauma or improper motion resulting in damage to the tendons and meridians, with subsequent localized obstruction of *qi* and blood.

Differentiation of syndromes

Acute soft tissue injury is differentiated according to meridian theory. For example, trauma of the neck is related to the Small Intestine, San Jiao, Gallbladder, Urinary Bladder and Du meridians; trauma in the chest and hypochondriac region is related to the Liver, Gallbladder and San Jiao meridians; mid-back injury is related to the Du meridian; injury of the bilateral sides of the back is related to the Urinary Bladder meridian. Injury of the extremities is also differentiated according to associated meridians.

Treatment

Body acupuncture

Main acupuncture points:

   Ashi points
   Shouxiaojie   (Ex53)
   Zuxiaojie   (Ex54)

Shouxiaojie (Ex53) and Zuxiaojie (Ex54) are clinically effective points for treating soft tissue injury above and below the lumbus respectively. These points are punctured after withdrawing the *ashi* and auxiliary point needles to dredge the meridians and relieve swelling and pain. The needles should be retained for 20–30 minutes and manipulated every 3–5 minutes using the even method, while the patient moves the injured region.

Auxiliary points are selected from distal points according to meridian theory.

● For soft tissue injury of the neck, Houxi (SI3) and Zhongzhu (SJ3) are added.
● For soft tissue injury of the chest and hypochondriac region, Taichong (Liv3) Yanglingquan (G34) and Zhigou (SJ6) are added.
● For soft tissue injury of the mid-back, Shuigou (Du26) and Baihui (Du20) are added.
● For soft tissue injury of the bilateral sides of the back, Weizhong (B40) and Kunlun (B60) are added.

Treat once or twice a day during the acute stage; treat once a day or once every other day during remission. Five treatments constitute one course.

Electroacupuncture

Points used are the same as for body acupuncture. Select one or two pairs of points each time. Puncture the points until a needling sensation is achieved, then connect the needles to an electrical stimulator. Apply moderate continuous wave stimulation for 30 minutes, once a day or once every other day. Three treatments constitute one course.

Point injection therapy

Ashi points are injected with 2–4 ml of procaine, hydroprednisone, dexamethasone or vitamin B_{12} once every three days. Three treatments constitute one course.

Auricular therapy

Auricular points:

Areas corresponding to the injured regions: regulate the flow of *qi* and blood. Locate

positive points; tape both frontal and dorsal surfaces to increase stimulation.

Ear Shenmen: main point for relieving pain.

Liver: nourishes the tendons and regulates the flow of *qi* to relieve pain.

Spleen: nourishes the muscles; produces and reinforces *qi* and blood.

Heart: improves the circulation of blood.

Use auricular taping with strong manipulation, once every other day. Five treatments constitute one course.

Remarks

- Traditional therapies are very effective for treating acute soft tissue injury; in many cases there will be great improvement in such symptoms as pain and swelling after one to three treatments.
- It is essential to establish a diagnosis prior to treatment. Cases of fracture and dislocation may not be punctured.
- The patient should rest during the acute stage and engage in appropriate exercise during remission.

7 Acute tonsillitis

Acute tonsillitis is an acute non-specific inflammation of the tonsils. It occurs mainly in the spring and autumn and primarily in children and teenagers. Manifestations include chills, fever, headache, sore throat aggravated by swallowing and general soreness of the body. Because acute tonsillitis may develop into chronic tonsillitis or develop accompanying complications such as otitis media, endocarditis, nephritis or rheumatic arthritis, immediate and proper treatment is essential.

Aetiology

According to traditional Chinese medicine, acute tonsillitis is caused either by exogenous

wind-heat invading the throat through the mouth and nose, or by endogenous pathogenic fire from the lungs and stomach flaring up along the meridians and accumulating in the throat.

Differentiation of syndromes

- Wind-heat type acute tonsillitis.
  Characterized by red, swollen and painful throat; accompanied by headache, fever, aversion to cold, cough with profuse sticky sputum, thin dry whitish tongue coating and rapid superficial pulse.

● Acute tonsillitis due to accumulation of heat in the lungs and stomach.
Characterized by red, swollen and painful throat; accompanied by high fever, thirst with a preference for cold beverages, headache, halitosis, scanty urine, constipation, thick dry yellowish tongue coating and rapid forceful pulse.

Treatment

Body acupuncture

Main acupuncture points:

Shaoshang	(L11)
Hegu	(LI4)
Yifeng	(SJ17)

The Lung meridian connects with the throat, which is the door to the lungs, so Shaoshang (L11), the *jing* (well) point of the Lung meridian, is pricked with a three-edged needle to draw several drops of blood and dispel heat. Treating this single point is sufficient in many cases. Hegu (LI4), the *yuan* (source) point of the Large Intestine meridian, functions to expel wind, dispel heat and relieve pain. Yifeng (SJ17) is a local point effective for treating tonsillitis.

Auxiliary points and appropriate manipulation are chosen according to differentiation of syndromes.

● For wind-heat type acute tonsillitis, Fengchi (G20) is added and punctured using the reducing method to expel wind-heat.
● For acute tonsillitis due to accumulation of heat in the lungs and stomach, Quchi (LI11) and Neiting (S44) are added and punctured using the reducing method to dispel heat.
● For cases with high fever, Dazhui (Du14) is added and pricked with a three-edged needle and then cupped for 15–20 minutes to dispel heat.

Treat once a day. Five treatments constitute one course.

Blood-letting puncturing

Acupuncture and auricular points:

Group1:
Shaoshang	(L11)
Shangyang	(LI1)
Lidui	(S45)

Group 2:
Shixuan	(Ex1)

Group 3:
Apex of Ear

Select one group each time. Prick the selected points with a three-edged needle to draw several drops of blood. Treat once a day. Five treatments constitute one course.

Auricular therapy

Auricular points:

Tonsil, Throat: correspond to the affected area. Tape Tonsil on both frontal and dorsal surfaces to increase stimulation.

Lung, Stomach, Large Intestine: expel endogenous heat.

Adrenal Gland, Endocrine: relieve inflammation.

Apex of Ear, Helix 1 to Helix 6: blood-letting puncturing of these points in rotation with a three-edged needle dispels heat.

Use auricular taping with strong manipulation and blood-letting puncturing where indicated, once every other day. Five treatments constitute one course.

Remarks

☯ Traditional therapies are very effective for treating acute tonsillitis. They are especially suitable for people who are allergic to medication and for pregnant women.
☯ These methods are also suitable for treating acute laryngopharyngitis.

8 Alcohol withdrawal

Long-term excessive consumption of alcohol may damage the heart, liver and brain, as well as increase the morbidity of various refractory problems such as hepatitis, hepatocirrhosis, hepatic cancer, cardiocerebral arteriosclerosis and peptic ulcer.

Aetiology and differentiation of syndromes

According to traditional Chinese medicine, excessive consumption of alcohol, which is hot and peppery, produces damp-heat which accumulates in the liver, gallbladder, spleen and stomach. Acupuncture can regulate the function of the *zangfu* organs to eliminate pathogenic damp-heat, as well as tranquillize the mind to relieve symptoms of alcohol withdrawal such as paroxysmal trembling, sweating, hallucinations and convulsions.

Treatment

Body acupuncture

Acupuncture points:

Baihui	(Du20)
Neiguan	(P6)
Danzhong	(Ren17)
Zhongwan	(Ren12)
Zhongji	(Ren3)
Zusanli	(S36)
Tianshu	(S25)
Sanyinjiao	(Sp6)
Yinlingquan	(Sp9)

The therapeutic principles for treating alcohol withdrawal are to open the chest, tranquillize the mind and eliminate pathogenic damp-heat. Baihui (Du20), the meeting point of the Du, Liver and six Yang Hand and Foot meridians, is one of the most important points for tranquillizing the mind. It is always punctured in alternation with Sishencong (Ex26). Neiguan (P6), the *luo* (collateral) point of the Pericardium meridian and one of the eight confluence points connecting with the Yinwei meridian, functions to open the chest and

tranquillize the mind. Danzhong (Ren17), the *hui* (influential) point of *qi*, functions to open the chest and promote the flow of *qi*. Zhongwan (Ren12), the *hui* (influential) point of the *fu* organs and the front-*mu* point of the stomach, is treated to regulate the Middle Jiao. Zhongji (Ren3), the front-*mu* point of the urinary bladder, eliminates pathogenic damp-heat. Zusanli (S36), the *he* (sea) and lower *he* (confluent) point of the Stomach meridian; Tianshu (S25), the front-*mu* point of the large intestine; and Sanyinjiao (Sp6), the meeting point of the three Foot Yin meridians and Yinlingquan (Sp9), the *he* (sea) point of the Spleen meridian, are treated in combination to strengthen the stomach and spleen in order to eliminate pathogenic damp-heat.

● For cases accompanied by convulsions, Shuigou (Du26), Hegu (LI4) and Taichong (Liv3) are added to extinguish endogenous wind and arrest convulsions.

All points are punctured using the reducing method, once a day or every other day. Ten treatments constitute one course.

Electroacupuncture

Points used are the same as for body acupuncture. Choose one or two pairs of points each time. Puncture until a needling sensation is achieved, then connect the needles with an electrical stimulator. Apply continuous wave stimulation of the highest endurable intensity for 20–30 minutes. Treat once a day or every other day. Ten treatments constitute one course.

Auricular Therapy

Auricular points:

Mouth, Stomach: inhibit the craving for alcohol.

Spleen, San Jiao: strengthen the spleen and discharge dampness.

Endocrine: regulates the endocrine function.

Liver, Chest: open the chest and promote the flow of *qi*.

Ear Shenmen, Occiput, Subcortex: calm the mind.

Apex of Ear: blood-letting puncturing of this point with a three-edged needle dispels heat and tranquillizes the mind.

Use auricular taping with strong manipulation and blood-letting puncturing where indicated, twice a week. Five treatments constitute one course.

Remarks

☯ Traditional therapies are effective for treating alcohol withdrawal; auricular therapy is used the most often due to its simplicity and painlessness.

☯ Traditional therapies are effective only for people who are actively motivated to stop drinking.

9 Allergic rhinitis

Allergic rhinitis is an allergic reaction of the nasal mucosa characterized by rhinocnesmus, persistent paroxysmal sneezing, dilute nasal discharge and intermittent or persistent nasal obstruction. There is usually a history of other allergic problems or a family history of allergy.

Aetiology

According to traditional Chinese medicine, allergic rhinitis is caused internally by deficiency of the lung *qi* and externally by invasion of wind-cold or wind-heat. The combination of deficient antipathogenic *qi* and excessive pathogenic *qi* results in dysfunction of the lungs' function of dispersal and descent and subsequent accumulation of bodily fluid which obstructs the nasal passages.

Differentiation of syndromes

● Wind-cold type allergic rhinitis.
  Characterized by nasal obstruction, dilute or sticky whitish nasal discharge and sneezing; accompanied by headache, cough, aversion to cold, whitish tongue coating and soft superficial pulse.
● Wind-heat type allergic rhinitis.
  Characterized by nasal obstruction with sticky yellowish nasal discharge; accompanied by headache, dry mouth, red tongue tip and yellowish tongue coating and rapid slippery pulse.
● Allergic rhinitis due to *qi* deficiency of the lungs and spleen.
  Characterized by long-standing nasal obstruction, sneezing and dilute nasal discharge; accompanied by susceptibility to the common cold, aversion to wind or cold on the back, dizziness, lassitude, pale complexion, poor appetite, pale tongue with whitish coating and weak pulse.

Treatment

Body acupuncture

Main acupuncture points:

Yingxiang	(LI20)
Hegu	(LI4)
Baihui	(Du20)
Yintang	(Ex27)
Zusanli	(S36)
Fengchi	(G20)

Main points for treating allergic rhinitis are selected from the Du, Large Intestine and Stomach meridians, since these meridians are closely connected with the nose. Yingxiang (LI20) (Welcoming Fragrance in Chinese) is a local point of the Large Intestine meridian effective for treating nasal problems. Hegu (LI4), the *yuan* (source) point of the Large Intestine meridian, functions to activate the meridians and open the nose. Baihui (Du20), the meeting point of the Du, Liver and six

Hand and Foot Yang meridians, functions to activate antipathogenic *qi* and expel exogenous pathogens. Yintang (Ex27) is a clinically effective local point for treating various nasal problems. It is punctured subcutaneously downward to a depth of 0.5–1.0 *cun*. Zusanli (S36), the *he* (sea) and lower *he* (confluent) point of the Stomach meridian, functions to strengthen antipathogenic *qi*. Fengchi (G20), an important point of the Gallbladder meridian located at the base of the skull, expels wind and opens the nose.

Auxiliary points and appropriate manipulation are chosen according to differentiation of syndromes.

● For wind-cold type allergic rhinitis, wind-cold is expelled by adding and puncturing Tongtian (B7) using the reducing method and applying moxibustion as needed.
● For wind-heat type allergic rhinitis, Neiting (S44) is added and punctured using the reducing method to dispel wind-heat.
● For allergic rhinitis due to *qi* deficiency of the lungs and spleen, antipathogenic *qi* is strengthened by adding and puncturing Feishu (B13) and Pishu (B20) using the reinforcing method and applying moxibustion as needed.

Treat once a day or once every other day. Ten treatments constitute one course.

Electroacupuncture

Points used are the same as for body acupuncture. Select one or two pairs of points each time. Puncture until a needling sensation is achieved, then connect the needles to an electrical stimulator. Apply moderate continuous wave stimulation for 20–30 minutes, once a day or once every other day. Ten treatments constitute one course.

Moxibustion

Acupuncture points:

Feishu	(B13)
Yingxiang	(LI20)
Yintang	(Ex27)
Shangxing	(Du23)
Baihui	(Du20)
Fengchi	(G20)

Apply moxa roll moxibustion for 15–20 minutes to two or three points each time. Treat once or twice a day. Ten treatments constitute one course.

This method is suitable for treating wind-cold type allergic rhinitis and allergic rhinitis due to *qi* deficiency of the lungs and spleen.

Auricular Therapy

Auricular points:

Internal Nose, External Nose: correspond to the affected area.

Lung: the lungs open into the nose, so Lung is taped to regulate the lungs' function of dispersal and descent and clear the nose.

Spleen: strengthens the spleen to transform and transport water and dampness.

Kidney: reinforces antipathogenic *qi*.

Endocrine, Adrenal Gland, Wind Stream: relieve inflammation and allergic reactions.

Apex of Ear: blood-letting puncturing of this point with a three-edged needle relieves inflammation and allergic reactions.

Use auricular taping with strong manipulation and blood-letting puncturing where indicated, twice a week. Five treatments constitute one course.

Remarks

● Traditional therapies are effective for treating allergic rhinitis, but long-term treatment should be given in order to consolidate results and prevent relapse.
● Two or more therapies are usually combined to increase stimulation.
● Nasal self-massage helps to consolidate results and prevent relapse. Using the index and middle fingers of each hand, first massage downward along both sides of the nose from the top to Yingxiang (LI20) twenty to thirty times, until the local area is hot. Then massage from Yingxiang (LI20) to bilateral Taiyang (Ex30) twenty to thirty times, until the local area is hot. Finally, rub Yingxiang (LI20), Yintang (Ex27), Taiyang (Ex30) and Fengchi (G20) for three to five minutes on each point. Massage two or three times a day. This method promotes the local flow of *qi* and blood to strengthen antipathogenic *qi* and open the nose.
● These methods are also suitable for treating chronic rhinitis.

10 Alopecia areata

Alopecia areata refers to the sudden occurrence of localized circular or elliptical patches of areata baldness on the head, with smooth and shiny skin and clearly defined borders. There are no subjective symptoms on the affected areas. In addition to baldness on the head, in some severe cases hair may be lost from the eyebrows, eyelashes, axillary or pubic hair, or even the body hair of the arms, legs, chest, etc. The causes of alopecia areata are various, including psychic factors, endocrine disturbance, dysbolism, local infection, autoimmune abnormality or genetic factors.

Aetiology

According to traditional Chinese medicine, the hair is the terminal of the blood and the blood functions to moisten and nourish the hair. Therefore hair loss may occur if the blood is insufficient or stagnant liver *qi* affects its flow.

Differentiation of syndromes

- Alopecia areata due to deficiency of the blood.
  Characterized by dizziness, pale complexion, insomnia, palpitation, lassitude, red tongue with thin whitish coating and weak thready pulse.
- Alopecia areata due to stagnation of the liver *qi*.
  Characterized by a feeling of fullness in the chest and hypochondriac region, frequent sighing, insomnia, bad dreams, depression or restlessness, poor appetite, purple spots on the edge of the tongue and wiry pulse.

Treatment

Body acupuncture

Main acupuncture points:

Local bald areas
Baihui   (Du20)
Fengchi   (G20)
Geshu   (B17)

Two methods may be used to stimulate the local bald areas. The affected areas may be tapped with a plum blossom needle, first spirally from the border to the centre and then concentrically, until the skin becomes congested or there is slight oozing of blood. Alternatively, three or four filiform needles may be applied subcutaneously from the border to the centre of the affected areas.

Baihui (Du20), the meeting point of the Du, Liver and six Hand and Foot Yang meridians located on the top of the head, and Fengchi (G20), an important point of the Gallbladder meridian located on the head, are punctured to activate the meridians and tranquillize the mind. Geshu (B17), the *hui* (influential) point of the blood, functions to nourish the blood and promote its flow.

Auxiliary points and appropriate manipulation are chosen according to differentiation of syndromes.

- For deficiency of blood, Zusanli (S36) and Sanyinjiao (Sp6) are added and punctured using the reinforcing method to strengthen the spleen and stomach.
- For stagnation of the liver *qi*, Taichong (Liv3), Neiguan (P6) and Danzhong (Ren17) are added and punctured using the even method to open the chest and promote the flow of the liver *qi*.

Treat once a day or once every other day. Ten treatments constitute one course.

Moxibustion

Apply moxa roll moxibustion to affected areas for 15–20 minutes until localized redness appears. Treat once a day or every other day. Ten treatments constitute one course.

Auricular therapy

Auricular points:

Corresponding areas: tap with a plum blossom needle or prick with a three-edged needle to cause mild bleeding in order to activate the meridians and clear the collaterals.

Lung, Spleen, Kidney: the lungs function to nourish the skin and hair and the spleen transports and transforms food to produce blood;

the kidneys store essence which is transformed into blood and back again. Therefore Lung, Spleen and Kidney are treated to nourish the skin and promote regeneration of the hair.

Liver: promotes the flow of the liver *qi*.

Ear Shenmen, Subcortex: regulate the nervous system to tranquillize the mind.

Endocrine, Adrenal Gland: regulate the endocrine system.

Use auricular taping with strong manipulation and blood-letting puncturing where indicated. Treat once or twice a week. Ten treatments constitute one course.

Remarks

☯ Traditional therapies are effective for treating alopecia areata, but long-term treatment using a combination of two or more therapies should be undertaken in order to increase stimulation.

☯ Blood-letting puncturing of the affected areas is an effective treatment for alopecia areata, functioning to improve local blood circulation and promote regeneration of the hair.

☯ It is useful to rub the affected areas with fresh ginger until they feel hot and become flushed, once or twice a day.

11 Amenorrhoea

Normal menstruation depends on coordination among the hypothalamus, pituitary gland and ovaries, which produce periodic changes in the endometria in response to changing levels of sex hormones. Organic or functional disturbance of any aspect may result in amenorrhoea. Amenorrhoea is classified into primary and secondary types. Primary amenorrhoea refers to lack of onset of menstruation, even after 18 years of age; secondary amenorrhoea refers to cessation of previously normal menstruation for more than three months.

Aetiology

Traditional Chinese medicine classifies amenorrhoea into excessive and deficient types. The excessive type is due to stagnation of *qi* and blood; it may be caused by mental injury resulting in stagnation of the liver *qi*, invasion of the uterus by exogenous cold, or obstruction of the meridians by phlegm-dampness. The deficient type is due to depletion of the blood; it may be caused either by congenital insufficiency, postpartum exhaustion resulting from frequent pregnancies, or improper diet or overstrain which damage the spleen and stomach. Primarily affected are the liver, kidneys and spleen.

Differentiation of syndromes

● Amenorrhoea due to stagnation of the liver *qi*.
Characterized by cessation of previously normal menstruation for more than three months; accompanied by depression, restlessness, feeling of fullness in the chest and hypochondriac region, distending pain in the lower abdomen, purple or purple-spotted tongue and wiry pulse.

● Amenorrhoea due to invasion of the uterus by exogenous cold.
Characterized by sudden cessation of previously normal menstruation following attack of cold during menstruation; accompanied by pain and feeling of cold in the lower abdomen aggravated by cold and alleviated by warmth, sensation of cold in the extremities, poor appetite, thin whitish tongue coating and slow deep pulse.

● Amenorrhoea due to blockage of the meridians by phlegm-dampness.
Characterized by cessation of previously normal menstruation or lack of onset of menstruation; accompanied by lassitude, obesity, feeling of fullness in the chest and epigastric region, profuse whitish leukorrhoea, greasy whitish tongue coating and slippery pulse.

● Amenorrhoea due to *yin* deficiency of the liver and kidneys.

Characterized by lack of onset of menstruation or cessation of previously normal menstruation for more than three months; accompanied by dizziness, tinnitus, dry mouth and throat, sore and weak back and knees, red tongue with little coating and wiry thready pulse.

- Amenorrhoea due to deficiency of the spleen and stomach.
  Characterized by gradual cessation of menstruation; accompanied by lassitude, shortness of breath, palpitation, pale complexion, poor appetite, loose stool, pale tongue with whitish coating and weak pulse.

Treatment

Body acupuncture

Main acupuncture points:

Guanyuan	(Ren4)
Sanyinjiao	(Sp6)
Guilai	(S29)

Guanyuan (Ren4), the meeting point of the Ren and three Foot Yin meridians, is an important point for treating gynaecological and genital problems. Sanyinjiao (Sp6), the meeting point of the three Foot Yin meridians, functions to strengthen the liver, spleen and kidneys. Guilai (S29), a point of the Stomach meridian located on the lower abdomen, is effective for treating menstrual problems.

Auxiliary points and proper manipulation are chosen according to differentiation of syndromes.

- For amenorrhoea due to stagnation of the liver *qi*, Taichong (Liv3), Diji (Sp8), Neiguan (P6) and Danzhong (Ren17) are added and punctured using the reducing method to promote the flow of *qi* and blood.
- For amenorrhoea due to invasion of the uterus by exogenous cold, Zhongji (Ren3), Diji (Sp8) and Xuehai (Sp10) are added and punctured using the reducing method and moxibustion is applied to warm the meridians and relieve pain.
- For amenorrhoea due to blockage of the meridians by phlegm-dampness, Zhongwan (Ren12), Fenglong (S40) and Zusanli (S36) are added and punctured using the even method to strengthen the spleen and eliminate phlegm-dampness.

- For amenorrhoea due to *yin* deficiency of the liver and kidneys, Taixi (K3), Ganshu (B18), Shenshu (B23) and Qihai (Ren6) are added and punctured using the even method to nourish the liver and kidneys.
- For amenorrhoea due to deficiency of the spleen and stomach, Pishu (B20), Weishu (B21), Zusanli (S36) and Zhongwan (Ren12) are added and punctured using the reinforcing method to strengthen the spleen and stomach.

Treat once a day or once every other day. Ten treatments constitute one course.

Moxibustion

Guanyuan	(Ren4)
Guilai	(S29)
Zhongji	(Ren3)
Sanyinjiao	(Sp6)

Apply moxa roll moxibustion for 15–20 minutes, or three to five medium-sized moxa cones, to one or two points each time. Treat once a day. Ten treatments constitute one course.

Moxibustion functions to warm the meridians and strengthen antipathogenic *qi*; it is therefore suitable for treating amenorrhoea due to invasion of the uterus by exogenous cold or deficiency of the spleen and stomach.

Electroacupuncture

Points used are the same as for body acupuncture. Select one or two pairs of points each time. Puncture until a needling sensation is achieved, then connect the needles to an electrical stimulator. Apply moderate continuous wave stimulation for 30 minutes. Treat once a day or once every other day. Ten treatments constitute one course.

Auricular therapy

Auricular points:

Internal Genitals, Pelvis, Abdomen: correspond to the affected regions.

Subcortex, Midpoint of Rim, Endocrine: regulate endocrine function.

Kidney, Spleen: strengthen both congenital and acquired essence.

Liver: regulates the flow of blood and *qi*.

Use auricular taping, twice a week. Five treatments constitute one course.

Remarks

☯ The causes of amenorrhoea are complicated; it is necessary to establish diagnosis prior to treatment.

☯ Traditional therapies are very effective for treating secondary amenorrhoea.

☯ Amenorrhoea may occur as a side effect of oral contraceptives. In this case, another type of oral contraceptive should be prescribed, or usage of oral contraceptives discontinued and another type of contraception substituted.

12 Angina pectoris

Angina pectoris is a type of coronary heart disease caused by coronary spasm or coronary arteriosclerosis which results in temporary or long-term myocardial ischaemia and subsequent damage to the cardiac muscle. Angina pectoris is typically marked by paroxysmal constrictive pain in the retrosternal region or left chest, radiating to the left arm and shoulder. It is usually induced by physical activity, mental injury, overeating, or attack by cold. In some cases it may occur while resting. The pain recedes spontaneously after a short time, or may be relieved by the administration of nitroglycerin.

Aetiology

Traditional Chinese medicine refers to angina pectoris as *xiongbi* (stagnation of *qi* and blood in the chest) or genuine cardiac pain. It is considered to have several primary causes. Mental injury may result in stagnation of the liver *qi* and subsequent stasis of blood in the heart collaterals; the heart collaterals may be obstructed by turbid phlegm; or deficiency of *qi* may fail to promote the flow of blood in the meridians. The pathogenesis of angina pectoris is primarily deficient in origin, including deficiency of *qi*, blood and *yang* and excessive in expression, including excess stagnant *qi*, blood and turbid phlegm. Primarily affected are the heart, liver and spleen.

Differentiation of syndromes

● Angina pectoris due to obstruction of stagnant blood in the heart collaterals.
Characterized by fixed stabbing pain in the precordial region, worsening at night or aggra-

vated by anger or grief; purple or purple-spotted tongue and thready or uneven pulse.

● Angina pectoris due to blockage of the heart collaterals by turbid phlegm.
Characterized by choking feeling and pain in the precordial region, sometimes radiating to the back; shortness of breath, a heavy feeling of the body, tooth prints and thick greasy coating on tongue and wiry or slippery pulse.

● Angina pectoris due to deficiency of the heart *qi*.
Characterized by dull pain and feeling of fullness in the chest, palpitation, lassitude, pale complexion, spontaneous sweating, pale or purple-spotted tongue and weak thready pulse.

● Angina pectoris due to deficiency of the heart *yang*.
Characterized by pain in the precordial region aggravated by cold, palpitation, feeling of coldness in the extremities, spontaneous sweating, pale tongue with whitish coating and deep, thready, slow pulse.

Treatment

Body acupuncture

Main acupuncture points:

Danzhong	(Ren17)
Jueyinshu	(B14)
Neiguan	(P6)

Danzhong (Ren17), the *hui* (influential) point for *qi* and the front-*mu* point of the pericardium and Jueyinshu (B14), the back-*shu* point of the pericardium, are treated in combination to promote the flow of *qi* and blood and relieve pain. Danzhong (Ren14) is punctured horizontally downward to Jiuwei (Ren15) or horizontally to the left to Rugen

(S18). Neiguan (P6), the *luo* (collateral) point of the Pericardium meridian and one of the eight confluence points connecting with the Yinwei meridian, is an important point for treating all heart problems.

Auxiliary points and appropriate manipulation are added according to differentiation of syndromes.

● For angina pectoris due to obstruction of stagnant blood in the heart collaterals, Geshu (B17) and Yinxi (H6) are added and punctured using the even method to improve the circulation of blood and relieve pain.
● For angina pectoris due to blockage of the heart collaterals by turbid phlegm, Fenglong (S40) and Zhongwan (Ren12) are added and punctured using the even method to strengthen the spleen and remove turbid phlegm.
● For angina pectoris due to deficiency of the heart *qi*, Zusanli (S36), Guanyuan (Ren4) and Sanyinjiao (Sp6) are added and punctured using the reinforcing method to tonify *qi* and promote the flow of blood.
● For angina pectoris due to deficiency of the heart *yang*, moxibustion is added on the main points to warm the heart *yang* and promote the flow of *qi* and blood.

Treat once a day or once every other day. Ten treatments constitute one course.

Electroacupuncture

Points used are the same as for body acupuncture. Select one or two pairs of points each time. Puncture using the even method until a needling sensation is achieved; then connect the needles to an electrical stimulator. Apply moderate intermittent wave stimulation for 30 minutes, once a day or once every other day. Ten treatments constitute one course.

Auricular Therapy

Auricular points:

Heart, Chest: correspond to the affected regions of the body; widen the chest to regulate the flow of *qi* and activate the meridians to remove stagnant blood.

Liver: regulates the liver *qi* to improve blood circulation.

Small Intestine: assists the heart to improve blood circulation.

Subcortex: regulates the circulation.

Spleen, Stomach: strengthen the spleen and stomach to remove turbid phlegm from the collaterals.

Use auricular taping, twice a week. Ten treatments constitute one course. Strong stimulation should be avoided to prevent aggravating the condition.

Remarks

☯ Acupuncture can effectively alleviate the symptoms of angina pectoris. Physical examinations such as electrocardiogram, echocardiogram and phonocardiogram may show improvement of the left side of the heart and of the blood supply to the cardiac muscles. However, long-term treatment should be given to consolidate the results.
☯ Animal experiments demonstrate that acupuncture can increase the blood supply to the coronary arteries, strengthen myocardial contractions, regulate ion imbalance of the myocardial cells and improve the electrical balance of the cardiac muscle.

13 Appendicitis

Appendicitis is an acute or chronic inflammation of the appendix. Acute appendicitis is marked in the initial stage by shifting abdominal pain, starting in the upper abdomen or umbilical region. After several hours the pain moves to the right

lower abdomen, becoming persistent with paroxysmal exacerbation. A small number of cases may experience pain in the lower right abdomen at onset. Other manifestations include nausea, vomiting, poor appetite, constipation, diarrhoea and fever. Chronic appendicitis is marked by frequently recurring or persistent dull pain in the right lower abdomen, usually induced or aggravated by exertion or improper diet and accompanied by distending pain or discomfort in the upper abdomen, constipation or frequent defecation. There is often a history of acute appendicitis.

Aetiology

Traditional Chinese medicine classifies appendicitis as abdominal pain and considers it to be caused primarily by improper diet, such as overindulgence in raw or cold food; overexertion after eating, or emotional injury. These conditions may affect the intestines' function of transportation and transformation and the flow of *qi* and blood, with resulting accumulation of damp-heat or stagnation of *qi* and blood in the interior. Mainly affected are the large intestine and the stomach.

Differentiation of syndromes

- Appendicitis due to severe dampness and slight heat.
  Characterized by sudden onset of shifting abdominal pain, starting in the upper abdomen or umbilical region and moving after several hours to the right lower abdomen, becoming persistent with paroxysmal exacerbation; accompanied by abdominal distension, nausea, vomiting, greasy yellowish tongue coating and rapid slippery pulse.
- Appendicitis due to severe heat and slight dampness.
  Manifestations in the initial stage are similar to appendicitis due to severe dampness and slight heat, but the pain in the right lower abdomen is more severe, with concurrent muscular tension and localized lumpiness. It is accompanied by fever, dry mouth with a desire for cold beverages, constipation, scanty yellowish urine, red tongue with greasy yellowish coating and rapid slippery pulse.
- Appendicitis due to toxic heat.
  Usually develops from either of the above two types. Characterized by severe pain in the entire abdomen with concurrent muscular tension and diffuse tenderness; accompanied by high fever and/or chills, dry lips and mouth, flushed face, red eyes, vomiting, constipation, rough tongue

with yellowish coating and full pulse. Toxic shock may occur in some cases.
- Appendicitis due to stagnant *qi* and blood.
  Characterized by frequently recurring or persistent dull pain in the right lower abdomen, usually induced or aggravated by exertion or improper diet; accompanied by distending pain or discomfort in the upper abdomen, constipation or frequent defecation. In some cases there may be no accompanying symptoms.

Treatment

Body acupuncture

Main acupuncture points:

Zusanli	(S36)
Shangjuxu	(S37)
Tianshu	(S25)

Zusanli (S36) and Shangjuxu (S37), the lower *he* (confluent) points of the Stomach and Large Intestine meridians respectively, are punctured to clear the intestines and stomach and relieve pain. If there is tenderness between Zusanli (S36) and Shangjuxu (S37) (a common occurrence) Lanweixue (Ex22) may be substituted. Tianshu (S25), the front-*mu* point of the large intestine, is punctured to clear the large intestine and eliminate pathogens.

Auxiliary points and appropriate methods of manipulation are chosen according to differentiation of syndromes.

- For appendicitis due to severe dampness and slight heat, Neiguan (P6) and Zhongwan (Ren12) are added and punctured using the reducing method to remove dampness and stop vomiting.
- For appendicitis due to severe heat and slight dampness, Hegu (LI4), Quchi (LI11) and Dazhui (Du14) are added and punctured using the reducing method, or Dazhui (Du14) is pricked with a three-edged needle and then cupped for 15–20 minutes to draw blood and clear away heat.
- For appendicitis due to toxic heat, auxiliary points and methods are the same as for appendicitis due to severe heat and slight dampness. Additional measures may also be undertaken concurrently.
- For appendicitis due to stagnant *qi* and blood, Shousanli (LI10) and Liangqiu (S34) are added and punctured using the reducing method to

promote the flow of *qi* and blood and relieve pain.

Treat three to four times a day for acute cases; three days constitute one course. Treat once a day for chronic cases and acute cases during the remission stage; five treatments constitute one course.

Electroacupuncture

Points used are the same as for body acupuncture. Select one or two pairs of points each time. Puncture using the reducing method until a needling sensation is achieved, then connect the needles to an electrical stimulator. Apply moderate continuous wave stimulation for one hour. Treat two or three times a day for acute cases; three days constitute one course. Treat once a day for chronic cases; ten treatments constitute one course.

Auricular therapy

Auricular points:

Appendix, Abdomen: correspond to the affected region of the body. Locate positive points; tape both frontal and dorsal surfaces to increase stimulation.

Liver: soothes the liver *qi* to relieve pain.

Spleen, Stomach: regulate the spleen and stomach.

San Jiao, Middle of Superior Concha: regulate the flow of *qi* to relieve abdominal pain.

Ear Shenmen, Sympathesis: main points for relieving pain.

Endocrine, Adrenal Gland: relieve inflammation.

Apex of Ear: blood-letting puncturing of this point with a three-edged needle relieves inflammation and pain.

Use auricular taping with strong manipulation and blood-letting puncturing where indicated, twice a week. Five treatments constitute one course.

Remarks

☯ The above therapies can immediately alleviate symptoms of appendicitis such as abdominal pain and vomiting; they are suitable for treating acute simple appendicitis, minor suppurative appendicitis, periappendicular abscess and chronic appendicitis.

☯ During the course of treatment, it is important to observe whether improvement occurs in symptoms and signs including abdominal pain, tenderness and rebound tenderness in the right lower abdomen and fever. Acupuncture should be continued if improvement occurs after two to three treatments; if the condition worsens, other measures should be undertaken.

☯ Acupuncture should be continued for nine to ten days following disappearance of signs and symptoms in order to prevent relapse.

14 Arrhythmia

Arrhythmia refers to abnormalities of either the rhythm or rate of the heartbeat, including tachycardia, bradycardia, premature beat, auricular fibrillation, etc. It is a common symptom of various organic diseases or functional disorders of the heart. Some cases show only abnormal ECG (electrocardiogram) with no subjective symptoms. General manifestations include palpitation, panic and sudden acceleration or brief cessation of the heartbeat; usually accompanied by dizziness, shortness of breath, feeling of

fullness in the chest and even loss of consciousness.

Aetiology and differentiation

Traditional Chinese medicine classifies arrhythmia as palpitation or chest pain. Due to its complex contributing factors, it is difficult to standardize syndromes for arrhythmia. However, the basic pathogenesis is either turbid phlegm, stagnant *qi* or blood, or deficiency of *qi*, blood, *yin* or *yang*, with resulting insufficient nourishment of the heart.

Treatment

Body acupuncture

Main acupuncture points:

Neiguan	(P6)
Shenmen	(H7)
Danzhong	(Ren17)
Xinshu	(B15)
Jueyinshu	(B14)

Neiguan (P6), the *luo* (collateral) point of the Pericardium meridian and one of the eight confluence points connecting with the Yinwei meridian, functions to activate the meridians and calm the mind. Shenmen (H7), the *yuan* (source) point of the Heart meridian, is a main point for treating all heart problems. Danzhong (Ren17), the front-*mu* point of the pericardium and the *hui* (influential) point of *qi*, is treated in combination with Jueyinshu (B14) and Xinshu (B15), the back-*shu* points of the pericardium and heart respectively, to promote the flow of *qi* and blood and tranquillize the mind.

Auxiliary points and appropriate manipulation are added according to differentiation of syndromes.

- For arrhythmia due to obstruction of stagnant blood in the heart collaterals, Geshu (B17) and Yinxi (H6) are added and punctured using the even method to improve the circulation of blood and relieve pain.
- For arrhythmia due to blockage of the heart collaterals by turbid phlegm, Fenglong (S40) and Zhongwan (Ren12) are added and punctured using the even method to strengthen the spleen and remove turbid phlegm.
- For arrhythmia due to deficiency of the heart *qi*, Zusanli (S36), Guanyuan (Ren4) and Sanyinjiao (Sp6) are added and punctured using the reinforcing method to tonify *qi* and promote the flow of blood.
- For arrhythmia due to deficiency of the heart *yang*, moxibustion is added on the main points to warm the heart *yang* and promote the flow of *qi* and blood.

Treat once a day or once every other day. Ten treatments constitute one course.

Electroacupuncture

Points used are the same as for body acupuncture. Select one or two pairs of points each time. Puncture until a needling sensation is achieved, then connect the needles to an electrical stimulator. Apply moderate intermittent wave stimulation for 15–20 minutes, once a day. Ten treatments constitute one course.

Auricular therapy

Main auricular points:

Heart, Chest: correspond to the affected areas of the body. Locate positive points; tape both frontal and dorsal surfaces to increase stimulation.

Liver: promotes the flow of *qi* and blood.

Subcortex: harmonizes the nervous function.

Auxiliary auricular points:

For tachycardia, Sympathesis, Ear Shenmen, Occiput, or Root of Ear Vagus are added.

For bradycardia, Adrenal Gland and San Jiao are added.

Use auricular taping twice a week, or massage using the even method twice a day. Ten treatments constitute one course.

Remarks

- The above therapies function biphasically in treating arrhythmia; i.e. they can both lower heart rate in cases of tachycardia and raise it in cases of bradycardia.
- Traditional therapies can not only alleviate the symptoms of arrhythmia, but also treat the diseases which cause it.
- The above therapies are more effective for arrhythmia due to ectopic cardiac rhythm than for arrhythmia due to disturbance of impulse conduction.
- Strong stimulation should be avoided in order to prevent aggravating the condition.

15 Bacillary dysentery

Bacillary dysentery is a communicable disease of the intestinal tract caused by the *Bacillus dysenteriae* bacteria. It occurs mainly in the summer and autumn. It is classified clinically into acute and chronic types. The acute type is marked by sudden onset of paroxysmal abdominal pain, bloody and pussy diarrhoea and rectal tenesmus, accompanied by systemic symptoms including high fever, chills, nausea, vomiting, general malaise, dehydration, acidosis, electrolyte disturbance or lowered blood pressure. The chronic type usually develops from acute bacillary dysentery which has not been treated promptly and correctly. It is marked by repeated attacks of bloody pussy diarrhoea and tenesmus, with no accompanying systemic symptoms.

Aetiology

According to traditional Chinese medicine, bacillary dysentery is caused primarily by consumption of contaminated food or invasion of the intestines by damp-heat, damp-cold, or epidemic pathogens, resulting in injury to the collaterals of the intestines.

Differentiation of syndromes

- Bacillary dysentery of the damp-heat type.
  Characterized by paroxysmal abdominal pain, bloody pussy stool, burning sensation in the anus and tenesmus; accompanied by fever, chills, headache, nausea or vomiting, feeling of fullness in the chest and abdomen, scanty yellowish urine, greasy yellowish tongue coating and rapid slippery pulse.
- Bacillary dysentery of the damp-cold type.
  Characterized by severe abdominal pain, bloody pussy stool and tenesmus; accompanied by chills, mild fever, feeling of heaviness in the head and body, feeling of fullness in the epigastric region, poor appetite, greasy whitish tongue coating and soft pulse.
- Bacillary dysentery due to epidemic pathogens.
  Characterized by sudden onset of high fever, nausea, vomiting, severe abdominal pain, frequent bloody pussy stool and severe tenesmus; accompanied by headache, restlessness, feeling of fullness in the chest, anorexia, thirst, deep red tongue with dry yellowish coating and rapid slippery pulse.
- Recurrent bacillary dysentery.
  Characterized by repeated attacks of dysentery, usually induced by improper diet, overexertion, mental injury or invasion by exogenous pathogens. Manifestations include bloody pussy stool, tenesmus, abdominal distension or pain, poor appetite, lassitude, drowsiness, pale or red tongue with greasy coating and soft loose pulse.

Treatment

Body acupuncture

Main acupuncture points:

Tianshu	(S25)
Shangjuxu	(S37)
Sanyinjiao	(Sp6)
Hegu	(LI4)

Tianshu (S25) and Shangjuxu (S37), the front-*mu* and lower *he* (confluent) points respectively of the large intestine, are treated in combination to strengthen the large intestine's function of transportation. These points are used for treating all problems of the large intestine. Sanyinjiao (Sp6), the meeting point of the three Foot Yin meridians, is punctured to strengthen the spleen and eliminate dampness. Hegu (LI4), the *yuan* (source) point of the Large Intestine meridian, functions to promote the flow of *qi* and relieve pain.

Auxiliary points and appropriate methods of manipulation are selected according to differentiation of syndromes and symptoms:

- For bacillary dysentery of the damp-heat type, Quchi (LI11) and Xuehai (Sp10) are added and punctured using the reducing method to dispel heat and cool the blood.
- For bacillary dysentery of the damp-cold type, dampness is removed and cold expelled by adding and puncturing Zhongwan (Ren12) and Yinlingquan (Sp9) using the reducing method and adding moxibustion as needed.

- For bacillary dysentery due to epidemic pathogens, toxic pathogens are eliminated by adding and puncturing Dazhui (Du14), Quchi (LI11) and Neiting (S44) using the reducing method, or pricking Dazhui (Du14) with a three-edged needle and then cupping for 15–20 minutes.
- For recurrent bacillary dysentery, anti-pathogenic *qi* is strengthened and pathogens eliminated by adding and puncturing Zusanli (S36), Dachangshu (B25) and Qihai (Ren6) using the even method and adding moxibustion as needed.
- For cases with severe vomiting, Neiguan (P6) is added and punctured using the reducing method to subdue rebellious rising of the stomach *qi* and arrest vomiting.

Treat acute cases once or twice a day; five treatments constitute one course. Treat chronic cases once a day or once every other day; ten treatments constitute one course.

Electroacupuncture

Points used are the same as for body acupuncture. Select two or three pairs of points each time. Puncture until a needling sensation is achieved, then connect the needles to an electrical stimulator. Apply moderate continuous wave stimulation for 30–40 minutes. Treat once or twice a day for acute cases; five treatments constitute one course. Treat once a day or once every other day for chronic cases; ten treatments constitute one course.

Auricular therapy

Main auricular points:

Large Intestine, Rectum, Abdomen: correspond to the affected areas of the body. Locate positive points; tape both frontal and dorsal surfaces to increase stimulation.

Spleen, San Jiao, Middle of Superior Concha: strengthen the spleen and eliminate dampness.

Endocrine, Adrenal Gland: relieve inflammation.

Sympathesis, Subcortex: relieve pain.

Auxiliary auricular points:

For cases with severe vomiting, Stomach and Cardia are added to subdue rebellious rising of the stomach *qi* and arrest vomiting.

For cases with high fever, Apex of Ear is punctured with a three-edged needle to draw blood and dispel heat.

Use auricular taping and blood-letting puncturing where indicated, once every other day for acute cases and twice a week for chronic cases. Ten treatments constitute one course.

Remarks

- Strong stimulation should be used and needles retained for 40 minutes to increase stimulation and improve effectiveness of treatment.
- Clinical studies indicate that acupuncture can effectively inhibit intestinal hyperperistalsis and angiectasis, thus providing a scientific explanation for the efficacy of acupuncture in alleviating symptoms of dysentery and providing an eventual cure.

16 *Bi* syndrome

Bi refers to obstruction of *qi* and blood. *Bi* syndrome is characterized by joint pain, usually accompanied by muscle soreness, swelling or deformity of joints and limitation of movement. It includes various diseases and disorders of modern medicine such as rheumatic arthritis, rheumatoid arthritis, spondylitis and senile osteoarthritis.

Aetiology

According to traditional Chinese medicine, *bi* syndrome is caused by internal deficiency of *qi* and blood and external invasion by wind, cold, damp or heat. The combination of internal and external factors results in obstruction of *qi* and blood and insufficient nourishment of the muscles, tendons and bones. Exogenous pathogens usually attack the body in combination, although one may be dominant in specific cases. For example, in 'wandering *bi* syndrome' pathogenic wind, the nature of which is to move, predominates. In 'painful *bi* syndrome' pathogenic cold predominates, causing contraction of the meridians. In 'heavy *bi* syndrome' pathogenic dampness, the nature of which is heavy and sticky, predominates. In 'febrile *bi* syndrome' pathogenic damp-heat, either transformed from pathogenic wind, damp or cold, or invading directly from the exterior, predominates.

Bi syndrome is characterized in the initial stage by excessive exogenous pathogens. Since the main pathogenesis during this stage is obstruction of *qi* and blood, the reducing method is applied to eliminate exogenous pathogens. As the syndrome develops, the body's *qi*, blood, *yin* and *yang* may be damaged. Pathogenesis in this stage is characterized by a combination of excessive exogenous pathogens and deficient *qi*, blood, *yin* and *yang*, so the even or reinforcing method is applied to eliminate exogenous pathogens and tonify the *qi*, blood, *yin* and *yang*.

Differentiation of syndromes

- Wind type, or wandering *bi* syndrome.
  Characterized by wandering pain and swelling of joints, occurring mainly in the joints of the upper limbs and back. In the initial stage, there may be exterior symptoms and signs such as aversion to wind, fever, thin and whitish tongue coating and superficial pulse.
- Cold type, or painful *bi* syndrome.
  Characterized by severe and fixed pain in the involved joints, relieved by heat and aggravated by cold, worsening at night and alleviated during the day. In the initial stage, there may be external symptoms and signs including aversion to cold, feeling of cold in the limbs, whitish tongue coating and tense wiry pulse.
- Damp type, or heavy *bi* syndrome.
  Characterized by swelling and fixed pain of the involved joints, occurring primarily in the joints of the lower limbs, alleviated by warmth or massage and aggravated by cold and damp. Additional manifestations include a feeling of heaviness in the body, lassitude, poor appetite, abdominal distension, greasy whitish tongue coating and soft slippery pulse.

- Heat type, or febrile *bi* syndrome.
  Characterized by redness, swelling, pain and sensation of heat in the involved joints, aggravated by heat and alleviated by cold. Additional manifestations include fever, restlessness, thirst with preference for cold drinks, red tongue with dry yellowish coating and rapid slippery pulse.
- *Bi* syndrome due to deficient *qi* and blood.
  Characterized by long-term intermittent mild or severe pain in the involved joints; accompanied by pale complexion, palpitation, shortness of breath, lassitude, spontaneous sweating, poor appetite, loose stool, pale tongue and weak thready pulse.
- *Bi* syndrome due to deficient *yang*.
  Characterized by long-standing pain and sensation of cold in the involved joints, aggravated by cold and alleviated by warmth. Joints may be rigid or deformed with accompanying muscular atrophy. Accompanied by pale complexion, feeling of coldness in the limbs, sore and weak back and knees, loose stool, pale thin tongue with slimy whitish coating and deep weak pulse.
- *Bi* syndrome due to deficient *yin*.
  Characterized by long-standing pain of involved joints with accompanying deformity and contracture; pain aggravated by heat and alleviated by cold, worsening at night and lessening during the day. Accompanied by emaciation, dizziness, tinnitus, flushed cheeks, dry mouth, restlessness, night sweating, sensation of heat in the palms and soles, thin red tongue with little coating and rapid thready pulse.

Treatment

Body acupuncture

Main acupuncture points:

Shoulder joint

Local points:	Jianyu	(LI15)
	Jianliao	(SJ14)
	Naoshu	(SI10)
	Tianzong	(SI11)
Distal points:	Hegu	(LI4)
	Waiguan	(SJ5)
	Houxi	(SI3)

Elbow joint

Local points:	Quchi	(LI11)
	Shousanli	(LI10)
	Xiaohai	(SI8)
	Tianjing	(SJ10)

Distal points:	Hegu	(LI4)
	Waiguan	(SJ5)
	Yanglao	(SI6)

Wrist joint

Local points:	Yangxi	(LI5)
	Wangu	(SI4)
	Yangchi	(SJ4)
	Yanglao	(SI6)
Distal points:	Hegu	(LI4)
	Waiguan	(SJ5)
	Houxi	(SI3)

Metacarpophalangeal and interphalangeal joints of the hands

Local points:	Baxie	(Ex6)
	Houxi	(SI3)
	Hegu	(LI4)
Distal points:	Quchi	(LI11)
	Waiguan	(SJ5)

Hip joint

Local points:	Huantiao	(G30)
	Zhibian	(B54)
Distal points:	Weizhong	(B40)
	Fengshi	(G31)

Knee joint

Local points:	Heding	(Ex19)
	Xiyan	(Ex20)
	Zusanli	(S36)
Distal points:	Kunlun	(B60)
	Xiaxi	(G43)

Ankle joint

Local points:	Jiexi	(S41)
	Kunlun	(B60)
	Shenmai	(B62)
	Qiuxu	(G40)
	Zhaohai	(K6)
Distal points:	Zusanli	(S36)
	Xuanzhong	(G39)
	Sanyinjiao	(Sp6)

Metatarsophalangeal and interphalangeal joints of the feet

Local points:	Bafeng	(Ex23)
	Zutonggu	(B66)
	Taibai	(Sp3)
Distal points:	Zusanli	(S36)
	Xuanzhong	(G39)

Spinal joints

Local points:	Huatuojiaji	(Ex46)
	Yaoyanggguan	(Du3) to
		Dazhui
		(Du14)

	Baliao	(B31–B34)
Distal points:	Weizhong	(B40)
	Renzhong	(Du26)
	Houxi	(SI3)

Both local and distal points are selected as main points for treating joint pain. Points of the Yang meridians are used to improve the flow of *qi* and blood and nourish the muscles, tendons and joints. Points of the Yang meridians of the hands are selected to treat the joints of the upper limbs; points of the Yang meridians of the feet are selected to treat the joints of the lower limbs; and points of the Du meridian are selected to treat joints of the spine.

Auxiliary points and appropriate methods of manipulation are chosen according to differentiation of syndromes.

- For wind type, or wandering *bi* syndrome, Fengchi (G20) and Hegu (LI4) are added and punctured using the reducing method to expel exogenous wind.
- For cold type, or painful *bi* syndrome, the meridians are warmed and exogenous wind expelled by adding and puncturing Dazhui (Du14) and Shenshu (B23) using the reducing method, or adding moxibustion or cupping as needed.
- For damp type, or heavy *bi* syndrome, the spleen is strengthened and exogenous dampness eliminated by adding and puncturing Sanyinjiao (Sp6), Yinjiao (Ren7) and Shuifen (Ren9) using the even method, or adding moxibustion as needed.
- For heat type, or febrile *bi* syndrome, Dazhui (Du14) and Quchi (LI11) are added and pricked with a three-edged needle, then cupped for 10–15 minutes to draw blood and expel heat. Alternatively, the *jing* (well) points may be pricked with a three-edged needle to let several drops of blood, expel heat and relieve pain.
- For *bi* syndrome due to deficient *qi* and blood, the spleen and stomach are strengthened by adding and puncturing Zusanli (S36), Zhongwan (Ren12) and Guanyuan (Ren4) using the reinforcing method and adding moxibustion as needed.
- For *bi* syndrome due to deficient *yang*, the meridians are warmed and exogenous wind expelled by adding and puncturing Mingmen (Du4) and Shenshu (B23) using the reinforcing method, and adding moxibustion as needed.

● For *bi* syndrome due to deficient *yin*, Taixi (K3) and Sanyinjiao (Sp6) are added and punctured using the even method to tonify the kidney *yin* and dispel deficient heat.

Treat once a day or once every other day; ten treatments constitute one course.

Moxibustion

Apply moxa roll moxibustion to selected *ashi* and local points for 10–15 minutes to each point each time. Treat once a day or every other day. Ten treatments constitute one course.

Moxibustion is suitable for treating cold type, wind type and damp type *bi* syndromes as well as *bi* syndrome due to deficient *qi* and blood or deficient *yang*. It is usually used in combination with body acupuncture to increase effectiveness.

Electroacupuncture

Points used are the same as for body acupuncture. Choose two to three pairs of points each time. Puncture until a needling sensation is achieved, then connect the needles to an electrical stimulator. Apply moderate continuous wave stimulation for 30 minutes each time. Treat once a day or once every other day. Ten treatments constitute one course.

Electroacupuncture can effectively relieve inflammation and pain and is suitable for treating all types of *bi* syndrome.

Point injection therapy

Both *ashi* and local points of the affected joints are selected. Commonly used injections include hydroprednisone, procaine and vitamin B_1 and B_{12}. Inject 0.5–1.0 ml into each point, once every other day. Ten treatments constitute one course.

Cupping therapy

For wind, cold and damp type *bi* syndrome, both *ashi* and local points are cupped for 10 minutes to warm the meridians and improve the flow of *qi* and blood. For heat type *bi* syndrome, local and *ashi* points are pricked with a three-edged needle and then cupped for 10 minutes to draw blood and clear away heat.

Moving cupping therapy is used for spinal joint pain. Coat both sides of the spine with a lubricant such as massage oil. Apply and move the cup from top to bottom and then bottom to top. Repeat several times, until purple spots (ecchymoses) appear on the cupped areas.

Cup twice a week. Five treatments constitute one course.

Auricular therapy

Auricular points:

Areas corresponding to the affected joints: locate positive points; tape both frontal and dorsal surfaces to increase stimulation.

Liver, Spleen, Kidney: soothe the liver, strengthen the spleen and tonify the kidneys to nourish the tendons, muscles and bones.

Endocrine, Adrenal Gland, Wind Stream: main anti-rheumatism, anti-inflammation and anti-allergy points.

Ear Shenmen: main point for pain relief.

Apex of Ear: blood-letting puncturing of this point with a three-edged needle expels exogenous pathogens to relieve pain.

Use auricular taping with strong manipulation and blood-letting puncturing where indicated, twice a week. Ten treatments constitute one course.

Remarks

☯ Acupuncture can improve the circulation of *qi* and blood and is therefore effective for treating all types of *bi* syndrome.

☯ Many points may be used for treating *bi* syndrome, but the following basic principles for point selection are always followed:
  – Select *ashi* and local points.
  – Select distal points according to meridian theory.
  – Select points according to differentiation of syndromes.

☯ The various therapies discussed in this section are usually applied in combination in order to increase stimulation and improve effectiveness.

17 Brandy nose

Brandy nose refers to chronic inflammation of the skin of the nasal, paranasal, glabellar or buccal regions. It is caused by gastrointestinal disturbance, endocrine disorder, food sensitivities or chronic local infection. Its stages are marked by erythema, pimples, pustules and rhinophyma successively. It usually occurs in adults.

Aetiology and differentiation of symptoms

According to traditional Chinese medicine, brandy nose is caused primarily by overindulgence in alcohol or greasy or spicy foods, leading to accumulation of damp-heat in the interior and its subsequent evaporation upward. There are usually no general symptoms.

Treatment

Body acupuncture

Main acupuncture points:

Suliao	(Du25)
Yingxiang	(LI20)
Hegu	(LI4)
Quchi	(LI11)
Zusanli	(S36)
Shaoshang	(L11)

Points are selected according to meridian theory. The Du meridian distributes to the nose and the Yangming meridians of the Large Intestine and Stomach distribute to the bilateral sides of the nose, so points of these meridians are punctured to activate the meridians and expel pathogens. Suliao (Du25) is pricked with a three-edged needle or tapped with a plum blossom needle to draw blood. The lungs open into the nose, so Shaoshang (L11), the *jing* (well) point of the Lung meridian, is pricked with a three-edged needle to draw several drops of blood and dispel heat.

All points are punctured using the reducing method, once a day or once every other day. Ten treatments constitute one course.

Auricular therapy

Auricular points:

Areas corresponding to the affected regions: tap with a plum blossom needle to draw blood.

Lung: expels pathogens from the skin.

Spleen, Stomach: strengthen the spleen and stomach to remove dampness.

Large Intestine, San Jiao: drain damp-heat.

Endocrine, Adrenal Gland: relieve inflammation.

Apex of Ear: blood-letting puncturing of this point with a three-edged needle dispels heat.

Use auricular taping with strong manipulation and blood-letting puncturing where indicated, twice a week. Five treatments constitute one course.

Remarks

- Both body acupuncture and auricular therapy are effective for treating brandy nose.
- Wash the face frequently with warm water and avoid greasy and spicy foods.

18 Bronchial asthma

Bronchial asthma is an allergic condition of the bronchi, usually occurring in the autumn and winter. It is marked by paroxysmal dyspnoea and wheezing in the throat, usually accompanied by a feeling of fullness in the chest, shortness of breath, productive cough, cyanosis and orthopnoea.

Aetiology

According to traditional Chinese medicine, bronchial asthma is caused by exogenous factors, improper diet, mental injury or overstrain which attack the interior phlegm, causing it to rise and obstruct the bronchi. Bronchial asthma is deficient in origin and excessive in expression.

Differentiation of syndromes

- Bronchial asthma due to blockage of phlegm and heat in the lungs.
  Characterized by dyspnoea, cough with sticky yellowish sputum, red tongue with sticky yellowish coating and rapid slippery pulse. Other symptoms may include restlessness, flushed face, fever, thirst with a preference for cold beverages and constipation.
- Bronchial asthma due to accumulation of phlegm-dampness in the lungs arising from deficiency of the spleen.
  Characterized by asthma, cough with profuse easily expectorated thin whitish sputum, feeling of fullness in the chest, slimy or greasy whitish tongue coating and soft slippery pulse. Other symptoms may include pale complexion, sensation of cold on the back, poor appetite and abdominal distension.
- Bronchial asthma due to failure of the kidneys to receive *qi*.
  Characterized by dyspnoea, shortness of breath and prolonged expiration aggravated by overstrain, pale tongue with whitish coating and deep weak pulse. Other symptoms may include dizziness, tinnitus, weak and sore back and knees and lassitude.

Treatment

Body acupuncture

Main acupuncture points:

Feishu	(B13)
Zhongfu	(L1)
Danzhong	(Ren17)
Tiantu	(Ren22)
Dingchuan	(Ex41)
Fenglong	(S40)

Feishu (B13) and Zhongfu (L1), the back-*shu* and front-*mu* points respectively of the lungs, are treated in combination to promote the flow of lung *qi* and

halt asthma. Danzhong (Ren17), the *hui* (influential) point of *qi*, functions to open the chest and regulate the flow of *qi*. Puncture horizontally downward for 1.0–1.5 *cun*; fix the needle with a piece of tape and retain for 24 hours to increase stimulation. Tiantu (Ren22), a local point for treating bronchial asthma, can effectively alleviate spasm of the bronchial smooth muscles to stop asthma. Dingchuan (Ex41) is a clinically effective point for treating asthma. Fenglong (S40), the *luo* (collateral) point of the Stomach meridian, functions to strengthen the spleen and stomach and dispel phlegm.

Auxiliary points and appropriate methods of manipulation are chosen according to differentiation of syndromes:

- For bronchial asthma due to blockage of phlegm and heat in the lungs, Dazhui (Du14), Kongzui (L7) and Yuji (L10) are added and punctured using the reducing method. Alternatively, Dazhui (Du14), Feishu (B13) and Danzhong (Ren17) may be pricked with a three-edged needle and then cupped for 15 minutes to draw blood and dispel heat.
- For bronchial asthma due to accumulation of phlegm-dampness in the lungs arising from deficiency of the spleen, the spleen is strengthened and phlegm dispelled by adding and puncturing Zusanli (S36), Zhongwan (Ren12) and Pishu (B20) using the even method, or adding moxibustion as needed.
- For bronchial asthma due to failure of the kidneys to receive *qi*, the kidneys are strengthened to help the lungs receive *qi* by adding and puncturing Shenshu (B23), Guanyuan (Ren4) and Qihai (Ren6) using the reducing method, adding moxibustion as needed.

Treat once a day or once every other day. Ten treatments constitute one course.

Moxibustion

Points on the front of the trunk:

Zhongfu	(L1)
Danzhong	(Ren17)
Zhongwan	(Ren12)
Guanyuan	(Ren4)
Qihai	(Ren6)

Points on the back of the trunk:

Dazhui	(Du14)
Dingchuan	(Ex41)
Feishu	(B13)

Pishu	(B20)
Shenshu	(B23)

The following three methods of moxibustion are utilized in clinical practice:

● Moxa roll moxibustion.
Select three to five points each time. Apply moxa roll moxibustion to each point for 10–15 minutes, once a day or once every other day. Ten treatments constitute one course. This method is usually used in combination with body acupuncture and is applied immediately after withdrawing the needles.
● Scarifying moxibustion.
Select two to three points each time. Apply a thin coating of garlic juice, then place a small moxa cone (0.5 cm high by 0.5 cm diameter) on each point. Ignite the cones and allow to burn out spontaneously. Remove ashes and repeat the garlic juice and moxa process five to eight times, until small blisters form. Carefully bandage with sterile gauze. After approximately seven days, aseptic post-moxibustion sores will appear on the moxa-ed areas. Debride with physiological saline and bandage with sterile gauze once a day. The sores will heal completely after approximately one month, leaving scars. If no aseptic post-moxibustion sores appear, treatment should be repeated until they do. In the event of secondary infection, additional treatment should be undertaken.

This method is quite painful, so additional analgesic measures may be utilized concurrently with treatment. The area surrounding the points may be tapped with the fingers during moxibustion to relieve pain, or 1.0–2.0 ml of 2% procaine solution may be injected subcutaneously as a local anaesthetic.

Scarifying moxibustion may be utilized during either the attack or remission stages of bronchial asthma. A course of three successive treatments should be given in mid-summer in order to prevent winter onset of asthma.
● Crude herb moxibustion, also called medicinal vesiculation.
Raw mustard seed (*semen sinapsi albae*), which functions to promote the flow of lung *qi* and dispel phlegm, is ground into powder and then mixed with sufficient water or ginger juice to make a paste. Apply the paste to three to five points for 2–4 hours each time. A sensation of burning or pain may occur and local skin will become flushed and blisters may appear in some cases. Debride lesions with physiological saline and bandage with sterile gauze once a day to avoid secondary infection.

This method is usually applied in mid-summer, during the remission stage. Treat three times, at 10 day intervals, once a year. Repeat for three successive years.

Crude herb moxibustion is suitable for treating all kinds of asthma.

Point implantation therapy

Points used are the same as for body acupuncture. Select two or three points each time. Use a triangular needle to implant surgical catgut on each point. (See Appendix.) Treat once every 20 to 30 days. Three treatments constitute one course.

Blood-letting puncturing

Acupuncture point:

Sifeng	(Ex2)

Prick the point with a three-edged needle until several drops of thick whitish or yellowish serum appear. Treat once a week. Three treatments constitute one course. This method is especially suitable for treating children.

Electroacupuncture

Points used are the same as for body acupuncture. Select one or two pairs of points each time. Puncture until a needling sensation is achieved, then connect the needles to an electrical stimulator. Apply moderate continuous wave stimulation for 20–30 minutes, once a day or once every other day. Ten treatments constitute one course.

Auricular therapy

Auricular points:

Trachea, Lung, Chest: correspond to the affected region of the body; ease the lungs and open the chest to relieve asthma.

Spleen: strengthens the spleen to remove phlegm.

Kidney: reinforces the kidneys' ability to receive *qi*.

Large Intestine: helps the lungs to perform their function of dispersal and descent of *qi*.

Sympathesis: alleviates spasm of the bronchial smooth muscle to relieve asthma.

Apex of Antitragus, Adrenal Gland, Endocrine, Wind Stream: relieve inflammation and allergic reactions.

Ear Shenmen, Occiput: tranquillize the mind and relieve inflammation.

Use auricular taping twice a week. Ten treatments constitute one course.

Remarks

☯ Bronchial asthma is a refractory problem with a tendency to relapse. There is no definitive cure. However, numerous clinical studies have shown that scarifying moxibustion and point implantation therapy produce good long-term results. Further clinical study and theoretical research concerning these therapies is therefore indicated.

☯ Body acupuncture, used either singly or in combination with electrical stimulation or auricular therapy, is the method of choice during the attack stage; moxibustion, point implantation and point pricking are usually utilized during the remission stage.

☯ Therapeutic results are related to the duration and stage of the illness and age of the patient. Results are better for those under 30 and those with a history of less than ten years of the illness. Traditional therapies are less effective in cases with complications such as infection, pulmonary emphysema or pulmonary heart disease.

☯ Long-term mild moxibustion or scarifying moxibustion on Zusanli (S36) can be self-administered in order to increase immunity, prevent relapse and achieve a radical cure.

☯ Direction and depth must be carefully monitored when puncturing Tinatu (Ren22) in order to avoid damage to the lungs or blood vessels. First puncture perpendicularly for 0.2 *cun*, then directly downward along the back of the sternum for 1.0–1.5 *cun*.

19 Calcaneodynia

Calcaneodynia is a common manifestation of various heel disorders, including calcaneal spur, calcaneal bursitis, epiphysitis of the calcaneum and calcaneitis. It is marked by pain in the calcaneal region, aggravated by walking or standing. There is usually a tender point on the tuberosity of the calcaneum, but no redness or swelling. Calcaneodynia occurs mainly in the elderly and more often in females than in males.

Aetiology and differentiation of syndromes

According to traditional Chinese medicine, calcaneodynia is caused primarily by deficiency of the kidneys due to age, with resulting insufficient nourishment of the bones. There are usually no general symptoms, although soreness and weakness of the back and knees may occur.

Treatment
Body acupuncture

Acupuncture points

Ashi points:
Taixi   (K3)
Kunlun   (B60)

The functioning of the bones and the condition of the kidney essence are closely related, since the marrow which nourishes the bones is formed from vital essence stored by the kidneys. Therefore, Taixi (K3), the *yuan* (source) point of the Kidney meridian and also a local point for heel problems, is punctured to tonify the kidney essence and nourish the bones. Kunlun (B60), the *jing* (river) point of the Urinary Bladder meridian, is also a local point for treating heel problems.

Puncture the points on the affected side using the reinforcing method, once a day or once every other day. Five treatments constitute one course.

Electroacupuncture

Points used are the same as for body acupuncture. Select one or two pairs of points each time. Puncture the points until a needling sensation is achieved, then connect the needles to an electrical stimulator. Apply moderate intermittent wave stimulation for 30 minutes. Treat once a day or once every other day. Five treatments constitute one course.

Moxibustion

Locate tender point; apply a 0.3–0.5 cm thick slice of lacerated fresh ginger to the point. Place a moxa cone on the ginger, ignite and allow to burn down. Burn three to five cones on the point. Rub the local area with fresh ginger following treatment. Moxa roll moxibustion may be used if no fresh ginger is available. Treat once a day. Five treatments constitute one course.

Auricular therapy

Auricular points:

Heel: corresponds to the affected area of the body. Tape both frontal and dorsal surfaces to increase stimulation.

Kidney: tonifies the kidney essence to nourish the bones.

Liver: tonifies the liver blood to reinforce the kidney essence.

Subcortex, Ear Shenmen: relieve pain.

Use auricular taping with strong manipulation, twice a week. Five treatments constitute one course.

Remarks

☯ Traditional therapies are effective for treating calcaneodynia. Two or more methods are usually combined to increase stimulation and improve effect.

20 Cardiac neurosis

Cardiac neurosis, also called neurocirculatory asthenia or effort syndrome, is a functional disorder of the cardiovascular system caused by disturbance of the central nervous system. This disorder occurs mainly in adults and more often in females than in males. It is characterized by dull precordial pain lasting several hours or days, or stabbing pain in the apical region of the heart lasting one to five seconds. Other symptoms may include lassitude, palpitation, shortness of breath, anxiety, restlessness, mild fever, perspiration, or trembling or numbness of the hands. Cardiac neurosis is induced or aggravated primarily by exertion or mental injury.

Aetiology

Traditional Chinese medicine classifies cardiac neurosis as chest pain or palpitation. It is considered to be caused by mental injury such as extreme grief which damages the heart and spleen, leading to insufficient heart blood; by fright which disturbs the kidneys, with resulting imbalance between the heart and kidneys; or by anger or anxiety resulting in stagnation of the liver *qi* which affects the mind. Primarily affected are the heart, spleen, kidneys and liver.

Differentiation of syndromes

● Cardiac neurosis due to deficiency of the heart and spleen.
   Characterized by dull pain in the precordial region, palpitation, shortness of breath, lassitude, poor appetite, pale complexion, pale tongue with whitish coating and weak thready pulse.

- Cardiac neurosis due to imbalance of the heart and kidneys.
  Characterized by dull pain in the precordial region, panic, insomnia, bad dreams, feeling of heat in the palms and soles, night sweating, flushed cheeks, red tongue tip with little coating and rapid thready pulse.
- Cardiac neurosis due to stagnation of the liver *qi*.
  Characterized by stabbing pain in the apical region of the heart, feeling of fullness in the chest, depression, frequent sighing, poor appetite, pale or purple-spotted tongue with whitish coating and wiry pulse.

Treatment

Body acupuncture

Main acupuncture points:

Shenmen	(H7)
Neiguan	(P6)
Danzhong	(Ren17)
Jueyinshu	(B14)
Xinshu	(B15)

Back-*shu* points of the heart and pericardium and points of the Heart and Pericardium meridians are selected to relieve pain and calm the mind. Shenmen (H7), the *yuan* (source) point of the Heart meridian, is effective for treating heart diseases. Neiguan (P6), the *luo* (collateral) point of the Pericardium meridian and one of the eight confluence points connecting with the Yinwei meridian, is an important point for treating all heart problems. Danzhong (Ren17), the front-*mu* point of the pericardium and the *hui* (influential) point of *qi*; Jueyinshu (B14), the back-*shu* point of the pericardium; and Xinshu (B15), the back-*shu* point of the heart are treated in combination to strengthen the heart and relieve pain.

Auxiliary points and appropriate methods of manipulation are chosen according to differentiation of syndromes:

- For cardiac neurosis due to deficiency of the heart and spleen, Zusanli (S36), Sanyinjiao (Sp6) and Pishu (B20) are added and punctured using the reinforcing method to strengthen the spleen and stomach.
- For cardiac neurosis due to imbalance of the heart and kidneys, Taixi (K3) and Sanyinjiao (Sp6) are added and punctured using

the even method to harmonize the heart and kidneys.
- For cardiac neurosis due to stagnation of the liver *qi*, Taichong (Liv3) and Yanglingquan (G34) are added and punctured using the even method to promote the flow of the liver *qi*.

Treat once a day or once every other day. Ten treatments constitute one course.

Auricular therapy

Main auricular points:

Heart, Chest: tranquillize the mind and widen the chest.

Liver: regulates the flow of liver *qi* to relieve pain.

Subcortex: regulates the nervous and cardiovascular functions.

Ear Shenmen, Occiput: tranquillize the mind and relieve pain.

Apex of Ear: blood-letting puncturing of this point with a three-edged needle activates the meridians to relieve pain.

Auxiliary auricular points:

For deficiency of the heart and spleen, Spleen and Stomach are added.

For imbalance of the heart and kidneys, Kidney is added.

Use auricular taping and blood-letting puncturing where indicated, twice a week. Five treatments constitute one course.

Remarks

- The above methods are very effective for treating cardiac neurosis.
- Explaining the pathogenesis of cardiac neurosis will relieve patients' anxiety, as well as encourage a positive attitude and confidence that traditional therapies can provide a cure.

21 Central retinitis

Central retinitis is an eye disease caused by spasm of the capillaries of the macula lutea retinae. Manifestations include hypopsia, metamorphopsia, micropsia and fixed area opaca in the centre of the visual field. Tests of visual acuity will reveal central scotoma. The condition may recur following recovery.

Aetiology

According to traditional Chinese medicine, central retinitis has two causes. Stagnation of the liver *qi* and deficiency of the spleen may result in accumulation of phlegm and dampness in the interior, or deficiency of the liver and kidneys may lead to insufficient nourishment of the eyes.

Differentiation of syndromes

● Central retinitis due to stagnation of the liver *qi* and deficiency of the spleen.
   Characterized by blurred vision; accompanied by dizziness, headache, feeling of fullness in the chest and hypochondriac region, depression, restlessness, poor appetite, abdominal distension, loose stool and deep wiry pulse.
● Central retinitis due to deficiency of the liver and kidneys.
   Characterized by blurred vision; accompanied by dizziness, tinnitus, poor memory, sore and weak back and knees, pale tongue with whitish coating and deep thready pulse.

Treatment

Body acupuncture

Main acupuncture points:

Fengchi	(G20)
Guangming	(G37)
Taiyang	(Ex30)
Qiuhou	(Ex31)

The liver opens into the eyes and the Liver meridian connects with the eyes. The Liver and Gallbladder meridians are connected both externally and internally, so main points for treating eye problems are selected from the Gallbladder meridian. Fengchi (G20), an important point of the Gallbladder meridian located at the base of the skull, functions to sharpen the eyesight and is effective for treating various eye problems. Guangming (G37) (Brightness in Chinese) is the *luo* (collateral) point of the Gallbladder meridian. It is an effective distal point for treating eye problems.

Taiyang (Ex30) and Qiuhou (Ex31) are two extraordinary local points for treating eye problems. When puncturing Qiuhou (Ex31), support the eyeball with the thumb or index finger, then slowly puncture the point below the eyeball to a depth of 1.0–1.5 *cun*. Use no twisting, thrusting or lifting.

Auxiliary points and appropriate manipulation are chosen according to differentiation of syndromes.

● For central retinitis due to stagnation of the liver *qi* and deficiency of the spleen, Taichong (Liv3), Neiguan (P6) and Zusanli (S36) are added and punctured using the even method to promote the flow of the liver *qi* and strengthen the spleen.
● For central retinitis due to deficiency of the liver and kidneys, Ganshu (B18), Shenshu (B23) and Taixi (K3) are added and punctured using the reinforcing method to strengthen the liver and kidneys.

Treat once a day or once every other day. Ten treatments constitute one course.

Auricular therapy

Auricular points:

Eye: corresponds to the affected area. Locate positive points; tape both frontal and dorsal surfaces to increase stimulation.

Liver, Kidney: strengthen the liver and kidneys to nourish the eyes.

Spleen: reinforces the spleen to remove dampness and phlegm.

Sympathesis: relaxes vasospasm.

Subcortex, Occiput: regulate the optic nerve function.

Apex of Ear: blood-letting puncturing of this point with a three-edged needle brightens the eyes.

Use auricular taping with strong manipulation and blood-letting puncturing where indicated, twice a week. Five treatments constitute one course.

Scalp acupuncture

Scalp lines:

Zhenshang Pangxian (MS13)

Puncture the contralateral side. Twirl the needles using the even method for 5 minutes, or connect the needles to an electrical stimulator and apply moderate intermittent wave stimulation for 20–30 minutes. The needles should be retained for up to 24 hours to increase stimulation.

Treat once a day or once every other day. Ten treatments constitute one course.

Remarks

☯ Traditional therapies are effective for treating central retinitis, but long-term treatment should be given to maximize effects.
☯ In order to avoid bleeding, use mild manipulation when puncturing Qiuhou (Ex31) and press the point briefly after withdrawing the needle.
☯ These methods are also suitable for treating optic atrophy.

22 Cervical spondylopathy

Cervical spondylopathy is caused by degeneration and hyperosteogeny of the cervical intervertebral discs with resulting compression of the cervical root nerves or the spinal cord. It occurs primarily in people over 40 years old. There is often a history of cervical trauma, strain or stiff neck.

Cervical spondylopathy is classified clinically into five types:

● Neck type.
  Marked by severe intermittent pain in the cervical region radiating to the upper back and aggravated by forward or backward bending or rotation of the neck. The condition persists for three to five days, with a remission stage between attacks.
● Nerve root type, further classified into three types:
  – Pain type.
    Marked by sudden onset of pain and soreness in the neck, shoulder, forearm and hand, usually on only one side, aggravated by coughing and at night.
  – Numb type.
    Marked by chronic numbness, possibly with mild pain in the shoulder, forearm, upper chest and back, aggravated at night. There

may be no symptoms during the day.
  – Atrophic type.
    Marked by weakness and atrophy of the upper limb on the affected side, but with no numbness or pain.
● Spinal compression type.
  Marked by gradually worsening feeling of heaviness in the affected limb, frequent falling and even paralysis in the advanced stage. Incontinence of urine or stool may also occur.
● Vertebroarterial type.
  Marked by vertigo, headache, restlessness, unstable gait, tinnitus or hypoacusis.
● Sympathetic type.
  Manifestations are various, including weak eyelids, distended and painful eyes, lacrimation and tinnitus or hypoacusis; discomfort in the throat and nausea; hypohidrosis or hyperhidrosis; or intermittent high or low blood pressure and tachycardia. Sympathetic type cervical spondylopathy is rarely seen in clinical practice.

Aetiology

According to traditional Chinese medicine, cervical spondylopathy is caused by a combination of internal deficiency of the liver and kidneys and external trauma or invasion by wind-cold or wind-damp. The internal and external factors combine to result in obstruction of *qi* and blood and insufficient nourishment of the muscles and bones.

Differentiation of syndromes

- Cervical spondylopathy due to stagnation of *qi* and blood.
  Characterized by severe pain in the neck and shoulder which may radiate to the unilateral or bilateral forearms and fingers, aggravated by coughing and worsening at night; purple-spotted tongue and uneven pulse.
- Cervical spondylopathy due to deficiency of the liver and kidneys.
  Characterized by numbness in the shoulder, forearm and upper chest, or weakness and atrophy of the upper limbs, with no accompanying numbness or pain. Paralysis, feeling of cold in the extremeties and incontinence of stool and urine may occur in some cases.
- Cervical spondylopathy due to hyperactivity of the liver *yang*.
  Characterized by vertigo, headache, restlessness, irritability, distended and painful eyes, tinnitus or hypoacusis, purple tongue and thready wiry pulse.

Treatment

Body acupuncture

Main acupuncture points:

Ashi points
Dazhui	(Du14)
Fengchi	(G20)
Houxi	(SI3)
Xuanzhong	(G39)

Ashi points, Dazhui (Du14) and Fengchi (G20) are local points for treating cervical spondylopathy. Specific *Ashi* points are first determined by X-ray examination or by locating tender points. They are then punctured obliquely towards the spinous process of the cervical vertebrae until the tip of the needle touches the periosteum of the spinous process and a needling sensation radiates to the affected arm. Houxi (SI3), one of the eight confluence points connecting with the Du meridian, is an important point for treating neck problems. Xuanzhong (G39), one of the eight *hui*

(influential) points related to the marrow, is an important point for treating bone diseases.

Auxiliary points and appropriate methods of manipulation are chosen according to differentiation of syndromes:

- For cervical spondylopathy due to stagnation of *qi* and blood, the flow of blood and *qi* are promoted and pain relieved by adding and puncturing Tianzong (SI11), Jianjing (G21), Jianyu (LI15) and Waiguan (SJ5) using the reducing method, or by pricking local points with a three-edged needle and then cupping for 15–20 minutes.
- For cervical spondylopathy due to deficiency of the liver and kidneys, the upper limbs are treated using the same auxiliary points as for cervical spondylopathy due to stagnation of *qi* and blood (see above). The lower limbs are treated by adding and puncturing Huantiao (G30), Yanglingquan (G34) and Zusanli (S36) using the reinforcing method.
- For cervical spondylopathy due to hyperactivity of the liver *yang*, Baihui (Du20), Taiyang (Ex30), Taichong (Liv3) and Taixi (K3) are added and punctured using the even-method to subdue hyperactive liver *yang*.

Treat once a day or once every other day. Ten treatments constitute one course.

Electroacupuncture

Points used are the same as for body acupuncture. Select two to three pairs of points each time. Puncture the points until a needling sensation is achieved, then connect the needles to an electrical stimulator. Apply continuous wave stimulation of the highest bearable intensity for thirty minutes. Treat once a day or once every other day. Ten treatments constitute one course.

Point injection therapy

Specific local *ashi* points are determined by X-ray examination or by locating tender points. The points are first punctured obliquely towards the spinous process of the cervical vertebrae until the tip of the needle touches the periosteum of the spinous process and a needling sensation radiates to the affected arm. They are then injected with 2–4 ml of vitamin B_1, vitamin B_{12}, or dexamethasone. Treat once a day or once every other day. Ten treatments constitute one course.

Cupping

Local *ashi* points and Dazhui (Du14) are pricked with a three-edged needle and then cupped for 10–15 minutes to draw a small amount of blood.

Cupping can effectively promote the flow of *qi* and blood and is suitable for treating cervical spondylopathy due to stagnation of *qi* and blood.

Moxibustion

Apply moxa roll moxibustion for 15–20 minutes to *ashi* points and Dazhui (Du14) once a day. Ten treatments constitute one course.

Moxibustion functions to warm the meridians and relieve pain and is suitable for treating cervical spondylopathy due to stagnation of *qi* and blood or deficiency of the liver and kidneys.

Auricular therapy

Main auricular points:

Cervical Vertebrae: correspond to the affected areas of the body. Locate positive points; tape both frontal and dorsal surfaces to increase stimulation.

Liver, Kidney: the liver nourishes the tendons and the kidneys the bones, so Liver and Kidney are taped to strengthen the tendons and bones.

Ear Shenmen: main point for relieving pain.

Auxiliary auricular points:

For dizziness, Occiput is added.

For numbness and pain of the arms and fingers, positive points on the scaphoid fossa are added.

Use auricular taping, twice a week. Five treatments constitute one course.

Remarks

- The above therapies are very effective for treating cervical spondylopathy of the neck and nerve root types. For spinal compression type cervical spondylopathy, additional measures such as surgery should also be considered.
- Cervical spondylopathy is a refractory problem that recurs easily. It is therefore essential to continue treatment even after symptoms have disappeared.
- Keeping the neck warm, using a comfortable pillow and doing the following exercises will help consolidate the effect of treatment and prevent relapse:
  - Neck stretching.
    Sitting on a chair with the eyes slightly closed, bend the head forwards, backwards, to the left and to the right. Rotate the head in clockwise and counterclockwise circles. Turn the head to the left and right to look up at the moon; turn the head to the left and right to look out at the sea. Repeat the series of motions slowly and deliberately 10–15 times, three to four times a day.
  - Neck massage.
    Rub the hands together until they feel hot. First massage along the bilateral sides of the neck from Fengchi (G20) to Dazhui (Du14) 15–20 times; then press Fengchi (G20) and Dazhui (Du14) 15–20 times; finally use both hands to rub the ears, especially the body of the antihelix and the earlobes, 15–20 times. Repeat two to three times a day.

The above exercises can be done singly or in combination.

23   Childhood anorexia

Childhood anorexia is a common digestive disorder that occurs primarily in children one to ten years old. It is characterized by long-standing poor appetite or even refusal to eat, usually accompanied by pale complexion, emaciation and retardation of growth and development.

Aetiology and differentiation of syndromes

According to traditional Chinese medicine, childhood anorexia is caused primarily by improper dietary habits, such as overeating or drinking, inappropriate food preferences or irregular meals, which result in injury to the spleen and stomach and their subsequent dysfunction. Manifestations include poor appetite, preference for certain foods, pale complexion, emaciation, susceptibility to the common cold, pale tongue with thin whitish coating and weak thready pulse.

Treatment

Body acupuncture

Acupuncture points:

Pishu	(B20)
Weishu	(B21)
Zhongwan	(Ren12)
Tianshu	(S25)
Zusanli	(S36)
Sanyinjiao	(Sp6)

Pishu (B20) and Weishu (B21), the back-*shu* points of the spleen and stomach respectively, are punctured to strengthen the spleen and stomach. The functions of the stomach and intestines are regulated by selecting Zhongwan (Ren12), the *hui* (influential) point of the *fu* organs and the front-*mu* point of the stomach; Tianshu (S25), the front-*mu* point of the large intestine; and Zusanli (S36), the *he* (sea) and lower *he* (confluent) point of the Stomach meridian. Sanyinjiao (Sp6), the meeting point of the three Foot Yin meridians, is treated to strengthen the spleen.

All points are punctured using the reinforcing method, with the needles removed immediately. Treat once a day or every other day. Five treatments constitute one course.

Moxibustion

Acupuncture points:

Zhongwan	(Ren12)
Shenque	(Ren8)
Guanyuan	(Ren4)
Zusanli	(S36)
Pishu	(B20)
Weishu	(B21)

Select two or three points each time. Apply moxa roll moxibustion to each point for 15–20 minutes, once a day. Ten treatments constitute one course.

This method functions to strengthen the spleen and stomach and can be undertaken at home by the children's parents.

Chiropractic

See Appendix 5.

Auricular therapy

Auricular points:

Stomach, Spleen: correspond to the affected areas of the body; strengthen the spleen and stomach to improve digestion and absorption.

Small Intestine: improves the absorption of nutrients.

Liver: regulates the flow of *qi* to improve transportation and transformation by the spleen and stomach.

Abdomen: promotes peristalsis.

Endocrine, Subcortex: regulate the digestive function.

Use auricular taping, twice a week. Five treatments constitute one course.

Blood-letting puncturing

Acupuncture point:

Sifeng	(Ex2)

Treat Sifeng (Ex2) of the right and left hands alternately. Prick the points with a three-edged needle, then press to express some yellowish fluid or blood. Treat once every other day. Five treatments constitute one course.

Remarks

☙ Traditional therapies are very effective for treating childhood anorexia. There is usually marked improvement in appetite, peristalsis and willingness to eat after only one or two treatments.

☙ Severe cases may be treated with several therapies in combination to increase stimulation and improve effectiveness.

24 Childhood hyperkinetic syndrome

Childhood hyperkinetic syndrome, also called minimal brain dysfunction, is a common developmental problem of childhood. It is characterized by hyperactivity, distractibility, excessive mood swings and cognitive difficulty. However, intelligence is close to or completely normal and sometimes superior. Minimal dysfunction of the central nervous system may be present. In most cases, all symptoms diminish or disappear with maturation. Common causes include heredity, abnormal or difficult labour resulting in oxygen deprivation, or disease in infancy.

Aetiology and differentiation of syndromes

According to traditional Chinese medicine, childhood hyperkinetic syndrome is caused by congenital insufficiency or acquired malnutrition, both of which may affect childhood development. Primarily affected are the heart, spleen, liver and kidneys.

Treatment

Body acupuncture

Acupuncture points:

Baihui	(Du20)
Fengchi	(G20)
Taiyang	(Ex30)
Neiguan	(P6)
Sanyinjiao	(Sp6)
Taixi	(K3)
Zusanli	(S36)
Taichong	(Liv3)
Hegu	(LI4)

Baihui (Du20), the meeting point of the Du, Liver and six Hand and Foot Yang meridians located on the top of the head and Fengchi (G20), a main point of the Gallbladder meridian located at the base of the skull, are punctured to refresh the brain and tranquillize the mind. Taiyang (Ex30) functions to brighten the eyes and strengthen the brain. Neiguan (P6), the *luo*

(collateral) point of the Pericardium meridian and one of the eight confluence points connecting with the Yinwei meridian, is treated to open the chest and calm the mind. Sanyinjiao (Sp6), the meeting point of the three Foot Yin meridians, strengthens the spleen, liver and kidneys. Taixi (K3), the *yuan* (source) point of the Kidney meridian, tonifies the kidneys. Zusanli (S36), the *he* (sea) and lower *he* (confluent) point of the Stomach meridian, is treated to strengthen the spleen and stomach in order to nourish the mind. Taichong (Liv3) and Hegu (LI4), the *yuan* (source) points of the Liver and Large Intestine meridians respectively, are usually treated in combination to regulate the flow of *qi* and calm the mind.

Select four to six points each time. Puncture using even manipulation, once every other day. Ten treatments constitute one course.

Electroacupuncture

Points used are the same as for body acupuncture. Select one or two pairs of points each time. Puncture until a needling sensation is achieved, then connect the needles to an electrical stimulator. Apply moderate intermittent wave stimulation for 20–30 minutes. Treat once every other day. Ten treatments constitute one course.

Chiropractic

See Appendix 5.

Auricular therapy

Auricular points:

Kidney: strengthens the congenital essence.

Liver, Heart: calm the mind.

Spleen, Stomach: strengthen the spleen and stomach to tonify the *qi* and blood.

Subcortex, Forehead: nourish the brain.

Ear Shenmen, Occiput: tranquillize the mind.

Use auricular taping, twice a week. Auricular massage is very useful for children with hyperkinetic syndrome and should be given by their parents or caregivers twice a day.

Remarks

☯ Traditional therapies are effective for treating childhood hyperkinetic syndrome. Two or more therapies are usually combined to increase stimulation.

☯ It is essential to undertake appropriate psychological counselling in addition to traditional treatment in order to shorten the course of the treatment.

25 Chloasma

Chloasma refers to acquired, localized, cutaneous melanosis. It may be caused by chronic illness, endocrine disorder, irregular menstruation, or overexposure to the sun, leading to hyperfunction of the cutaneous melanocytes. Adult women are especially susceptible to this problem. Affected skin is marked by light or dark brown patches with a clearly delineated border, symmetrically distributed in the shape of a butterfly covering the forehead and zygomatic, buccal, nasal and perioral regions.

Aetiology and differentiation of syndromes

According to traditional Chinese medicine, chloasma is caused either by deficiency of the kidney essence or stagnation of the liver *qi*, either of which may lead to insufficient nourishment of the face. There are usually no general symptoms accompanying localized manifestations.

Treatment

Auricular therapy

Auricular points:

Areas corresponding to the affected regions: tap with a plum blossom needle to cause mild bleeding.

Liver: improves the flow of *qi* and blood.

Spleen, Stomach: strengthen the spleen and stomach to improve digestion and nourish the face.

Kidney: tonifies the kidneys to nourish the face.

Endocrine, Adrenal Gland, Midpoint of Rim: regulate endocrine function.

Use auricular taping with strong manipulation and blood-letting puncturing where indicated, twice a week. Ten treatments constitute one course.

Remarks

☯ Auricular therapy is effective for treating chloasma, but extended treatment (usually three courses) should be given to achieve results.

☯ Maintain a positive psychological attitude and avoid overexposure to the sun.

26 Cholecystitis

Cholecystitis is an acute or chronic inflammation of the gallbladder. The acute type is marked by sudden persistent pain in the right upper abdomen with paroxysmal exacerbation and radiation to the right shoulder and back, usually accompanied by nausea, vomiting and fever. It occurs primarily in middle-aged people, more often in women than in men. It is usually induced by overindulgence in greasy foods. Cases of chronic cholecystitis are usually preceded by a history of acute cholecystitis. The manifestations of an attack of chronic cholecystitis are similar to those of acute cholecystitis. The remission stage of chronic cholecystitis is marked by distension and discomfort in the upper abdomen after eating, eructation and aversion to greasy foods, usually accompanied by dull pain in the right shoulder and back aggravated by standing, motion or cold showers.

Aetiology

Traditional Chinese medicine classifies cholecystitis as hypochondriac pain or jaundice. It is considered to be caused by mental injury resulting in stagnation of the liver *qi* and subsequent accumulation of bile in the gallbladder; by exogenous or endogenous damp-heat which accumulates in the liver and gallbladder with resulting disturbance of bile secretion; or by stones or ascarides which obstruct bile secretion. In protracted cases the spleen and stomach may be damaged, or stones may be formed by vaporization of the bile accumulated by damp-heat, further aggravating the condition. Primarily affected are the liver, spleen, gallbladder and stomach.

Differentiation of syndromes

- Cholecystitis due to accumulation of damp-heat in the liver and gallbladder.
  Characterized by sudden onset or repeated attack of severe pain in the upper abdomen and hypochondriac region, aggravated by pressure and eating; accompanied by fever or intermittent fever with chills; nausea, vomiting, yellowish eyes or skin, dry throat and bitter taste in the mouth, poor appetite, aversion to greasy food, constipation, scanty yellowish urine, red tongue with greasy yellowish coating and rapid wiry slippery pulse.
- Cholecystitis due to stagnation of the liver *qi*.
  Characterized by dull or distending pain in the right upper abdomen with paroxysmal exacerbation and radiation to the right shoulder and back; accompanied by feeling of fullness in the chest, depression, frequent sighing, poor appetite, abdominal distension, eructation, whitish tongue coating and wiry pulse.
- Cholecystitis due to combined deficiency of the spleen and stagnation of the liver *qi*.
  Characterized by distension and discomfort in the upper abdomen after eating, eructation,

aversion to greasy food, poor appetite, loose stool, lassitude, sallow complexion, pale tongue with greasy whitish coating and soft pulse.

Treatment

Body acupuncture

Main acupuncture points:

Riyue	(G24) (right)
Danshu	(B19)
Yanglingquan	(G34)
Neiguan	(P6)
Zusanli	(S36)

Cholecystitis is a disorder of the gallbladder and stomach. Therefore Riyue (G24) and Danshu (B19), the front-*mu* and back-*shu* points respectively of the gallbladder and Yanglingquan (G34), the *he* (sea) and lower *he* (confluent) point of the Gallbladder meridian, are treated to regulate the function of the gallbladder. Neiguan (P6), the *luo* (collateral) point of the Pericardium meridian and one of the eight confluence points connecting with the Yinwei meridian and Zusanli (S36), the *he* (sea) point of the Stomach meridian, are treated in combination to harmonize the stomach.

Auxiliary points and appropriate methods of manipulation are chosen according to differentiation of syndromes.

- For cholecystitis due to accumulation of damp-heat in the liver and gallbladder, Zhongji (Ren3), Yinlingquan (Sp9) and Xingjian (Liv2) are added and punctured using the reducing method to eliminate damp-heat.
- For cholecystitis due to stagnation of the liver *qi*, Taichong (Liv3), Hegu (LI4) and Zhigou (SJ6) are added and punctured to promote the flow of *qi* and relieve pain.
- For cholecystitis due to combined deficiency of the spleen and stagnation of the liver *qi*, Zhongwan (Ren12), Tianshu (S25) and Sanyinjiao (Sp6) are added and punctured using the reinforcing method to strengthen the spleen and stomach.

Electroacupuncture

Points used are the same as for body acupuncture. Select one or two pairs of points each time. Puncture the points until a needling sensation is achieved, then connect the needles to an electrical stimulator. Apply moderate intermittent wave stimulation for 20–30 minutes. Treat once a day or once every other day. Ten treatments constitute one course.

Auricular therapy

Auricular points:

Pancreas & Gallbladder: corresponds to the affected organs. Locate positive points; tape both frontal and dorsal surfaces to increase stimulation. Concentrate on treating the right auricle.

Liver: soothes the liver and gallbladder.

Abdomen, Thoracic Vertebrae: locate positive points; tape both frontal and dorsal surfaces to increase stimulation. The Thoracic Vertebrae positive point is usually found between Thoracic Vertebrae and the scaphoid fossa.

Spleen, Stomach: strengthen the spleen and stomach to transport and transform water and dampness.

San Jiao: dispels damp-heat.

Root of Ear Vagus: clinically effective point for treating cholecystitis.

Endocrine: regulates the endocrine function.

Apex of Ear: blood-letting puncturing of this point with a three-edged needle dispels damp-heat.

Use auricular taping with strong manipulation and blood-letting puncturing where indicated, twice a week. Five treatments constitute one course.

Remarks

- Traditional therapies can effectively relieve the pain and inflammation of both acute and chronic cholecystitis. There will often be great improvement in symptoms such as pain in the upper right abdomen and vomiting after one or two treatments.
- When puncturing Yanglingquan (G34) it is essential to locate and puncture tender points near it. A tender point will generally be found on Dannangxue (Ex21), located one to two *cun* below Yanglingquan (G34).
- For cases of suppurative gangrenous cholecystitis or perforated gallbladder, concurrent emergency treatment should be undertaken.

27 Cholelithiasis

Cholelithiasis, or gallstones, is a commonly seen acute abdominal condition. The formation of stones in the gallbladder or biliary ducts is due primarily to cholestasis, infection of the biliary tract, or metabolic cholesterol disturbance. It occurs mainly in the middle-aged and more often in females than in males. There is usually a history of frequently recurring persistent dull pain in the upper abdomen. During remission, there may be no symptoms or mild dull pain in the right upper abdomen; during the active stage, manifestations differ according to the location of the stones. The most common symptom is paroxysmal colicky pain in the right upper abdomen radiating to the right shoulder. Other commonly seen symptoms include aversion to greasy food, nausea, vomiting, bitter taste in the mouth, poor appetite and fever.

Aetiology

Traditional Chinese medicine classifies cholelithiasis as hypochondriac pain. It is considered to be caused by exogenous or endogenous damp-heat which leads to dampness and heat in the gallbladder and liver; the accumulated dampness subsequently vaporizes and forms stones.

Differentiation of syndromes

- Cholelithiasis due to accumulation of damp-heat in the liver and gallbladder.
  Characterized by sudden onset or repeated attack of severe pain in the upper abdomen and hypochondriac region, aggravated by pressure

and eating; accompanied by fever or intermittent fever with chills; nausea, vomiting,
yellowish eyes or skin, dry throat and bitter taste
in the mouth, poor appetite, aversion to greasy
food, constipation, scanty yellowish urine, red
tongue with greasy yellowish coating and wiry,
slippery and rapid pulse.

● Cholelithiasis due to stagnation of the liver *qi*.
Characterized by dull or distending pain in the
right upper abdomen with paroxysmal exacerbation and radiation to the right shoulder and back;
accompanied by feeling of fullness in the chest,
depression, frequent sighing, poor appetite,
abdominal distension, eructation, whitish tongue coating and wiry pulse.

● Cholelithiasis due to combined deficiency of the
spleen and stagnation of the liver *qi*.
Characterized by distension and discomfort in
the upper abdomen after eating, eructation,
aversion to greasy food, poor appetite, loose
stool, lassitude, sallow complexion, pale tongue
with greasy whitish coating and soft pulse.

Treatment

Body acupuncture

Main acupuncture points:

Riyue	(G24) (right)
Danshu	(B19)
Yanglingquan	(G34)
Neiguan	(P6)
Zusanli	(S36)

Cholelithiasis is a disorder of the gallbladder and
stomach. Therefore Riyue (G24) and Danshu
(B19), the front-*mu* and back-*shu* points respectively of the gallbladder and Yanglingquan (G34),
the *he* (sea) and lower *he* (confluent) point of the
Gallbladder meridian, are treated to regulate the
function of the gallbladder. Neiguan (P6), the *luo*
(collateral) point of the Pericardium meridian and
one of the eight confluence points connecting with
the Yinwei meridian and Zusanli (S36), the *he*
(sea) point of the Stomach meridian, are treated in
combination to harmonize the stomach.

Auxiliary points and appropriate methods of
manipulation are chosen according to differentiation of syndromes:

● For cholelithiasis due to accumulation of damp-
heat in the liver and gallbladder, Zhongji
(Ren3), Yinlingquan (Sp9) and Xingjian (Liv2)
are added and punctured using the reducing
method to eliminate damp-heat.

● For cholelithiasis due to stagnation of the liver
qi, Taichong (Liv3), Hegu (LI4) and Zhigou
(SJ6) are added and punctured to promote the
flow of *qi* and relieve pain.

● For cholelithiasis due to combined deficiency of
the spleen and stagnation of the liver *qi*,
Zhongwan (Ren12), Tianshu (S25) and Sanyinjiao (Sp6) are added and punctured using the
reinforcing method to strengthen the spleen and
stomach.

Electroacupuncture

Points used are the same as for body acupuncture.
Select one or two pairs of points each time.
Puncture the points until a needling sensation is
achieved, then connect the needles to an electrical
stimulator. Apply moderate intermittent wave stimulation for 20–30 minutes. Treat once a day or
once every other day. Ten treatments constitute one
course.

Auricular therapy

Auricular points:

Pancreas & Gallbladder: corresponds to the
affected organs. Locate positive points; tape
both frontal and dorsal surfaces to increase
stimulation. Concentrate on treating the right
auricle.

Liver: soothes the liver and gallbladder.

Abdomen, Thoracic Vertebrae: locate positive
points; tape both frontal and dorsal surfaces to
increase stimulation. The Thoracic Vertebrae
positive point is usually found between Thoracic
Vertebrae and the scaphoid fossa.

Spleen, Stomach: strengthen the spleen and
stomach to transport and transform water and
dampness.

San Jiao: dispels damp-heat.

Root of Ear Vagus: clinically effective point for
treating cholelithiasis.

Endocrine: regulates the endocrine function.

Apex of Ear: blood-letting puncturing of this
point with a three-edged needle dispels damp-
heat.

Use auricular taping with strong manipulation
and blood-letting puncturing where indicated,
twice a week. Five treatments constitute one
course.

Remarks

☯ Acupuncture can effectively relieve the colicky pain of cholelithiasis, as well as its other symptoms.

☯ Clinical studies indicate that treating certain acupuncture points, including Yanglingquan (G34), Riyue (G24), Zusanli (S36) and Danshu (B19), can increase bile secretion, promote contractility of the gallbladder and decrease tonicity of Oddi's sphincter to promote the discharge of gallstones.

☯ Discharge of the stones depends on their size, shape and location. Smooth stones less than 1 cm in diameter are easily discharged; stones located in the common bile duct are more easily discharged than those in the gallbladder or intrahepatic duct.

☯ Comprehensive programme for discharging gallstones:

Time	Treatment
10.15 a.m.	40 ml 33% Epsom salt solution (oral administration)
10.25 a.m.	High fat meal (2–3 fried eggs)
10.30 a.m.	Electroacupuncture Acupuncture points: Riyue (G24) Danshu (B19) Yanglingquan (G34) Zusanli (S36) Puncture until a needling sensation is achieved, then connect the needles to an electrical stimulator. Apply intermittent wave stimulation of the strongest bearable intensity for 30–60 minutes.

The three methods combined in this comprehensive programme function to both increase contraction of the gallbladder and relax Oddi's sphincter in order to rapidly and effectively promote the discharge of gallstones.

Treat once every other day for people with strong constitutions and mild reactions and once a week for those with weak constitutions and severe reactions. Four to six treatments constitute one course. Allow a one month interval between courses.

28 Chronic bronchitis

Chronic bronchitis is a chronic non-specific inflammation of the mucosa and peripheral tissues of the trachea and bronchi caused by bacterial or viral infection, or by irritation due to physical or chemical factors or allergenic pathogens. It is marked by long-standing intermittent cough with sputum, induced or aggravated by cold or over-strain and usually accompanied by a feeling of fullness in the chest, shortness of breath and lassitude.

Aetiology

Traditional Chinese medicine classifies chronic bronchitis as endogenous cough. Primarily affected are the lungs, spleen and kidneys. The lungs govern dispersal and descent of *qi*; cough results when the lungs are affected and the *qi* cannot

descend. The spleen governs transportation and transformation of dampness; phlegm is produced when the spleen is deficient. The kidneys govern reception of *qi*; respiratory difficulty occurs if the kidneys are deficient and the *qi* cannot be received.

Differentiation of syndromes

● Chronic bronchitis due to *qi* deficiency of the lungs and spleen.
 Characterized by cough with profuse thin sputum, shortness of breath, feeling of fullness in the chest, lassitude, poor appetite, spontaneous sweating, aversion to wind, susceptibility to the common cold, pale tongue with whitish coating and weak pulse.

- Chronic bronchitis due to accumulation of phlegm-damp in the lungs.
  Characterized by cough with easily expectorated, profuse thin whitish sputum; feeling of fullness in the chest, poor appetite, abdominal distension, feeling of heaviness and weakness of the body and limbs, greasy whitish tongue coating and soft loose pulse.
- Chronic bronchitis due to *yin* deficiency of the lungs and kidneys.
  Characterized by dry cough or cough with scanty bloody sputum, afternoon fever, night sweating, flushed cheeks, feeling of heat in the palms and soles, dry throat with hoarseness, emaciation, dry reddish tongue with little coating and rapid thready pulse.
- Chronic bronchitis due to *yang* deficiency of the spleen and kidneys.
  Characterized by cough with thin whitish sputum, dizziness, palpitation, aversion to cold, feeling of cold in the limbs, weak or sore back and knees, oedema, swollen tongue with tooth prints and whitish coating and deep slippery pulse.

Treatment

Body acupuncture

Main acupuncture points:

Feishu	(B13)
Zhongfu	(L1)
Danzhong	(Ren17)
Tiantu	(Ren22)
Bailao	(Ex38)
Dingchuan	(Ex41)

Feishu (B13) and Zhongfu (L1), the back-*shu* and front-*mu* points respectively of the lung, are usually tender in cases of chronic bronchitis and are punctured to regulate the lung *qi*. Danzhong (Ren17), the *hui* (influential) point of *qi*, is punctured horizontally downward for 1.0–1.5 *cun* to regulate the flow of *qi* and open the chest to stop cough. To increase stimulation, the needle may be retained on the point by taping the handle to the skin. Tiantu (Ren22), a local point for treating bronchial problems, can effectively alleviate spasm of the bronchial smooth muscle to relieve cough. It is punctured perpendicularly for 0.2 *cun*, then vertically downward along the posterior wall of the sternum for 1.0–1.5 *cun*. Bailao (Ex38) and Dingchuan (Ex41) are both clinically effective points for treating lung diseases.

Auxiliary points and appropriate methods of manipulation are chosen according to differentiation of syndromes.

- For chronic bronchitis due to *qi* deficiency of the lungs and spleen, Pishu (B20), Qihai (Ren6) and Zusanli (S36) are added and punctured using the reinforcing method to strengthen the spleen and tonify *qi*.
- For chronic bronchitis due to accumulation of phlegm-dampness in the lungs, Zhongwan (Ren12), Pishu (B20) and Fenglong (S40) are added and punctured using the even method to strengthen the spleen and eliminate phlegm.
- For chronic bronchitis due to *yin* deficiency of the lungs and kidneys, Yuji (L10), Taixi (K3) and Sanyinjiao (Sp6) are added and punctured using the even method to nourish the kidney *yin* and moisten the lungs.
- For chronic bronchitis due to *yang* deficiency of the spleen and kidneys, the spleen and kidneys are warmed by adding and puncturing Pishu (B20), Shenshu (B23), Guanyuan (Ren4) and Mingmen (Du4) using the reinforcing method and adding moxibustion as needed.

Treat once a day or once every other day. Ten treatments constitute one course.

Moxibustion

Acupuncture points on the back:

Feishu	(B13)
Gaohuang	(B43)
Shenzhu	(Du12)
Dazhui	(Du14)
Pishu	(B20)
Shenshu	(B23)
Mingmen	(Du4)

Acupuncture points on the front:

Danzhong	(Ren17)
Zhongfu	(L1)
Guanyuan	(Ren4)
Qihai	(Ren6)

Three types of moxibustion may be employed:

- Moxa roll moxibustion.
  Select three to five points each time. Apply moxa roll moxibustion for 10–15 minutes to each point. Treat once a day; ten treatments constitute one course.
- Ginger moxibustion.
  Select three to five points each time. Puncture 3 mm thick pieces of fresh ginger several times

with a needle. Place one piece of ginger on each point; place moxa cones on top of the ginger and ignite. Use three to five moxa cones on each point. Treat once a day or once every other day; ten treatments constitute one course.

● Scarifying moxibustion.
Select two to three points each time. After applying a thin layer of garlic juice to each point, place moxa cones on the points, let them burn completely down and remove the ashes. Repeat the process five to eight times until small blisters form. Bandage with sterile gauze. After seven days, aseptic post-moxibustion sores will appear on the points. The sores should be debrided once a day with physiological saline solution and bandaged with sterile gauze. After about one month the sores will disappear, leaving scars. If no post-moxibustion sores appear following moxibustion, repeat the process. If secondary infection occurs, additional treatment should be undertaken.

The following methods may be used to alleviate the pain of scarifying moxibustion: tap the area surrounding the points with the palm of the hand, or inject 1–2 ml of 0.2% procaine solution subcutaneously as a local anaesthetic.

Scarifying moxibustion is usually applied in the summer. Treat once a year. Three treatments constitute one course.

Cupping

Apply moving cupping along the first and second lines of the Urinary Bladder meridian on the back using the following method. Apply a thin layer of lubricant such as Vaseline, then apply the cup moving it from top to bottom while rotating. Repeat several times until purple spots appear. Treat twice a week. Ten treatments constitute one course.

Point implantation therapy

Acupuncture points:

Feishu	(B13)
Pishu	(B20)
Shenshu	(B23)
Gaohuang	(B45)
Dingchuan	(Ex41)
Zhongwan	(Ren12)
Danzhong	(Ren12)

Select three to four points each time. For procedure see Appendix 9. Treat once every two weeks. Five treatments constitute one course.

Electroacupuncture

Points used are the same as for body acupuncture. Select one or two pairs of points each time. Puncture until a needling sensation is achieved, then connect the needles to an electrical stimulator. Apply moderate continuous wave stimulation for 20 minutes, once a day or once every other day. Ten treatments constitute one course.

Auricular therapy

Auricular points:

Trachea, Lung, Chest: correspond to the affected areas of the body, regulate the flow of *qi* to widen the chest and relieve cough.

Spleen: strengthens the spleen to reduce phlegm.

Kidney: reinforces the kidneys to improve the reception of *qi*.

Large Intestine: the large intestine is connected both internally and externally with the lungs, so Large Intestine is treated to improve the lungs' function of dispersal and descent.

Endocrine: relieves inflammation.

Ear Shenmen, Occiput: tranquillize the mind and relieve inflammation.

Use auricular taping, twice a week. Ten treatments constitute one course.

Remarks

☯ The auricular area corresponding to the bronchi is located between Trachea and Lung; auricular palpation is used to locate positive points precisely.
☯ Traditional therapies can effectively relieve the symptoms of chronic bronchitis, including cough, shortness of breath and feeling of fullness in the chest.
☯ Modern experimental research has shown that moxibustion can raise the immune level of the human body and harmonize the autonomic nervous system; this is consistent with clinical reports that moxibustion, particularly scarify-

ing moxibustion, can not only alleviate the symptoms of chronic bronchitis, but also prevent relapse and even achieve a radical cure following long-term treatment.

☯ Scarifying moxibustion is applied primarily in midsummer in order to prevent winter onset of chronic bronchitis. This method is referred to as 'treating winter's disease in the summer.'

29 Chronic diarrhoea

Chronic diarrhoea is a chronic problem of the digestive system characterized by persistent diarrhoea lasting for over two months and usually accompanied by abdominal distension or pain and poor appetite. It is a common symptom of many diseases and disorders such as chronic enteritis, intestinal tuberculosis, functional disturbance of the intestines and colonitis.

Aetiology

According to traditional Chinese medicine, chronic diarrhoea may be caused either by severe impairment of the spleen *yang* arising from improperly treated acute diarrhoea, or by deficient kidney *yang* insufficient to warm the spleen and separate liquid and solid.

Differentiation of syndromes

● Chronic diarrhoea due to deficiency of the spleen *yang*.
  Characterized by persistent diarrhoea containing undigested food, aggravated by intake of cold or greasy food; poor appetite, lassitude, sallow complexion, pale tongue with whitish coating and weak pulse.
● Chronic diarrhoea due to deficiency of the kidney *yang*.
  Characterized by pre-dawn diarrhoea, aggravated by cold or exertion; accompanied by coldness of the limbs and body, sore and weak back and knees, pale tongue with whitish coating and deep thready pulse.
● Chronic diarrhoea due to blockage of the collaterals by stagnant blood.
  Characterized by bloody diarrhoea, fixed stabbing abdominal pain aggravated by pressure, dark complexion, dry mouth and little thirst,

tongue purple or with ecchymosis and uneven pulse.

Treatment

Body acupuncture

Main acupuncture points:

Tianshu	(S25)
Shangjuxu	(S37)
Zusanli	(S36)

Tianshu (S25), the front-*mu* point of the large intestine and Shangjuxu (S37), the lower *he* (confluent) point of the Large Intestine meridian, are treated in combination to strengthen the large intestine's function of transportation. These points are used for treating all problems of the large intestine. Zusanli (S36), the *he* (sea) and lower *he* (confluent) point of the Stomach meridian, is punctured to strengthen the spleen and stomach and arrest diarrhoea.

Auxiliary points and appropriate methods of manipulation are selected according to differentiation of syndromes:

● For chronic diarrhoea due to deficiency of the spleen *yang*, Pishu (B20) and Zhongwan (Ren12) are added and punctured using the reinforcing method to strengthen the spleen.
● For chronic diarrhoea due to deficiency of the kidney *yang*, the kidneys are warmed by adding and puncturing Guanyuan (Ren4) and Mingmen (Du4) using the reinforcing method and adding moxibustion to Guanyuan (Ren4), Mingmen (Du4) and Shenque (Ren8).
● For chronic diarrhoea due to blockage of the collaterals by stagnant blood, Diji (Sp8), Xuehai (Sp10) and Sanyinjiao (Sp6) are added and punctured using the even method to promote circulation of blood and relieve pain.

Treat once a day or once every other day. Ten treatments constitute one course.

Electroacupuncture

Points used are the same as for body acupuncture. Select one or two pairs of points each time. Puncture the points until a needling sensation is achieved, then connect the needles to an electric stimulator. Apply moderate intermittent wave stimulation for 20 minutes. Apply moderate continuous wave stimulation for 30 minutes. Treat once a day or once every other day. Ten treatments constitute one course.

Hot salt compress therapy

Points:

Shenque	(Ren8)
Tianshu	(S25)
Guanyuan	(Ren4)

Heat 500–1000 g of salt in a hot dry pan. Fill small bags half full with the hot salt. Apply the bags to either Shenque (Ren8) and Tianshu (S25), or Guanyuan (Ren4) (choose one set of points each time). Protect the skin by placing a towel under the bags while they are very hot; when they start to cool down the towel can be removed. Change to new hot bags when the first ones are no longer hot. Apply for 30–60 minutes, once or twice a day. Ten treatments constitute one course. This method can warm the spleen and kidney *yang* and is therefore an ideal treatment for chronic diarrhoea.

Auricular therapy

Main auricular points:

Large Intestine, Small Intestine, Rectum, Abdomen: correspond to the affected areas of the body.

Spleen: the spleen governs transportation and transformation of water and dampness, so Spleen is treated to strengthen the spleen and eliminate dampness.

Endocrine, Subcortex: regulate the function of the digestive system.

Ear Shenmen, Occiput: tranquillize the mind and relieve pain.

Auxiliary auricular points:

For deficiency of the kidney *yang*, Kidney is added.

Use auricular taping twice a week, or auricular pressure and self-massage twice a day. Ten treatments constitute one course.

Remarks

- Traditional therapies are very effective for treating all types of chronic diarrhoea.
- In cases of severe dehydration due to frequent diarrhoea, additional measures should be undertaken concurrently.
- Raw, cold, spicy and greasy foods should be avoided during treatment.

30 Chronic pelvic inflammatory disease

Chronic pelvic inflammatory disease refers to chronic inflammation of the internal genitals, pelvis, peritoneum and pelvic connective tissues in women. There is often a history of infertility or menstrual disorder. Manifestations include mild fever, fatigue, sinking pain in the lower abdomen, lower back pain and profuse vaginal discharge.

Aetiology

Traditional Chinese medicine classifies chronic pelvic inflammatory disease as lower abdominal pain. It is considered to be caused by exogenous or endogenous damp-cold or damp-heat which accumulates in the Lower Jiao and blocks the flow of *qi* and blood.

Primarily affected are the liver, spleen and kidneys.

Differentiation of syndromes

- Chronic pelvic inflammatory disease of the damp-cold type.
  Characterized by pain and sensation of cold in the lower abdomen, soreness or pain in the lumbosacral region, profuse thin clear vaginal discharge, pale complexion, dark red tongue with whitish coating and soft deep pulse.
- Chronic pelvic inflammatory disease of the damp-heat type.
  Characterized by pain in the lower abdomen and lumbosacral region, profuse sticky yellowish vaginal discharge, scanty yellowish urine, red tongue with greasy yellowish coating and rapid slippery pulse.
- Chronic pelvic inflammatory disease due to stagnation of the *qi* and blood.
  Characterized by stabbing pain in the lower abdomen and lumbosacral region, possible mass in the lower abdomen, dark red or purple-spotted tongue with thin whitish coating and uneven pulse.

Treatment

Body acupuncture

Main acupuncture points:

Zhongji	(Ren3)
Guilai	(S29)
Sanyinjiao	(Sp6)
Baliao	(B31–34)

The main pathogenesis of pelvic inflammatory disease is accumulation of dampness in the Lower Jiao. Therefore Zhongji (Ren3), the front-*mu* point of the urinary bladder and the meeting point of the Ren and three Foot Yin meridians, is punctured to remove dampness. Guilai (S29), a point of the Stomach meridian located on the lower abdomen, functions to activate the meridians and promote the flow of *qi* and blood. Sanyinjiao (Sp6), the meeting point of the three Foot Yin meridians, is treated to strengthen the spleen, liver and kidneys.

Baliao (B31–34), four pairs of bilateral points of the Urinary Bladder meridian located in the posterior sacral foramina, are effective for treating pelvic problems and are usually tender in cases of chronic pelvic inflammatory disease. One or two bilateral pairs are punctured each time. It is essential that a needling sensation be felt in the lower abdomen when puncturing these points if good results are to be obtained.

Auxiliary points and proper manipulation are chosen according to differentiation of syndromes.

- For chronic pelvic inflammatory disease of the damp-cold type, cold is dispelled and dampness removed by adding and puncturing Yinlingquan (Sp9) and Guanyuan (Ren4) using the reducing method and adding moxibustion as needed.
- For chronic pelvic inflammatory disease of the damp-heat type, Ligou (Liv5) and Qugu (Ren2) are added and punctured using the reducing method to expel heat and remove dampness.
- For chronic pelvic inflammatory disease due to stagnation of the *qi* and blood, Diji (Sp8), Hegu (LI4) and Taichong (Liv3) are added and punctured using the reducing method to promote the flow of *qi* and blood, relieve pain and dissolve masses.

Treat once a day or once every other day. Ten treatments constitute one course.

Moxibustion

Points used are the same as for body acupuncture. Select three or four points each time. Apply moxa roll moxibustion for 20–25 minutes, or three to five medium sized moxa cones, to each point. Treat once a day. Ten treatments constitute one course.

Moxibustion functions to warm the meridians and promote the flow of *qi* and blood and is therefore especially suitable for treating chronic pelvic inflammatory disease of the damp-cold type and chronic pelvic inflammatory disease due to stagnation of the *qi* and blood.

Electroacupuncture

Points used are the same as for body acupuncture. Select one or two pairs of points each time. Puncture until a needling sensation is achieved, then connect the needles to an electrical stimulator. Apply continuous wave stimulation of the highest bearable intensity for 30 minutes, once a day or once every other day. Ten treatments constitute one course.

Auricular therapy

Auricular points:

Pelvis, Internal Genitals, Abdomen: correspond to the affected regions. Locate positive points; tape both frontal and dorsal surfaces to increase stimulation.

San Jiao, Spleen: eliminate dampness.

Liver: the Liver meridian passes through the lower abdomen, so Liver is taped to activate the Liver meridian *qi*.

Endocrine,   Adrenal   Gland: relieve inflammation.

Ear Shenmen: relieves pain.

Apex of Ear: blood-letting puncturing of this point with a three-edged needle dispels damp-heat.

Use auricular taping and blood-letting puncturing where indicated, twice a week. Five treatments constitute one course.

Remarks

☯ Traditional therapies are effective for treating chronic pelvic inflammatory disease; two or more methods are usually used in combination in order to increase stimulation and improve effectiveness.
☯ These methods are also suitable for treating acute pelvic inflammation, vulvitis, bartholinitis and cervicitis.

31 Chronic pharyngitis

Chronic pharyngitis is a chronic and diffuse inflammation of the pharyngeal mucosa. It is characterized by long-term discomfort, the sensation of a foreign body or obstruction in the throat and itching dryness and mild soreness of the pharynx. Coughing and vomiting may occur if the pharynx is further irritated.

Aetiology and differentiation of syndrome

According to traditional Chinese medicine, chronic pharyngitis is caused primarily by *yin* deficiency of the lungs and kidneys which allows deficient fire to flare up along the meridians and damage the throat.

In addition to local symptoms and signs, there may be general manifestations including flushed cheeks, a sensation of heat in the palms and soles, dry mouth, red tongue with little coating and rapid thready pulse.

Treatment
Body acupuncture

Main acupuncture points:

Taixi	(K3)
Zhaohai	(K6)
Lieque	(L7)
Hegu	(LI4)
Zusanli	(S36)
Tiantu	(Ren22)
Lianquan	(Ren23)

The main pathogenesis of chronic pharyngitis is deficient fire due to *yin* deficiency of the lungs and kidneys. Therefore, points of the Lung and Kidney meridians are selected to nourish *yin* and extinguish deficient fire. Taixi (K3), the *yuan* (source) point of the Kidney meridian, functions to nourish the kidney *yin*. Zhaohai (K6), one of the eight confluence points connecting with the Yinqiao meridian and Lieque (L7), one of the eight confluence points connecting with the Ren meridian, are usually treated in combination to nourish *yin* and extinguish deficient fire when treating throat problems. The Large Intestine and Stomach meridians also connect with the throat, so Hegu (LI4), the *yuan* (source) point of the Large Intestine meridian and Zusanli (S36), the *he* (sea) and lower *he* (confluent) point of the Stomach meridian, are treated in combination to strengthen *qi* and nourish *yin*. Tiantu (Ren22) and Lianquan (Ren23), two local points of the Ren meridian, are effective for treating throat problems. Tiantu (Ren22) is punctured first perpendicularly for 0.2 *cun* and then downward along the back of the sternum for 0.5–1.0 *cun* using mild manipulation. Lianquan (Ren23) is punctured obliquely toward the root of the tongue for 0.3–0.5 *cun*.

Treat once a day or once every other day. Ten treatments constitute one course.

Auricular therapy

Auricular points:

Throat, Mouth: correspond to the affected area.

Lung, Kidney: tonify the lung and kidney *yin* to moisten the throat.

San Jiao: regulates the flow of *qi*.

Adrenal Gland, Endocrine: relieve inflammation.

Ear Shenmen: relieves inflammation and pain.

Use auricular taping, twice a week. Five treatments constitute one course.

Remarks

- Traditional therapies are very effective for treating chronic pharyngitis, but extended treatment should be given in order to consolidate the effects.
- Use extreme care when puncturing Tiantu (Ren22) and Lianquan (Ren23) to avoid damage to the lungs and trachea. There have been reports of death resulting from improper manipulation of these points, especially Tiantu (Ren22).
- These methods are also suitable for treating chronic tonsillitis and laryngitis.

32 Competition syndrome

Competition syndrome refers to a series of symptoms caused by overstrain or tension before or during competitive events such as sports meets, exams or performances, with resulting imbalance between excitation and inhibition of the cerebral cortex. Manifestations include dizziness, insomnia, headache, restlessness, dry mouth, poor appetite, weakness, listlessness, nausea, vomiting, diarrhoea, constipation, dysmenorrhoea, irregular menstruation, trembling or even loss of consciousness.

Aetiology and differentiation of syndromes

According to traditional Chinese medicine, competition syndrome is caused by overstrain or

tension which affects the heart and spleen, resulting in various mental and digestive disorders.

Treatment

Body acupuncture

Main acupuncture points:

Baihui	(Du20)
Fengchi	(G20)
Zusanli	(S36)

Baihui (Du20), the meeting point of the Du, Liver and six Hand and Foot Yang meridians, functions to refresh the brain and tranquillize the mind. Fengchi (G20), an important point of the Gallbladder meridian at the base of the skull, is treated to activate the meridians, refresh the brain and calm the mind. Zusanli (S36), the *he* (sea) and lower *he* (confluent) point of the Stomach meridian, strengthens the spleen and stomach.

Auxiliary points are added according to symptoms:

- For dizziness and headache, Taiyang (Ex30) is added.
- For nausea and vomiting, Neiguan (P6) is added.
- For diarrhoea or constipation, Tianshu (S25) is added.
- For dysmenorrhoea or irregular menstruation, Sanyinjiao (Sp6) is added.
- For loss of consciousness, Shuigou (Du26) and Laogong (P8) are added in emergency situations.

All points are punctured using the even method, once a day or every other day. Five treatments constitute one course.

Auricular therapy

Main points:

Heart: the mind resides in the heart, so Heart is treated to calm the mind.

Spleen: strengthens the spleen's ability to produce *qi* and blood to nourish the heart.

Liver: improves the flow of *qi* to tranquillize the mind.

Subcortex: harmonizes excitation and inhibition of the cerebral cortex.

Auxiliary auricular points are added according to symptoms:

- For headache and dizziness, blood-letting puncturing of Apex of Ear is added.
- For insomnia, Occiput and Anterior Lobe are added.
- For poor appetite, Stomach and Abdomen are added.
- For nausea and vomiting, Cardia and Stomach are added.
- For diarrhoea or constipation, Large Intestine and Abdomen are added.
- For dysmenorrhoea or irregular menstruation, Internal Genitals, Endocrine and Abdomen are added.

Use auricular taping with strong manipulation and blood-letting puncturing where indicated, three to five days before competition. Auricular self-massage may also be practised two or three times a day.

Remarks

- Traditional therapies, particularly auricular therapy, are very effective and easily accepted methods for treating competition syndrome. Advance treatment can not only prevent the occurrence of the symptoms of competition syndrome, but can also raise the competititve level by improving mental concentration and physical ability.
- It is helpful to massage Taiyang (Ex30), Baihui (Du20) and Fengchi (G20) starting three to five days before competition, or at any time. Massage each point for three to five minutes, two or three times a day.

33 Constipation

Constipation refers to difficult and infrequent defecation. It is a common symptom of various diseases and disorders including chronic constipation, gastrointestinal neurosis, fever and problems of the rectum and anus. Additional symptoms may include abdominal distension, headache, dizziness, poor appetite, insomnia, nausea, vomiting and weakness.

Aetiology

Traditional Chinese medicine classifies constipation into excessive and deficient types. In both types, peristalsis of the large intestine is affected, resulting in lengthy retention of digested food in the intestines. Excessive type constipation is caused by accumulation of heat in the intestines which consumes the intestinal fluid and is characterized by difficult and infrequent defecation with hard stool. Deficient type constipation is caused by deficiency of *qi*, blood, or bodily fluid with resulting lack of moisture in the intestines and is characterized by difficult defecation with soft stool, usually accompanied by sweating, shortness of breath and weakness during defecation.

Differentiation of syndromes

- Constipation due to excessive heat.
  Characterized by constipation and abdominal pain or distension; accompanied by flushed face, headache, restlessness, dry mouth with foul breath, scanty yellowish urine, red tongue with dry yellowish coating and rapid slippery pulse.
- Constipation due to stagnation of the liver *qi*.
  Characterized by difficult defecation with hard or normally formed stool; accompanied by feeling of fullness in the chest and hypochondriac region; sighing, depression, or restlessness; greasy whitish tongue coating and wiry pulse.
- Constipation due to deficiency of *qi* and blood.
  Characterized by difficult defecation with either hard or soft stool; accompanied by sweating, lassitude, shortness of breath, pale complexion, pale tongue with thin whitish coating and weak thready pulse.
- Constipation due to deficiency of the kidney *yin*.
  Characterized by constipation, dizziness or tinnitus, weak and sore back and knees, emaciation, flushed cheeks, sensation of heat in the palms and soles, night sweating, thin red tongue with little coating and rapid thready pulse.
- Constipation due to deficiency of the kidney *yang*.
  Characterized by difficult defecation with either hard or soft stool; accompanied by pain and feeling of coldness in the abdomen, feeling of coldness in the limbs, pale complexion, profuse urine, pale tongue with whitish coating and slow deep pulse.

Treatment

Body acupuncture

Main acupuncture points:

Tianshu	(S25)
Dachangshu	(B25)

Shangjuxu	(S37)
Daheng	(Sp15)
Zhigou	(SJ6)

Tianshu (S25) and Dachangshu (B25), the front-*mu* and back-*shu* points respectively of the large intestine and Shangjuxu (S37), the lower *he* (confluent) point of the Large Intestine meridian, are treated in combination to promote peristalsis. Daheng (Sp15), a local point on bilateral sides of the abdomen, functions to improve peristalsis of the large intestine. Zhigou (SJ6), the *jing* (river) point of the San Jiao meridian, is a clinically effective point for treating constipation.

Auxiliary points and appropriate methods of manipulation are chosen according to differentiation of syndromes.

- For constipation due to excessive heat, Quchi (LI11) and Neiting (S44) are added and punctured using the reducing method to dispel heat and loosen the bowels.
- For constipation due to stagnation of the liver *qi*, Neiguan (P6), Taichong (Liv3) and Yanglingquan (G34) are added and punctured using the reducing method to soothe the liver *qi* and loosen the bowels.
- For constipation due to deficiency of *qi* and blood, Zusanli (S36) and Qihai (Ren6) are added and punctured using the reinforcing method to reinforce the *qi* and blood and moisten the bowels.
- For constipation due to deficiency of the kidney *yin*, Taixi (K3), Zhaohai (K6) and Sanyinjiao (Sp6) are added and punctured using the even method to 'fill the river to lift the ship,' i.e. to moisten the bowels and loosen the stool.
- For constipation due to deficiency of the kidney *yang*, Mingmen (Du4) and Guanyuan (Ren4) are added and punctured using the reinforcing method and moxibustion is applied to these points and Shenque (Ren8), to warm and restore the kidney *yang* and loosen the bowels.

Treat once a day or once every other day. Ten treatments constitute one course.

Electroacupuncture

Points used are the same as for body acupuncture. Select one or two pairs of points each time. Puncture until a needling sensation is achieved, then connect the needles to an electrical stimulator. Apply moderate continuous wave stimulation for 20–30 minutes. Treat once a day or once every other day. Ten treatments constitute one course.

Auricular therapy

Main auricular points:

Large Intestine, Rectum, Abdomen: correspond to the affected areas of the body; improve peristalsis.

San Jiao: improves the flow of *qi* and bodily fluid.

Middle of Superior Concha: clinically effective point for treating abdominal diseases and disorders.

Auxiliary auricular points:

For excessive cases, Stomach and Apex of Ear are added; Apex of Ear is punctured with a three-edged needle to draw blood and dispel heat.

For deficient cases, Lung and Spleen are added to produce and distribute bodily fluid to moisten the intestines.

For excessive cases use auricular taping and blood-letting puncturing where indicated, twice a week. Five treatments constitute one course. For deficient cases use auricular taping twice a week, or auricular pressure and self-massage twice a day. Ten treatments constitute one course.

Remarks

- Traditional therapies are very effective for treating constipation; in many cases there may be defecation after two or three treatments.
- The above methods may be applied singly or in combination.
- In cases of deficient type constipation, self-massage may be practised daily before defecation. Press and rub the abdomen, starting at the lower right and ascending clockwise following the colon, ending at the lower left. Repeat 10–15 times.
- For cases of constipation due to intestinal tumours or enterostenosis, the primary problem should be treated.
- These methods are also suitable for treating enteroparalysis.

34 Costal chondritis

Costal chondritis is a chronic non-specific inflammation of the costal cartilage. It occurs primarily in adults and is usually induced by chest trauma or respiratory tract infection. Usually affected is the costal cartilage of the second and third ribs. Manifestations include swelling and eminence of the affected costal cartilage and persistent dull pain aggravated by coughing, deep breathing, or movement of the chest or shoulders. The symptoms may disappear spontaneously after approximately one month, but recur easily.

Aetiology

Traditional Chinese medicine classifies costal chondritis as chest or hypochondriac pain and considers it to be caused by trauma, exogenous pathogens, or mental injury which result in stagna-

tion of *qi* and blood in the chest and hypochondriac regions. There are usually no general symptoms in addition to local pain, swelling and eminence. Primarily affected are the Gallbladder and San Jiao meridians.

Treatment

Body acupuncture

Acupuncture points:

Yanglingquan	(G34)
Qiuxu	(G40)
Zhigou	(SJ6)
Ashi points	

The Gallbladder meridian is closely related to the chest and hypochondriac regions, therefore Yanglingquan (G34) and Qiuxu (G40), the *he* (sea) and *yuan* (source) points respectively of the Gall-bladder meridian, are treated in combination to activate the Gallbladder meridian and promote the flow of *qi* and blood to relieve pain. Zhigou (SJ6) is a clinically effective point for treating diseases of the chest and hypochondriac regions.

Puncture using strong manipulation until a needling sensation is felt in the affected area. Treat once a day or once every other day. Five treatments constitute one course.

Point injection therapy

Ashi points are injected with 2–4 ml of procaine, vitamin B$_1$, vitamin B$_{12}$, or hydroprednisone, once every four days. Five treatments constitute one course.

Auricular therapy

Auricular points:

> Chest, Thoracic Vertebrae: correspond to the affected area of the body. Locate positive points; tape both frontal and dorsal surfaces to increase stimulation. Sensitive points are usually found between Thoracic Vertebrae and the scaphoid fossa.

> Liver, Pancreas & Gallbladder: both the Liver and Gallbladder meridians pass through the chest and hypochondriac region, so these points are taped to clear and activate the meridians and collaterals to relieve pain and swelling.

> Kidney: the kidneys nourish the bones and the Kidney meridian passes through the chest, so Kidney is taped to activate the Kidney meridian, nourish the bones and relieve pain.

> Ear Shenmen: main point for pain relief.

Use auricular taping with strong manipulation, twice a week. Five treatments constitute one course.

Remarks

- The above therapies are very effective for treating costal chondritis. They may be used singly or in combination.
- Do not puncture local points too deeply to avoid damaging the internal organs or blood vessels.

35 Cutaneous pruritus

Cutaneous pruritus is a common skin problem that may occur secondary to various diseases and disorders including endocrine dysfunction, parasitosis, diabetes mellitus, hepatic illness, nephritic disorders or tumours. In the elderly, it is referred to as pruritus senilis. Cutaneous pruritus is marked in the initial stage by paroxysmal itching without skin lesions. As the condition develops, scratch marks, scabs, pigmentation or lichenification due to extensive scratching may appear. The condition may be either localized, appearing mainly on the anus and scrotum or vulva, or general.

Aetiology

According to traditional Chinese medicine, cutaneous pruritus is caused either by excessive heat in the blood, or by deficiency of blood leading to endogenous wind and dryness.

Differentiation of syndromes

- Cutaneous pruritus due to excessive heat in the blood.
  Characterized by severe cutaneous itching, aggravated by heat and alleviated by cold; accompanied by thirst with a preference for cold beverages, restlessness, scanty urine, constipation, red tongue with yellowish coating and rapid pulse.
- Cutaneous pruritus due to deficiency of blood leading to endogenous wind and dryness.
  Characterized by long-term persistent or intermittent itching of the skin; accompanied by pale

complexion, palpitation, insomnia, restlessness, lassitude, pale tongue with thin whitish coating and weak thready pulse.

Treatment

Body acupuncture

Main acupuncture points:

Xuehai	(Sp10)
Quchi	(LI11)
Hegu	(LI4)
Sanyinjiao	(Sp6)
Fengchi	(G20)

Xuehai (Sp10) (Sea of Blood in Chinese) functions to stimulate the flow of blood and expel wind. It is a main point for treating various skin diseases. Quchi (LI11) and Hegu (LI4), the *he* (sea) and *yuan* (source) points respectively of the Large Intestine meridian, are treated in combination to expel wind and relieve itching. Sanyinjiao (Sp6), the meeting point of the three Foot Yin meridians, functions to strengthen the liver and spleen. Fengchi (G20) is an important point for expelling wind and relieving itching.

Auxiliary points and appropriate manipulation are chosen according to differentiation of syndromes and location of pruritus.

- For cutaneous pruritus due to excessive heat in the blood, Dazhui (Du14) and Feishu (B13) are added and pricked with a three-edged needle, then cupped for 10–15 minutes to draw a small amount of blood to dispel heat.
- For cutaneous pruritus due to deficiency of blood leading to endogenous wind and dryness, Geshu (B17), Feishu (B13), Zusanli (S36) and Taixi (K3) are added and punctured using the reinforcing method to tonify the blood and activate the meridians. Moxibustion may also by applied.
- For cutaneous pruritus of the vulva or scrotum, Ligou (Liv5), Qugu (Ren2) and Zhongji (Ren3) are added. Qugu (Ren2) and Zhongji (Ren3) are punctured obliquely downward until a needling sensation is experienced in the external genitals.
- For cutaneous pruritus of the anus, Changqiang (Du1) and Chengshan (B57) are added.

Treat once a day or once every other day. Ten treatments constitute one course.

Blood-letting puncturing

Acupuncture points:

Dazhui	(Du14)
Xuehai	(Sp10)
Quchi	(LI11)
Feishu	(B13)
Geshu	(B17)
Weizhong	(B40)

Select two or three points each time. Prick using a three-edged needle and then cup for 10–15 minutes to draw a small amount of blood. Puncture the points alternately, once every other day. Five treatments constitute one course.

This method functions to expel wind and dispel heat and is ideal for treating cutaneous pruritus.

Auricular therapy

Auricular points:

Areas corresponding to the affected regions: tap with a plum blossom needle to cause mild bleeding and dispel heat.

Lung: disperses the lung *qi* to expel wind-heat.

Liver: regulates the flow of blood and *qi*.

Spleen: strengthens the spleen *qi*.

Heart, Ear Shenmen, Occiput, Subcortex: calm the mind and relieve itching.

Centre of Ear: clinically effective point for relieving itching.

Apex of Ear: blood-letting puncturing of this point with a three-edged needle expels wind and dispels heat to relieve itching.

Use auricular taping with strong manipulation and blood-letting puncturing where indicated, twice a week. Long-term treatment should be given to consolidate the results.

Remarks

- Traditional therapies are effective for treating cutaneous pruritus; the various therapies may be used either singly or in combination.
- The causes of cutaneous pruritus are varied; diagnosis should be established before treatment in order to treat the condition appropriately.

36 Cystic hyperplasia of the breast

Cystic hyperplasia of the breast is caused by cystogenesis of the mammary tubes and acinar epithelia. It occurs primarily in women above 40 years old with a history of irregular menstruation, infertility or miscarriage. It is marked by periodic distending pain in the breast, aggravated by mental injury or before menstruation and alleviated after menstruation; and multiple masses in the breast which may be circular, oval or lobulated, with an indistinct border and adhesion to peripheral tissues. The masses may vary with the menstrual cycle and state of mind.

Aetiology

According to traditional Chinese medicine, cystic hyperplasia of the breast is caused primarily by mental injury which leads to stagnation of the liver *qi* and accumulation of phlegm in the interior. Usually affected are the liver, spleen and stomach.

Differentiation of syndromes

- Cystic hyperplasia of the breast due to stagnation of the liver *qi*.
  Characterized by distending pain and masses in the breast, aggravated by mental injury or before menstruation and alleviated after menstruation; usually accompanied by depression or irritability, feeling of fullness in the chest and hypochondriac region, frequent sighing, insomnia, bad dreams, poor appetite, abdominal distension, thin whitish tongue coating and wiry pulse.
- Cystic hyperplasia of the breast due to hyperactivity of the liver-fire.
  Characterized by distending or burning pain and masses in the breast, sometimes with scanty dark brown or haematic secretion from the nipple; accompanied by restlessness, irritability, insomnia, bad dreams, dry mouth with bitter taste, irregular menstruation, scanty yellowish urine, red tongue with yellowish coating and rapid wiry pulse.
- Cystic hyperplasia of the breast due to injury of the spleen and stomach by hyperactive liver *qi*.

Characterized by distending pain and masses in the breast, aggravated by mental injury or before menstruation and alleviated after menstruation; accompanied by lassitude, pale complexion, scanty menses or amenorrhoea, poor appetite, abdominal distension, loose stool, pale tongue with whitish coating and weak pulse.

Treatment

Body acupuncture

Main acupuncture points:

Jianjing	(G21)
Taichong	(Liv3)
Neiguan	(P6)
Yingchuang	(S16)
Danzhong	(Ren17)
Rugen	(S18)

The main pathogenesis of cystic hyperplasia of the breast is stagnation of the liver *qi*. The flow of *qi* in the chest is therefore promoted by puncturing Taichong (Liv3), the *yuan* (source) point of the Liver meridian and Neiguan (P6), the *luo* (collateral) point of the Pericardium meridian and one of the eight confluence points connecting with the Yinwei meridian. Jianjing (G21), the meeting point of the Gallbladder meridian and the San Jiao, Stomach and Yangwei meridians, is punctured obliquely forward for 0.5–0.8 *cun* to promote the circulation of *qi* and blood in the Liver and Stomach meridians. Yingchuang (S16), Danzhong (Ren17) and Rugen (S18) are local points for treating problems of the breast.

Auxiliary points and appropriate manipulation are chosen according to differentiation of syndromes.

- For cystic hyperplasia of the breast due to stagnation of the liver *qi*, the reducing method is used to promote the flow of *qi* and dissolve the masses.
- For cystic hyperplasia of the breast due to hyperactivity of the liver fire, Xingjian (Liv2) and Zulinqi (G41) are added and punctured using the reducing method to dispel liver fire.
- For cystic hyperplasia of the breast due to injury of the spleen and stomach by hyperactive liver *qi*, Zusanli (S36), Sanyinjiao (Sp6) and Zhong-

wan (Ren12) are added and punctured using the reinforcing method to strengthen the spleen and stomach.

Treat once a day or once every other day. Ten treatments constitute one course.

Electroacupuncture

Points used are the same as for body acupuncture. Select one or two pairs of points each time. Puncture until a needling sensation is achieved, then connect the needles to an electrical stimulator. Apply moderate intermittent wave stimulation for 20–30 minutes, once a day or once every other day. Ten treatments constitute one course.

Auricular therapy

Auricular points:

Chest, Thoracic Vertebrae: correspond to the affected areas of the body. Locate positive points; tape both frontal and dorsal surfaces to increase stimulation. Auricular points corresponding to the breast are located between Chest and Thoracic Vertebrae and between Thoracic Vertebrae and the scaphoid fossa.

Stomach: the Stomach meridian passes through the breasts, so Stomach is taped to activate the meridian and dispel heat and toxins.

Liver: soothes the liver to regulate the flow of *qi* and strengthen the spleen.

Endocrine, Midpoint of Rim, Internal Genitals.

Subcortex: regulate the nervous and endocrine functions.

Ear Shenmen, Occiput: tranquillize the mind.

Auxiliary auricular points:

For cystic hyperplasia of the breast due to hyperactivity of the liver fire, Apex of Ear is punctured with a three-edged needle to draw several drops of blood and dispel liver fire.

Use auricular taping with strong manipulation and blood-letting puncturing where indicated, twice a week. Five treatments constitute one course.

Remarks

☯ Traditional therapies are very effective for treating cystic hyperplasia of the breast.
☯ It is essential to differentiate cystic hyperplasia of the breast from breast cancer prior to undertaking treatment with traditional therapies.

37 Cystitis

Cystitis is an acute or chronic bacteriologically caused inflammation of the internal wall of the urinary bladder. Acute cystitis is marked by sudden onset of lower abdominal pain and frequent, dripping and painful urination, accompanied by visible blood in the urine and pyuria. Frequency of urination is higher during the day than at night. The manifestations of chronic cystitis are similar to or milder than those of acute cystitis, recurring frequently.

Aetiology

Traditional Chinese medicine classifies cystitis as a *lin* syndrome and considers it to be caused by exogenous or endogenous damp-heat which descends and accumulates in the Lower Jiao.

Differentiation of syndromes

● Cystitis due to severe dampness and slight heat.

Characterized by frequent, dripping and painful urination with scanty turbid yellowish urine; accompanied by lumbar pain, nausea, vomiting, poor appetite, greasy yellowish tongue coating and rapid slippery pulse.

● Cystitis due to severe heat and slight dampness.
Characterized by frequent, dripping and painful urination with bloody urine which may contain blood clots; accompanied by pain in the lower abdomen and lumbar region, fever, thirst with desire for cold beverages, constipation, red tongue with yellowish coating and rapid forceful pulse.

Treatment

Body acupuncture

Main acupuncture points:

Zhongji	(Ren3)
Pangguangshu	(B28)
Sanyinjiao	(Sp6)

Zhongji (Ren3) and Pangguangshu (B28), the front-*mu* and back-*shu* points respectively of the urinary bladder, are treated in combination to strengthen the urinary bladder and remove damp-heat. Sanyinjiao (Sp6), the meeting point of the three Foot Yin meridians, is an important point for treating urogenital problems.

Auxiliary points and appropriate methods of manipulation are chosen according to differentiation of syndromes.

● For cystitis due to severe dampness and slight heat, Zhongwan (Ren12), Yinlingquan (Sp9) and Neiguan (P6) are added and punctured using the reducing method to remove dampness.
● For cystitis due to severe heat and slight dampness, Hegu (LI4), Dazhui (Du14) and Xuehai (Sp10) are added and punctured using the reducing method. Alternatively, Zhiyin (B67) may be pricked with a three-edged needle to draw 5–8 drops of blood in order to clear away heat and cool the blood.

Treat once a day. Five treatments constitute one course.

Electroacupuncture

Points used are the same as for body acupuncture. Select one or two pairs of points each time. Puncture using the reducing method until a needling sensation is achieved, then connect the needles to an electric stimulator. Apply moderate intermittent wave stimulation for 30 minutes. Treat once a day. Five treatments constitute one course.

Auricular therapy

Auricular points:

Urinary Bladder, Urethra, Abdomen, Pelvis: correspond to the affected regions of the body. Locate positive points; tape both frontal and dorsal surfaces to increase stimulation.

Kidney: tonifies the kidneys to drain dampness.

Spleen: strengthens the spleen to transport and transform water and dampness.

San Jiao: dispels heat and removes dampness.

Endocrine, Adrenal Gland: relieve inflammation.

Ear Shenmen: relieves pain.

Apex of Ear: blood-letting puncturing of this point with a three-edged needle dispels heat and relieves pain.

Use auricular taping with strong manipulation and blood-letting puncturing where indicated, twice a week. Five treatments constitute one course.

Remarks

☯ Acupuncture and auricular therapy are effective for treating cystitis; there is often great improvement in symptoms such as frequent, dripping, painful urination and pain in the lower abdomen and lumbar region after two or three treatments.
☯ The three methods discussed may be applied either singly, or in combination to increase stimulation and improve effectiveness.

38 Developmental disability

Developmental disability becomes apparent during early childhood. Intelligence lags behind other children of the same age group and never completely matures. Causes of developmental disability include birth trauma and heredity, but 40–75 per cent of cases have no clear and definite cause.

Aetiology and differentiation of syndromes

According to traditional Chinese medicine, the brain is the Sea of Marrow. Marrow is produced by the kidneys; if the kidney essence is insufficient, the brain will receive insufficient nourishment and developmental disability will occur.

Treatment

Body acupuncture

Acupuncture points:

Baihui	(Du20)
Shangxing	(Du23)
Fengchi	(G20)
Shenmen	(H7)
Neiguan	(P6)
Zusanli	(S36)
Sanyinjiao	(Sp6)
Pishu	(B20)
Shenshu	(B23)
Taixi	(K3)

Baihui (Du20) and Shangxing (Du23), points of the Du meridian located on the head, and Fengchi (G20), an important point of the Gallbladder meridian located at the base of the skull, are treated in combination to refresh the brain and promote mental development.

Neiguan (P6), the *luo* (collateral) point of the Pericardium meridian and one of the eight confluence points connecting with the Yinwei meridian and Shenmen (H7), the *yuan* (source) point of the Heart meridian, are treated in combination to strengthen the mind.

Zusanli (S36), the *he* (sea) and lower *he* (confluent) point of the Stomach meridian; Sanyinjiao (Sp6), the meeting point of the three Foot Yin meridians; and Pishu (B20), the back-*shu* point of the spleen, are treated in combination to strengthen the spleen and stomach, the basis of the acquired constitution.

Shenshu (B23), the back-*shu* point of the kidneys and Taixi (K3), the *yuan* (source) point of the Kidney meridian, are treated in combination to tonify the kidneys, the basis of the congenital constitution.

Select five to seven points each time. Puncture using the reinforcing method, once every other day. Ten treatments constitute one course.

Electroacupuncture

Points used are the same as for body acupuncture. Select one or two pairs of points each time. Puncture until a needling sensation is achieved, then connect the needles to an electrical stimulator. Apply moderate continuous wave stimulation for 20–30 minutes, once every other day. Ten treatments constitute one course.

Scalp Acupuncture

Scalp lines:

Dingzhongxian	(MS5)
Dingpangxian 1	(MS8)
Dingpangxian 2	(MS9)
Dingnie Qianxiexian	(MS6)

Puncture the lines using the reinforcing method for 5 minutes, or connect the needles with an electrical stimulator and apply intermittent wave stimulation for 20–30 minutes. Treat once a day or once every other day. Ten treatments constitute one course.

Point injection therapy

Select three to five acupuncture points each time. Inject each point with 1–2 ml of acetyl-glutamine. Treat once every other day. Ten treatments constitute one course.

Auricular therapy

Auricular points:

Kidney: reinforces the congenital essence to nourish the marrow and brain.

Liver: tonifies the liver-blood to nourish the tendons.

Spleen, Stomach, Abdomen: strengthen the acquired essence and stimulate intellectual development.

Subcortex, Adrenal Gland, Endocrine: regulate the nervous and endocrine functions.

Forehead, Temple, Occiput: tonify the brain.

Use auricular taping, twice a week. Ten treatments constitute one course. Auricular massage is very useful for children with developmental disability and should be given by their parents or caregivers twice a day.

Remarks

☯ Developmental disability is a refractory problem. Two or more therapies should be used in combination and long-term treatment undertaken in order to achieve results.

☯ The younger the child when treatment is instituted, the better the results will be.

☯ It is essential to combine additional rehabilitation measures with traditional therapies in order to increase effectiveness and maximize the child's abilities.

39 Diabetes mellitus

Diabetes mellitus is a disturbance of the carbohydrate metabolism caused by relative or absolute hypoinsulinism. Diabetes mellitus is typically marked by polydipsia, polyphagia, polyuria, emaciation and lassitude. Laboratory tests will reveal high blood sugar and glucose positive urine. Accompanying manifestations may include cutaneous pruritus, frequently recurring carbuncle or furuncle, multiple neuritis, sexual dysfunction, irregular menstruation, hypertension, arterial sclerosis and disorders of the eye.

Aetiology

According to traditional Chinese medicine, diabetes mellitus is caused either by overindulgence in greasy or spicy food which damages the spleen and stomach, with resulting accumulation of heat in the interior; by mental injury resulting in stagnation of the liver *qi* which subsequently turns into liver fire; or by excessive sexual activity which consumes the kidney *yin*. Any of these factors may result in *yin* deficiency and subsequent production of endogenous dry-heat. *Yin* deficiency and dry-heat may also interact, worsening the condition. Primarily affected are the lungs, spleen, stomach and kidneys.

Differentiation of syndromes

● Diabetes mellitus due to injury of the lungs and stomach by pathogenic dry heat.
  Characterized by excessive thirst, polydipsia, frequent hunger, polyphagia, profuse yellowish urine, frequent urination, constipation, red tongue with dry yellowish coating and rapid pulse.
● Diabetes mellitus due to *yin* deficiency of the liver and kidneys.
  Characterized by turbid, sugary, or creamy urine; frequent urination, dizziness, tinnitus, restlessness, sensation of heat in the palms and soles, dry throat and skin, emaciation, soreness and weakness of the back and knees, bad dreams, cutaneous pruritus, thin red tongue with little coating and rapid thready pulse.
● Diabetes mellitus due to *yang* deficiency of the spleen and kidneys.
  Characterized by turbid creamy urine, frequent urination, listlessness, lassitude, dark complexion, emaciation, soreness and weakness of the back and knees, sensation of cold in the limbs, loose stool, sexual dysfunction, pale tongue with dry whitish coating and deep, thready, weak pulse.

Treatment

Body acupuncture

Main acupuncture points:

Pishu	(B20)
Shenshu	(B23)
Zusanli	(S36)
Sanyinjiao	(Sp6)
Huatuojiaji	(Ex46) (T6-T8)

Diabetes mellitus is a disorder of the *zang* organs; therefore the back-*shu* points of the spleen and kidneys are selected as main points to reinforce the spleen and kidneys. Zusanli (S36), the *he* (sea) and lower *he* (confluent) point of the Stomach meridian, is punctured to strengthen the stomach and spleen. Sanyinjiao (Sp6), the meeting point of the Spleen, Liver and Kidney meridians, is punctured to tonify the three *zang* organs. Huatuojiaji (Ex46) (T6-T8) has been proven through clinical experience to be effective for treating diabetes mellitus.

Auxiliary points and appropriate manipulation are chosen according to differentiation of syndromes and symptoms.

- For diabetes mellitus due to injury of the lungs and stomach by pathogenic dry heat, Yuji (L10), Quchi (LI11), Tianshu (S25) and Neiting (S44) are added and punctured using the reducing method to treat symptoms and clear away dry-heat.
- For diabetes mellitus due to *yin* deficiency of the liver and kidneys, Guanyuan (Ren4), Taichong (Liv3) and Taixi (K3) are added and punctured using the even method to nourish the kidney and liver *yin*.
- For diabetes mellitus due to *yang* deficiency of the spleen and kidneys, Guanyuan (Ren4), Qihai (Ren6), Zhongwan (Ren12), Mingmen (Du4) and Taixi (K3) are added and punctured using the reinforcing method to warm the spleen and kidneys. Moxibustion may also be added as needed.
- For cases involving cutaneous pruritus, Quchi (LI11) and Xuehai (Sp10) are punctured to stop itching.

Point implantation therapy

Points chosen are the same as for body acupuncture. Select two to three points each time. Using a triangular suture needle, implant surgical catgut on each point. Points may be treated repeatedly or in turn. Treat once a week. Three treatments constitute one course.

Auricular therapy

Main auricular points:

Pancreas & Gallbladder: stimulate the pancreas to secrete insulin and lower blood sugar.

San Jiao: the mixed branches of the glossopharyngeal nerve, vagus nerve and facial nerve pass through this area, so San Jiao is treated to directly stimulate the vagus nerve and improve secretion of insulin by the pancreas.

Spleen, Kidney: tonify the bodily fluid and *yin* to moisten endogenous dry-heat.

Midpoint of Rim, Endocrine: regulate endocrine function to improve insulin secretion.

Subcortex: regulates digestive, nervous and endocrine functions.

Auxiliary auricular points are chosen corresponding to the location of complicating conditions:

For cutaneous pruritus, Wind Stream and Ear Shenmen are added.

For skin infections, Adrenal Gland and areas corresponding to the affected region of the body are added.

Use auricular taping, primarily on the left auricle, twice a week. Ten treatments constitute one course. Sterilize the auricle and press carefully in order to avoid auricular infection.

Remarks

- Experimental studies show that acupuncture can activate the islet ß cells to secrete insulin and lower blood sugar.
- Acupuncture is more effective when insulin dependence is not a factor.
- Dietary measures should be combined with acupuncture. In severe cases, hypoglycaemic agents should be added.
- In cases of insulin dependence, insulin dosage may be gradually decreased as symptoms improve and blood sugar approaches normal levels during the course of traditional therapy.
- Acupuncture points should be strictly sterilized during treatment in order to avoid skin infections.

40 *Dian* and *kuang* syndromes

Dian and *kuang* syndromes (depressive and manic in Chinese) are classified by traditional Chinese medicine as mental disorders. *Dian* syndrome encompasses a series of depressive mental disorders, including depression, apathy, mutism, excessive doubt, anxiety, paranoia, blanking out and visual or auditory hallucination. *Kuang* syndrome includes a series of manic mental disorders, including mania, restlessness, irritability, flight of ideas, hyperthymergasia and hyperactive behaviour. The two syndromes may appear either individually or in conjunction, transforming back and forth. Western medicine subsumes these syndromes into various psychoses, including schizophrenia, reactive psychosis, involutional psychosis, periodic psychosis, melancholy, mania and hypomania.

Aetiology

According to traditional Chinese medicine, both *dian* and *kuang* syndromes are closely related to emotional injuries and pathogenic phlegm. *Dian* syndrome is due to disturbance of the mind caused by stagnant *qi* and accumulated phlegm, which are produced when anger and brooding damage the liver and spleen. If *dian* syndrome is not properly treated in the initial stage, stagnant *qi* and phlegm gradually damage both the *qi* and blood. *Kuang* syndrome has two possible causes. First, endogenous fire produced by stagnant *qi* may vaporize the bodily fluid producing pathogenic phlegm; this phlegm fire then attacks the mind. Second, sudden or great terror may result in abnormal flow of *qi* which disturbs the mind. Consumption of the body's *yin* by endogenous fire in *kuang* syndrome results in phlegm fire in the initial stage and deficient fire in the advanced stage.

Differentiation of syndromes

- *Dian* syndrome due to disturbance of the mind by stagnant *qi* and pathogenic phlegm.
  Characterized by gradual onset of depression, apathy, excessive doubt and incoherence or irrational laughing or crying; accompanied by feeling of pressure in the chest and hypochon-

driac region, frequent sighing, anorexia, abdominal distension, greasy whitish tongue coating and wiry slippery pulse.
- *Dian* syndrome due to deficiency of the heart *qi* and spleen blood.
  Characterized by long-standing depression, blanking out, susceptibility to sorrow or fright, trance and incoherent speech; accompanied by lassitude, pale complexion, poor appetite, loose stool, pale and swollen tongue with tooth marks and weak thready pulse.
- *Kuang* syndrome due to attack on the mind by phlegm-fire.
  Characterized by sudden onset of mania, manifesting as shouting, tearing off of clothes, running about, smashing things and hitting people; insomnia; accompanied by restlessness, flushed face, pink eyes, anorexia, thirst with preference for cold drinks, constipation, scanty yellowish urine, dark red or spotted tongue with greasy yellowish coating and rapid wiry slippery pulse.
- *Kuang* syndrome due to hyperactivity of deficient fire.
  Characterized by long-standing manic mental disorders, manifesting as intermittent mania and mental fatigue, anxiety, mental stress, restlessness, susceptibility to fright and insomnia; accompanied by emaciation, flushed cheeks, sensation of heat on the palms and soles, dry red tongue with little or no coating and rapid, wiry, thready pulse.

Treatment

Body acupuncture
Dian syndrome

Main acupuncture points:

Points of the Ren meridian
Zhongwan	(Ren12)
Jiuwei	(Ren15)
Danzhong	(Ren17)

Points of the Stomach meridian
Huaroumen	(S24)
Tianshu	(S25)
Zusanli	(S36)
Fenglong	(S40)

Points of the Pericardium meridian

Jianshi	(P5)
Daling	(P7)

Additional points

Shenmen	(H7)
Baihui	(Du20)
Fengchi	(G20)

The main pathogenesis of *dian* syndrome is stagnation of *qi* and blockage of phlegm. Therefore points of the Ren, Stomach and Pericardium meridians are selected as main points to improve the flow of *qi*, remove phlegm and relieve depression. The mind is stimulated and depression relieved by puncturing Baihui (Du20) and Fengchi (G20) in combination with Shenmen (H7), the *yuan* (source) point of the Heart meridian, which is punctured toward Daling (P7).

● For cases involving deficiency of the heart *qi* and spleen-blood, Sanyinjiao (Sp6), Jueyinshu (B14), Xinshu (B15) and Pishu (B20) are added and punctured using the reinforcing method to strengthen the spleen and tonify the heart. Alternatively, moxibustion may be used on Zhongwan (Ren12) to strengthen the Middle Jiao and remove phlegm.

Select seven to eight main points each time. Puncture using the reducing method during the initial stage and the even method in the intermediate and advanced stages, unless otherwise indicated. Add auxiliary points according to differentiation of syndromes. Treat once a day. Ten treatments constitute one course.

Kuang syndrome

Main acupuncture points:

Points of the Du meridian

Shuigou	(Du26)
Shangxing	(Du23)
Baihui	(Du20)
Fengfu	(Du16)
Dazhui	(Du14)

Points of the Pericardium meridian

Jianshi	(P5)
Laogong	(P8)

Points of the Ren meridian

Zhongwan	(Ren12)
Juque	(Ren14)
Jiuwei	(Ren15)
Danzhong	(Ren17)

Additional points

Fengchi	(G20)
Taichong	(Liv3)
Yongquan	(K1)
Huaroumen	(S24)
Fenglong	(S40)

The main pathogenesis of *kuang* syndrome is disturbance of the mind by phlegm fire. Therefore, points of the Du, Ren and Pericardium meridians are selected as main points to dispel fire, eliminate phlegm and soothe the mind. Taichong (Liv3), the *yuan* (source) point of the Liver meridian, is punctured toward Yongquan (K1), the *jing* (well) point of the Kidney meridian, to calm the mind. Fengchi (G20), Fenglong (S40) and Huaroumen (S24) are punctured to soothe the mind and eliminate phlegm.

Select seven to eight main points each time; puncture using the reducing method.

Auxiliary points and methods are added according to symptoms or differentiation of syndromes.

● For manic attack, Shuigou (Du26), Baihui (Du20), Laogong (P8), Taichong (Liv3) and Yongquan (K1) are punctured using the reducing method to soothe the mind. Alternatively, the *jing* (well) points of the Hand meridians may be pricked with a three-edged needle to cause bleeding and dispel heat, or Dazhui (Du14), Quze (P3) and Weizhong (B40) may be punctured with a three-edged needle and then cupped for 10–15 minutes to draw blood and calm the mind.
● For cases involving deficient fire, Sanyinjiao (Sp6), Taixi (K3) and Neiguan (P6) are added and punctured using the even method to nourish the body's yin and reduce pathogenic fire.
● For cases involving visual hallucination, Taiyang (Ex30) and Fengchi (G20) are added; for cases involving auditory hallucination, Yifeng (SJ17), Ermen (SJ21) and Zhongzhu (SJ3) are added; for cases involving aphonia, Lianquan (Du23) and Tongli (H5)are added.

Treat once a day. Ten treatments constitute one course.

Electroacupuncture

Points used are the same as for body acupuncture. Select two to three pairs of points each time. Puncture until a needling sensation is achieved; then connect the needles to an electrical stimulator. Apply mild to moderate stimulation for 20–30 minutes, twice a day during the initial stage and once a day thereafter. Ten treatments constitute one course.

Remarks

☯ Acupuncture is effective for treating *dian* and *kuang* syndromes. The earlier treatment is instituted, the better the result will be.
☯ The method used when puncturing Dazhui (Du14) and Fengfu (Du16) is very important. With the patient's head lowered, puncture Dazhui (Du14) obliquely upward to a depth of 0.5–0.8 *cun*; puncture Fengfu (Du16) toward the base of the lower jaw to a depth of 0.5–0.8 *cun*. Manipulate both points using the even method for 3–5 minutes and then withdraw the needles.

  Some experienced practitioners assert that better therapeutic results may be attained by inserting the needle into the vertebral canal, even touching the spinal cord, to cause the patient to experience a sensation of electric shock. However, this method is extremely dangerous and cannot be advocated. If the needle should accidentally enter the vertebral canal, producing sensations of shock or even paralysis, it must be withdrawn immediately. Paralysis may recover spontaneously within several hours in mild cases. Proper treatment should be given in severe cases to aid the recovery process. However, damage to the spinal cord may be irreversible.
☯ Attention should be paid to avoiding accidents during acupuncture, especially bending or breaking needles while treating uncooperative patients experiencing *dian* or *kuang* syndrome.
☯ Baihui (Du20) and Sishencong (Ex 26) may be punctured alternately.

41 Drug withdrawal

Drug withdrawal refers to the physiological and psychological process of overcoming physical addiction to drugs such as heroin or other narcotics, barbiturates or amphetamines, by complete cessation of use. It has been shown that traditional therapies can relieve both the physical symptoms and psychological craving present during the withdrawal process.

Aetiology and differentiation of syndromes

According to traditional Chinese medicine, addictive drugs such as narcotics, amphetamines and barbiturates easily damage the body's *yang qi*, especially that of the heart, lungs, stomach and spleen. Therefore, when an addicted person suddenly stops taking the drug on which she or he is dependent, symptoms such as wracking chills, sweating, aching or burning bones, severe stomach cramps, abdominal pain or diarrhoea, restlessness, paranoia, poor appetite, lassitude, wheezing, coughing and runny nose invariably occur.

Treatment

Body acupuncture

Acupuncture points:

Baihui	(Du20)
Fengchi	(G20)
Neiguan	(P6)
Dazhui	(Du14)
Zhongwan	(Ren12)
Zusanli	(S36)
Sanyinjiao	(Sp6)
Danzhong	(Ren17)
Guanyuan	(Ren4)
Hegu	(LI4)

The general therapeutic principle for treating drug withdrawal is to tranquillize the mind, warm the body's *yang qi* and strengthen the spleen and stomach. Baihui (Du20), the meeting point of the Du, Liver and six Hand and Foot Yang meridians, functions to both tranquillize the mind and warm the body's *qi*. Fengchi (G20), an important point of the Gallbladder meridian located at the base of the skull, functions to calm the mind. Neiguan (P6), the *luo* (collateral) point of the Pericardium meridian and one of the eight confluence points connecting with the Yinwei meridian, functions to both calm the mind and relieve stomach pain. Dazhui (Du14), the meeting point of the Du and six Hand and Foot Yang meridians, functions to invigorate the body's *yang qi*.

The spleen and stomach are the *ben* (root) of the acquired constitution. They are strengthened by treating the following points in combination: Zhongwan (Ren12), the front-*mu* point of the stomach and the *hui* (influential) point of the *fu* organs; Zusanli (S36), the *he* (sea) and lower *he* (confluent) point of the Stomach meridian; and Sanyinjiao (Sp6), the meeting point of the Spleen, Liver and Kidney meridians.

Hegu (LI4), the *yuan* (source) point of the Large Intestine meridian, functions to relieve pain. Danzhong (Ren17), the *hui* (influential) point of *qi*, functions to widen the chest and relieve wheezing and coughing. Guanyuan (Ren4) is an important point for tonifying the body's *qi*.

Select four to six points each time. Puncture using the reinforcing method. Treat once or twice a day for the first three to four days and once a day or once every other day thereafter. Fifteen treatments constitute one course.

Moxibustion

Acupuncture points:

Baihui	(Du20)
Dazhui	(Du14)
Zhongwan	(Ren12)
Shenque	(Ren8)
Guanyuan	(Ren4)
Zusanli	(S36)

Select two or three points each time. Apply moxa roll moxibustion for 10–15 minutes or three to five medium size cones on each point. Treat once a day. Ten treatments constitute one course.

This method functions to both invigorate the body's *yang qi* and strengthen the spleen and stomach.

Electroacupuncture

Points used are the same as for body acupuncture. Select one to three pairs of points each time. Puncture until a needling sensation is achieved, then connect the needles to an electrical stimulator. Apply moderate intermittent wave stimulation for 30 minutes, once a day. Ten treatments constitute one course.

Auricular therapy

Auricular points:

Lung, Large Intestine, Kidney: promote drug excretion.

Stomach, Spleen: strengthen the stomach and spleen to reinforce antipathogenic *qi*.

Subcortex, Forehead: harmonize the central nervous system.

Liver, Chest: regulate the flow of *qi* to widen the chest.

Ear Shenmen, Occiput: tranquillize the mind.

Use auricular taping with strong manipulation twice a week. Ten treatments constitute one course.

Remarks

- The simplicity, effectiveness and lack of side effects of traditional drugless therapies make them ideal methods of treatment both during and after drug withdrawal.
- Normally six to eight weeks are required to restore normal function of the central nervous system following drug withdrawal, so treatment should be continued until this interval has passed.
- The above therapies may be used singly or in combination.
- Effectiveness may be improved and duration of treatment shortened by combining additional therapeutic measures, such as psychotherapy, social rehabilitation and retraining programmes, with traditional therapies.

42 Dysfunction of the temporomandibular joint

Dysfunction of the temporomandibular joint is a commonly seen oral problem, occurring primarily in adults. It is marked by pain in the temporomandibular joint when opening or closing the mouth, usually aggravated by speaking, chewing or yawning. Articular dyskinesia may also be present, with snapping or popping of the joint occurring when opening or closing the mouth.

Aetiology and differentiation of syndromes

Traditional Chinese medicine classifies dysfunction of the temporomandibular joint as toothache. It is considered to be caused by exogenous wind-cold, overstrain of the joint, or mental injury, any of which may lead to stagnation of *qi* and blood in the meridians. Primarily affected are the Stomach and Large Intestine meridians. There are usually no general symptoms.

Treatment

Body acupuncture

Main acupuncture points:

Xiaguan	(S7)
Jiache	(S6)
Zusanli	(S36)
Hegu	(LI4)
Tinggong	(SI19)

All points are selected according to meridian theory. Xiaguan (S7), Jiache (S6) and Tinggong (SI19) are local points used for treating dysfunction of the temporomandibular joint; Xiaguan (S6) is punctured perpendicularly to a depth of 0.8–1.0 *cun* with the mouth closed. Zusanli (S36) and Hegu (LI4), distal points of the Stomach and Large Intestine meridians respectively, are punctured to activate the meridians and relieve pain.

Treat once every day or once every other day. Ten treatments constitute one course.

Auricular therapy

Main auricular points:

Jaw, Teeth, Mouth: correspond to the affected areas of the body. Tape both frontal and dorsal surfaces to increase stimulation.

Stomach, Large Intestine, San Jiao: the Stomach, Large Intestine and San Jiao meridians distribute to the mandible, so these points are treated to clear and activate the meridians and collaterals.

Ear Shenmen and Occiput: tranquillize the mind and relieve pain.

Remarks

☯ Both body acupuncture and auricular therapy are very effective for treating dysfunction of the temporomandibular joint.

43 Dysfunctional uterine bleeding

Dysfunctional uterine bleeding refers to abnormal uterine bleeding caused by gonadal dysfunction, but with no accompanying organic or general genital problems. It is classified into anovulatory and ovulatory types. The anovulatory type occurs primarily during adolescence or the climacteric and is marked by irregular menstrual cycles and periods with unusually scanty or profuse menstrual blood. The ovulatory type occurs primarily during the reproductive period of life and is marked by short menstrual cycles with long periods, or normal length cycles and periods with unusually scanty or profuse menstrual blood.

Aetiology

According to traditional Chinese medicine, normal menstruation is closely linked to the Chong and Ren meridians. The Chong meridian is also called the Sea of Blood; the Ren meridian is the sea of all Yin meridians and functions to nourish the uterus and fetus. Injury to either of these meridians may result in dysfunctional uterine bleeding. Dysfunctional uterine bleeding is classified into excessive and deficient types in clinical practice. The excessive type has two possible causes. Mental injury may cause stagnation of the liver *qi* which transforms into pathogenic fire; or overindulgence in spicy foods or overprescription of 'hot' herbal medicine may damage the Chong or Ren meridians, resulting in overflow of blood. The deficient type is caused by deficiency of either the spleen *qi* or kidney *yang*, with resulting inability by the Chong and Ren meridians to control the blood of the meridians.

Differentiation of syndromes

- Dysfunctional uterine bleeding of the liver fire type.
  Characterized by dark red clotted menstrual blood and distending pain in the lower abdomen, aggravated by mental stress; accompanied by a feeling of fullness in the chest and hypochondriac region, depression or irritability, frequent sighing, bitter taste in the mouth, dark red or purple-spotted tongue and rapid wiry pulse.
- Dysfunctional uterine bleeding of the blood-heat type.
  Characterized by profuse thick red menstrual blood with a fetid odour; accompanied by flushed face, restlessness, thirst with a preference for cold drinks, red tongue with yellowish coating and rapid slippery pulse.
- Dysfunctional uterine bleeding due to deficiency of the spleen *qi*.
  Characterized by profuse or dripping reddish menstrual blood; accompanied by pale complexion, lassitude, shortness of breath, poor appetite, pale tongue with thin whitish coating and weak thready pulse.

- Dysfunctional uterine bleeding due to deficiency of the kidney *yang*.
  Characterized by reddish menstrual blood, pain and a feeling of cold in the lower abdomen; accompanied by sore and weak back and knees, feeling of cold in the extremities, aversion to cold and preference for warmth, pale tongue with whitish coating and deep thready pulse.

Treatment

Body acupuncture

Main acupuncture points:

Sanyinjiao	(Sp6)
Xuehai	(Sp10)
Yinbai	(Sp1)
Guanyuan	(Ren4)

The spleen functions to control blood in the meridians, therefore points of the Spleen meridian are primary points chosen for treating dysfunctional uterine bleeding. Sanyinjiao (Sp6), the meeting point of the three Foot Yin meridians, is punctured to strengthen the spleen, liver and kidneys. Xuehai (Sp10) (Sea of Blood in Chinese) is an important point for treating bleeding problems. Yinbai (Sp1), the *jing* (well) point of the Spleen meridian, is commonly used for treating dysfunctional uterine bleeding. For excessive type uterine bleeding, Yinbai (Sp1) is pricked with a three-edged needle to draw three to five drops of blood and expel heat; for the deficient type, Yinbai (Sp1) is treated with moxa roll moxibustion for 15–20 minutes to strengthen the spleen and arrest bleeding. Guanyuan (Ren4), the meeting point of the Ren and three Foot Yin meridians, is an important point for treating uterine and genital problems.

Auxiliary points and proper manipulation are chosen according to differentiation of syndromes.

- For dysfunctional uterine bleeding of the liver fire type, Xingjian (Liv2) and Yanglingquan (G34) are added and punctured using the reducing method to dispel liver fire.
- For dysfunctional uterine bleeding of the blood heat type, Quchi (LI11) and Dazhui (Du14) are added and punctured using the reducing method to dispel excessive heat.
- For dysfunctional uterine bleeding due to deficiency of the spleen *qi*, the spleen is strength-

ened by adding and puncturing Zusanli (S36) and Qihai (Ren6) using the reinforcing method and applying moxibustion as needed.

● For dysfunctional uterine bleeding due to deficiency of the kidney *yang*, the kidney *yang* is warmed by adding and puncturing Zigongxue (Ex45) and Mingmen (Du4) using the reinforcing method and applying moxibustion as needed.

Treat excesssive cases once a day; five treatments constitute one course. Treat deficient cases once a day or once every other day, ten treatments constitute one course.

Moxibustion

Points used are the same as for body acupuncture. Apply moxa roll moxibustion to two or three points for 15–20 minutes, once a day. Five treatments constitute one course.

Moxibustion functions to strengthen the spleen and warm the kidneys, so it is suitable for treating deficient types of dysfunctional uterine bleeding.

Electroacupuncture

Points used are the same as for body acupuncture. Select one or two pairs of points each time. Puncture until a needling sensation is achieved, then connect the needles to an electrical stimulator. Apply moderate continuous wave stimulation for 30 minutes. Treat excessive cases once a day; five treatments constitute one course. Treat deficient cases once a day or once every other day; ten treatments constitute one course.

Auricular therapy

Main auricular points:

Internal Genitals, Pelvis, Abdomen: correspond to the affected region. Locate positive points; tape both frontal and dorsal surfaces to increase stimulation.

Liver, Spleen: soothe the liver and strengthen the spleen.

Endocrine, Midpoint of Rim, Subcortex: regulate endocrine function.

Auxiliary auricular points:

For abdominal pain, Ear Shenmen and Occiput are added.

For restlessness and irritability, Chest is added and Apex of Ear is pricked with a three-edged needle to draw several drops of blood.

Use auricular taping and blood-letting puncturing where indicated, twice a week. Five treatments constitute one course.

Remarks

☯ Traditional therapies, especially moxibustion, are very effective for treating dysfunctional uterine bleeding. They may be used singly or in combination.

☯ For cases occurring during the climacteric, gynaecological examination is necessary to differentiate dysfunctional uterine bleeding from possible uterine tumour.

44 Dysmenorrhoea

Dysmenorrhoea is a commonly seen gynaecological disorder marked by pain in the lower abdomen before, during, or after menstruation. It is classified into primary and secondary types. In primary dysmenorrhoea, lower abdominal pain commences with onset of the menarche, with no organic genital conditions present. It is caused primarily by hypoplasia of the uterus, mental injury or endocrine disorder. In secondary dysmenorrhoea, lower abdominal pain commences some time after the menarche; it is caused primarily by organic problems of the internal genitals. Manifestations of both primary and secondary dysmenorrhoea include cramps in the lower abdomen during menstruation, sometimes radiating to the vulva, anus and back, often accompanied by nausea, vomiting, headache, dizziness, pale complexion and sweating and coldness of the hands and feet.

Aetiology

Traditional Chinese medicine classifies dysmenorrhoea into excessive and deficient types. Excessive dysmenorrhoea is caused either by mental injury or invasion of the uterus by exogenous cold, either of which may cause stagnation of blood and *qi* in the meridians. Deficient dysmenorrhoea is caused either by deficiency of the liver and kidneys leading to insufficient nourishment of the uterus, or by deficiency of the kidney *yang* which results in endogenous cold.

Differentiation of syndromes

- Dysmenorrhoea due to invasion of the uterus by exogenous cold.
  Characterized by pain and feeling of cold in the lower abdomen before or during menstruation, sometimes radiating to the lumbosacral region, aggravated by cold and alleviated by warmth; scanty dark red clotted menstrual blood, dark red or purple-spotted tongue and deep tense pulse.
- Dysmenorrhoea due to stagnation of the liver *qi*.
  Characterized by distending pain in the lower abdomen before or during menstruation, aggravated by mental stress; scanty dark clotted menstrual blood; accompanied by distending pain in the chest, breasts and hypochondriac region; restlessness or depression, frequent sighing, dark red or spotted tongue with thin whitish coating and wiry pulse.
- Dysmenorrhoea due to deficiency of the liver and kidneys.
  Characterized by dull pain in the lower abdomen during or after menstruation, alleviated by pressure; scanty dilute red menstrual blood; accompanied by dizziness, tinnitus, blurred vision, lassitude, sore and weak back and knees, pale tongue and deep thready pulse.
- Dysmenorrhoea due to deficiency of the kidney *yang* resulting in endogenous cold in the uterus.
  Characterized by feeling of cold and pain in the lower abdomen during or after menstruation, alleviated by warmth and pressure; scanty clotted red menstrual blood; accompanied by feeling of cold in the extremities, pale complexion, aversion to cold, sore and weak back and knees, pale thin tongue with whitish coating and deep thready slow pulse.

Treatment

Body acupuncture

Main acupuncture points:

Guanyuan	(Ren4)
Guilai	(S29)
Sanyinjiao	(Sp6)

Guanyuan (Ren4), the meeting point of the Ren and three Foot Yin meridians, is an important point for treating uterine and genital problems. Guilai (S29), a point of the Stomach meridian located on the lower abdomen, functions to regulate menstruation and relieve pain. Sanyinjiao (Sp6), the meeting point of the three Foot Yin meridians and Guanyuan (Ren4) are an important pair of points used in combination to treat gynaecological problems.

Auxiliary points and proper manipulation are chosen according to differentiation of syndromes.

- For dysmenorrhoea due to invasion of the uterus by exogenous cold, the meridians are warmed and exogenous cold expelled by adding and puncturing Xuehai (Sp10), Diji (Sp8) and Hegu (LI4) using the reducing method and applying moxibustion as needed.
- For dysmenorrhoea due to stagnation of the liver *qi*, Taichong (Liv3), Yanglingquan (G34) and Neiguan (P6) are added and punctured using the reducing method to promote the flow of the liver *qi*.
- For dysmenorrhoea due to deficiency of the liver and kidneys, Taichong (Liv3), Taixi (K3), Shenshu (B23) and Baihui (Du20) are added and punctured using the reinforcing method to strengthen the liver and kidneys.
- For dysmenorrhoea due to deficiency of the kidney *yang* resulting in endogenous cold in the uterus, the kidney *yang* is tonified by adding and puncturing Mingmen (Du4), Shiqizhui (Ex50) and Qihai (Ren4) using the reinforcing method and applying moxibustion as needed.

Start treatment three to five days before the menstrual period is expected. Treat once a day. Five treatments constitute one course.

Moxibustion

Acupuncture points:

Guanyuan	(Ren4)
Guilai	(S29)
Mingmen	(Du4)
Zhiyin	(B67)
Sanyinjiao	(Sp6)

Select one or two points each time. Treat each point with moxa roll moxibustion for 15–20 minutes, or three to five medium sized moxa cones. Start treatment three to five days before the menstrual period is expected. Treat once or twice a day. Five treatments constitute one course.

Moxibustion functions to warm the meridians and expel cold and is therefore especially suitable for treating dysmenorrhoea due to invasion of the uterus by exogenous cold and dysmenorrhoea due to deficiency of the kidney *yang* resulting in endogenous cold in the uterus.

Its simplicity and safety make moxibustion, especially moxa roll moxibustion, ideal for self-treatment at home. Apply moxa roll moxibustion to one point for 15–20 minutes each time.

Electroacupuncture

Points used are the same as for body acupuncture. Select one or two pairs of points each time. Puncture until a needling sensation is achieved, then connect the needles to an electric stimulator. Apply moderate intermittent wave stimulation for 30 minutes. Start treatment five to seven days before the menstrual period is expected. Treat once a day. Five treatments constitute one course.

Auricular therapy

Main auricular points:

Internal Genitals, Pelvis, Abdomen: correspond to the affected regions. Locate positive points; tape both frontal and dorsal surfaces to increase stimulation.

Liver: the Liver meridian passes through the lower abdomen, so Liver is taped to activate the Liver meridian *qi* and relieve pain.

Endocrine, Midpoint of Rim: regulate endocrine function.

Subcortex, Ear Shenmen: harmonize nervous function and relieve pain.

Auxiliary auricular points:

For excessive type dysmenorrhoea, strong manipulation is used.

For deficient type dysmenorrhoea, Spleen and Kidney are added.

Use auricular taping, twice a week. Treatment given three to five days before the menstrual period is due provides obvious relief of pain during menstruation.

Remarks

☯ Traditional therapies are very effective for treating primary dysmenorrhoea; in most cases there will be great improvement or even cure after treating through two or three menstrual cycles.

☯ In cases of secondary dysmenorrhoea it is necessary to treat the underlying problem concurrently in order to achieve good results.

45 Eczema

Eczema is an allergic skin condition marked by pleomorphic skin lesions accompanied by severe itching, with various internal and external causes. It is classified into acute and chronic types. Acute eczema affects primarily the craniofacial region and flexion aspect of the extremities. Skin lesions may exhibit oedematous erythema, pimples, vesi-

cles, oozing erosion, scabs, or infection. The condition usually lasts 2–3 weeks, but may recur after recovery. Chronic eczema affects mainly the hands, retroauricular region, scrotum or vulva and legs. Skin lesions may exhibit pachylosis, pachyderma, deep dermatoglyph, pigmentation with scales and scratch marks. Chronic eczema may occur primarily or may develop from acute eczema.

Aetiology

According to traditional Chinese medicine, eczema is caused either by exogenous damp-heat and pathogens leading to stagnation of *qi* and blood in the skin, or by deficiency of blood leading to insufficient nourishment of the skin.

Differentiation of syndromes

- Damp-heat eczema.
  Characterized by sudden onset of various skin lesions, including oedematous erythema, pimples, vesicles, oozing erosion and scabs; accompanied by itching, fever, thirst, restlessness, red tongue with yellowish coating and rapid slippery pulse.
- Eczema due to deficiency of blood.
  Characterized by frequently occurring or persistent skin lesions, including pachylosis, pachyderma, deep dermatoglyph, pigmentation with scales and scratch marks; accompanied by severe itching, restlessness, insomnia, poor appetite, pale tongue with thin whitish coating and weak thready pulse.

Treatment

Body acupuncture

Main acupuncture points:

Xuehai	(Sp10)
Sanyinjiao	(Sp6)
Hegu	(LI4)
Quchi	(LI11)

Xuehai (Sp10) (Sea of Blood in Chinese) functions to promote the flow of blood and expel wind and is one of the most important points for treating skin conditions. Sanyinjiao (Sp6), the meeting point of the three Foot Yin meridians, functions to dispel heat and clear away dampness. Hegu (LI4) and Quchi (LI11), the *yuan* (source) and *he* (sea) points respectively of the Large Intestine meridian, are treated in combination to stop itching. by expelling wind and dispelling heat.

Auxiliary points and appropriate manipulation are chosen according to both differentiation of syndromes and location of skin lesions.

- For damp-heat eczema, Dazhui (Du14) and Weizhong (B40) are added and pricked with a three-edged needle. They are then cupped for 10–15 minutes to draw a small amount of blood in order to expel damp-heat.
- For eczema due to deficiency of blood, Geshu (B17), Feishu (B13) and Zusanli (S36) are added and punctured using the reinforcing method to tonify the blood and extinguish endogenous wind. In addition, the areas of the skin lesions are sterilized and tapped lightly with a plum blossom needle until the skin reddens or small flecks of blood appear. (This method may not be used for eczema of the scrotum or vulva.)
- For eczema of the face or neck, Zusanli (S36) and Houxi (SI3) are added.
- For eczema of the flexion aspect of the extremities, Weizhong (B40) and Chize (L5) are added.
- For eczema of the hands, Yangchi (SJ4) and Baxie (Ex6) are added.
- For eczema of the feet, Jiexi (S41) and Bafeng (Ex23) are added.
- For eczema of the retroauricular region, Yifeng (SJ17) and Fengchi (G20) are added.
- For eczema of the scrotum or vulva, Ligou (Liv5) and Zhongji (Ren3) are added.
- For eczema of the legs, Weizhong (B40) and Fengshi (G31) are added.

Treat acute cases once a day; five treatments constitute one course. Treat chronic cases once every day or every other day; ten treatments constitute one course.

Moxibustion

Points:

Areas of skin lesions

Apply moxa roll moxibustion to the affected areas for 20–30 minutes. This method functions to promote the flow of blood and expel wind, so it can immediately relieve the severe itching of eczema. It is commonly used to treat infantile eczema.

Treat once or twice a day. Ten treatments constitute one course.

Blood-letting puncturing

Acupuncture points:

Xuehai	(Sp10)
Quchi	(LI11)
Dazhui	(Du14)
Weizhong	(B40)
Geshu	(B17)
Feishu	(B13)
Areas of skin lesions	

Select one or two points each time. Prick using a three-edged needle, then cup for 10–15 minutes to draw a small amount of blood. Treat different points each time. For chronic cases, areas of the skin lesions are sterilized and then tapped with a plum blossom needle, or pricked with a three-edged needle with mild manipulation, until the skin reddens and flecks of blood appear. (This method cannot be used for eczema of the scrotum or vulva.)

Blood-letting puncturing functions to dispel heat and promote the flow of blood, so it is suitable for treating both acute and chronic eczema.

Auricular therapy

Auricular points:

Areas corresponding to the affected regions: tap with a plum blossom needle to cause mild bleeding in order to dispel damp-heat and pathogens.

Lung: the lungs nourish the skin, so Lung is treated to dispel pathogens from the skin.

Spleen, San Jiao: remove dampness and heat.

Large Intestine: removes dampness and pathogens from stool.

Endocrine, Adrenal Gland, Wind Stream: relieve allergies.

Heart, Ear Shenmen, Occiput: calm the mind and relieve itching.

Centre of Ear: clinically effective point for relieving itching.

Auxiliary auricular points:

For acute eczema, Apex of Ear is added and punctured with a three-edged needle.

For chronic eczema, Liver and Kidney are added.

Use auricular taping with strong manipulation and blood-letting puncturing where indicated, twice a week. Five treatments constitute one course.

Remarks

☯ Traditional therapies are very effective for treating eczema; in many cases the severe itching may be relieved after just one or two treatments.
☯ The various traditional therapies may be used singly, or may be combined to increase stimulation.
☯ These methods are also suitable for treating dermatitis medicamentosa and contact dermatitis.

46 Epidemic keratoconjunctivitis

Epidemic keratoconjunctivitis is a communicable viral infection of the corneoconjunctival region, usually occurring in the summer and autumn. It is marked by burning pain or the sensation of a foreign object in the eye, palpebral oedema, conjunctival congestion and watery secretion. If the cornea is affected, pain, photophobia, lacrimation or hypopsia may occur.

Aetiology

According to traditional Chinese medicine, epidemic keratoconjunctivitis is caused either by exogenous wind-heat or by hyperactive fire in the liver and gallbladder, either of which may ascend to attack the eyes.

Differentiation of syndromes

● Epidemic keratoconjunctivitis due to exogenous wind-heat.
  Characterized by swelling and redness of the eyes, aversion to light and lacrimation; accompanied by headache, fever, aversion to wind and rapid superficial pulse.

● Epidemic keratoconjunctivitis due to hyper-active fire in the liver and gallbladder.
Characterized by swelling and redness of the eyes, aversion to light or hypopsia; accom-panied by headache, bitter taste in the mouth, dry mouth, restlessness, red tip and edges of the tongue and rapid wiry pulse.

Treatment

Body acupuncture

Main acupuncture points:

Fengchi	(G20)
Hegu	(LI4)
Taiyang	(Ex30)
Zanzhu	(B2)

Fengchi (G20), an important point of the Gall-bladder meridian located at the base of the skull, functions to expel wind-heat and is a main point for treating various eye problems. Hegu (LI4), the *yuan* (source) point of the Large Intestine merid-ian, functions to expel exogenous wind-heat. Taiyang (Ex30), an extraordinary local point for eye diseases, is pricked with a three-edged needle to let several drops of blood. Zanzhu (B2), also a local point for eye problems, is punctured towards Yuyao (Ex28).

Auxiliary points and appropriate manipulation are chosen according to differentiation of syndromes:

● For epidemic keratoconjunctivitis due to exoge-nous wind-heat, Guanchong (SJ1) is added and pricked with a three-edged needle to expel heat.
● For epidemic keratoconjunctivitis due to hyper-active fire in the liver and gallbladder, Xingjian (Liv2) and Xiaxi (G43) are added and punctured using the reducing method to dispel endogenous fire.

Treat once a day. Five treatments constitute one course.

Auricular therapy

Auricular points:

Eye, Eye2: correspond to the affected tissues. Locate positive points; tape both frontal and dorsal surfaces to increase stimulation.

Lung: according to Five Orbiculus theory (see Glossary), the lungs correspond to the con-junctiva, so Lung is taped to dispel heat in the conjunctiva.

Liver: the liver opens into the eyes and the Liver meridian connects with the eyes, so Liver is taped to dispel heat and brighten the eyes.

Apex of Ear: blood-letting puncturing of this point with a three-edged needle dispels heat and pathogens.

Use auricular taping with strong manipulation and blood-letting puncturing where indicated, twice a week.

Remarks

๛ Both body acupuncture and auricular therapy are very effective for treating epidemic kerato-conjunctivitis; in many cases there will be great improvement after only one or two treatments.
๛ For cases with no obvious general symptoms or signs, puncture only the main body acu-puncture points, or puncture Apex of Ear with a three-edged needle.
๛ These methods are also suitable for treating other types of conjunctivitis, keratitis and electric ophthalmitis.

47 Epididymitis

Epididymitis is an acute or chronic inflammation of the epididymides, caused primarily by spread of urogenital infection through the spermatic ducts. Acute epididymitis occurs primarily in adults, usually unilaterally. It is marked by sudden

swelling or sinking pain in the affected testicle, radiating to the lower abdomen and groin. Accom-panying general symptoms include chills and fever. Chronic epididymitis is marked by persistent dull sinking pain in the affected testicle, with periodic acute attacks. There is usually a history of acute epididymitis, chronic prostatitis, or long-term indwelling catheter.

Aetiology

According to traditional Chinese medicine, epididymitis is caused primarily by exogenous or endogenous damp-cold or damp-heat which descends and accumulates in the Lower Jiao.

Differentiation of syndromes

- Epididymitis due to damp-cold.
  Characterized by swelling and sinking pain in the affected testicle, aggravated by cold and alleviated by heat; accompanied by aversion to cold and preference for heat, feeling of cold in the lower abdomen, whitish tongue coating and deep pulse.
- Epididymitis due to damp-heat.
  Characterized by redness, swelling and pain in the affected testicle; accompanied by fever, bitter taste in the mouth, scanty yellowish urine, red tongue with greasy yellowish coating and rapid wiry pulse.
- Epididymitis due to deficient *qi* and stagnant blood.
  Characterized by persistent dull sinking pain in the affected testicle, aggravated by exertion; accompanied by distension in the lower abdomen, pale or purple-spotted tongue with whitish coating and thready pulse.

Treatment

Body acupuncture

Main acupuncture points:

Guanyuan	(Ren4)
Ligou	(Liv5)
Sanyinjiao	(Sp6)
Guilai	(S29)

The Liver and Ren meridians are closely related to the external genitals, therefore Guanyuan (Ren4), the meeting point of the Ren and three Foot Yin meridians and Ligou (Liv5), the *luo* (collateral) point of the Liver meridian, are chosen

as main points to puncture to activate the meridians and remove pathogens in the testicles. Sanyinjiao (Sp6), the meeting point of the three Foot Yin meridians, is an important point for treating urogenital problems. Guilai (S29) is a local point for treating epididymitis.

Auxiliary points and appropriate methods of manipulation are chosen according to differentiation of syndromes.

- For epididymitis due to damp-cold, moxibustion is added to expel cold.
- For epididymitis due to damp-heat, Dadun (Liv1) is added and pricked with a three-edged needle to let several drops of blood in order to clear away heat.
- For epididymitis due to deficient *qi* and stagnant blood, Xuehai (Sp10) and Taichong (Liv3) are added and punctured using the even method to reinforce *qi* and promote circulation of the blood.

Treat once a day or once every other day. Five treatments constitute one course.

Electroacupuncture

Points used are the same as for body acupuncture. Select one or two pairs of points each time. Puncture using the reducing method until a needling sensation is achieved, then connect the needles to an electrical stimulator. Apply moderate continuous wave stimulation for 30 minutes. Treat once a day or once every other day. Five treatments constitute one course.

Auricular therapy

Auricular points:

Internal Genitals, External Genitals: correspond to the affected area of the body. Locate positive points; tape both frontal and dorsal surfaces to increase stimulation.

Pelvis, Abdomen: relieve pain in the lower abdomen.

Liver: the Liver meridian connects with the external genitals, so Liver is taped to activate the Liver meridian *qi*.

San Jiao: dispels damp-heat.

Kidney: the kidneys open into both the external genitals and the anus, so Kidney is taped to dispel damp-heat in the testicles.

Endocrine, Adrenal Gland, Apex of Antitragus: relieve inflammation.

Apex of Ear: blood-letting puncturing of this point with a three-edged needle dispels heat and relieves pain.

Use auricular taping with strong manipulation and blood-letting puncturing where indicated, twice a week. Five treatments constitute one course.

Remarks

- Traditional therapies are very effective for treating epididymitis; in many cases there will be great improvement in symptoms and signs after two or three treatments.
- When puncturing Guanyuan (Ren4) and Guilai (S29), it is important that the needling sensation be felt in the external genitals.
- These methods are also suitable for treating spermatitis, spermophlebectasia and hydrocele of the tunica vaginalis.

48 Epilepsy

Epilepsy is caused by frequently recurring abnormal neurogenic firing leading to sudden and temporary dysfunction of the cerebrum. Clinically, epilepsy is classified into four types:

1. Grand mal epilepsy, marked by loss of consciousness and spasm of the entire body, lasting from 5 to 15 minutes;
2. Petit mal epilepsy, marked by temporary disturbance of consciousness lasting for less than a minute, with no accompanying spasm
3. Localized epilepsy, marked by temporary localized spasm lasting for less than a minute, with no disturbance of consciousness.
4. Psychomotor epilepsy, marked by temporary disturbance of consciousness and mental confusion, lasting from several minutes to half an hour.

Aetiology

According to traditional Chinese medicine, epilepsy is caused by mental injury, congenital insufficiency, improper diet, or head trauma. Mainly affected are the liver, kidney and spleen. Stagnant *qi*, accumulated phlegm and endogenous fire are the primary pathogenic factors.

Differentiation of syndromes

- Epilepsy due to liver fire and phlegm heat.
  Attacks are characterized by loss of consciousness, trismus, superduction of the eyes, spasm of the entire body, purple complexion, wheezing, excessive frothy salivation, or even incontinence of urine or stool. The resting stage is characterized by restlessness, irritability, insomnia, dry mouth with bitter taste, constipation, red tongue with greasy yellowish coating and rapid wiry pulse.
- Epilepsy due to stagnant liver *qi* and turbid phlegm.
  Attacks are characterized by disturbance of consciousness, dull eyes, cold feeling in the hands and feet, dark complexion, excessive frothy salivation, or localized convulsion. The resting stage is characterized by a feeling of stuffiness in the chest and hypochondriac region, depression, anxiety, frequent sighing, lassitude, fatigue, poor appetite, nausea or vomiting, loose stool, pale tongue with greasy whitish coating and wiry slippery pulse.
- Epilepsy due to *yin* deficiency of the liver and kidneys, resulting from long-term or frequent attacks of epilepsy due to liver fire and phlegm heat.
  Characterized by lassitude, dizziness, vertigo, dry eyes, thin auriculae, dark complexion, insomnia, poor memory, sore and weak back and knees, constipation, scanty yellowish urine, red tongue with no coating and rapid, wiry, thready pulse.
- Epilepsy due to *yang* deficiency of the spleen and kidneys, resulting from long-term or

frequent attacks of epilepsy due to stagnant liver *qi* and turbid phlegm.

Characterized by listlessness, fatigue, poor memory, emaciation, sensation of cold in the hands and feet, sallow complexion, anorexia, loose stool, sore and weak back and knees, pale and swollen tongue with tooth-marks and slow deep pulse.

Treatment

Body acupuncture
Epileptic attack

Main acupuncture points:

Renzhong	(Du26)
Baihui	(Du20)
Taichong	(Liv3)
Hegu	(LI4)

The main pathogenesis of epileptic attack is agitation of turbid phlegm by endogenous wind, which causes disturbance of mental activity. Therefore, according to the therapeutic principle of restoring consciousness and arresting convulsions, main points are chosen to dispel endogenous wind and turbid phlegm caused by stagnation of the liver *qi* and deficiency of the spleen and kidneys. Renzhong (Du26), the meeting point of the Du, Large Intestine and Stomach meridians, and Baihui (Du20), the meeting point of the Du meridian and the Hand and Foot Liver and Yang meridians, are effective for restoring consciousness and arresting convulsions, the two main disorders of the Du meridian. Treating Taichong (Liv3), the *yuan* (source) point of the Liver meridian and Hegu (LI4), the *yuan* (source) point of the Large Intestine meridian in combination is called 'opening the four passes', and functions both to restore consciousness and arrest convulsions.

Auxiliary points and appropriate manipulation are added according to differentiation of syndromes.

- For epileptic attack due to liver fire and phlegm heat, Shixuan (Ex1) is added and pricked with a three-edged needle to draw blood. The reducing method is used to dispel heat and restore consciousness.
- For epileptic attack due to *yin* deficiency of the liver and kidneys, Sanyinjiao (Sp6) and Taixi (K3) are added and punctured using the even method to reinforce the liver and kidneys.
- For epileptic attack due to *yang* deficiency of

the spleen and kidneys, Qihai (Ren6) and Zusanli (S36) are added and punctured using the reinforcing method and moxibustion is applied to Baihui (Du20) and Qihai (Ren6) to warm the spleen and kidneys.

Resting Stage

Main acupuncture points:

Points of the Du meridian
Changqiang	(Du1)
Jinsuo	(Du8)
Dazhui	(Du14)
Fengfu	(Du16)
Baihui	(Du20)

Points of the Ren meridian
Guanyuan	(Ren4)
Zhongwan	(Ren12)
Jiuwei	(Ren15)
Danzhong	(Ren17)

Additional points
Fengchi	(G20)
Neiguan	(P6)
Fenglong	(S40)
Yaoqi	(Ex51)

Points of the Du meridian are effective for tranquillizing the mind, those of the Ren meridian for regulating the flow of *qi* and removing phlegm. Therefore, points of the Du and Ren meridians are the main points selected for treating epilepsy. The gallbladder controls the power of decision and is linked internally and externally with the liver, which is responsible for stagnant *qi* and accumulated phlegm. Therefore Fengchi (G20), an important point of the Gallbladder meridian close to the brain, is chosen for its properties of dispelling endogenous wind and calming the mind. Neiguan (P6), the *luo* (collateral) point of the Pericardium meridian and one of the eight confluence points connecting with the Yinwei meridian, is selected for its effectiveness at widening the chest and tranquillizing the mind. Fenglong (S40), the *luo* (collateral) point of the Stomach meridian, is useful for strengthening the spleen and stomach and dispelling phlegm. Yaoqi (Ex51), located on the Du meridian, has been proven through clinical experience to be effective in the treatment of epilepsy.

Auxiliary points and appropriate manipulation are added according to differentiation of syndromes.

● For epilepsy due to liver fire and phlegm heat, pathogenic heat is removed by either adding and puncturing Xingjian (Liv2) using the reducing method, or pricking Dazhui (Du14) with a three-edged needle and then cupping for 10–15 minutes.

● For epilepsy due to stagnant liver *qi* and turbid phlegm, the liver *qi* is soothed and the spleen strengthened to remove turbid phlegm by adding and puncturing Taichong (Liv3), Sanyinjiao (Sp6) and Zusanli (S36) using the even method.

● For epilepsy due to *yin* deficiency of the liver and kidneys, the kidney *yin* is tonified by adding and puncturing Taichong (Liv3), (Taixi) (K3) and Sanyinjiao (Sp6) using the even method.

● For epilepsy due to *yang* deficiency of the spleen and kidneys, the spleen and kidneys are warmed by either adding and puncturing Pishu (B20), Shenshu (B23) and Mingmen (Du4) using the reinforcing method, or by applying moxibustion to Baihui (Du20), Mingmen (Du4), Guanyuan (Ren4) and Zhongwan (Ren12).

Select five to six main points and appropriate auxiliary points each time. Points of the Ren and Du meridians may be used alternately or concurrently. Treat once a day or every other day. Thirty treatments constitute one course.

Electroacupuncture

Points used are the same as for body acupuncture. Select two to three pairs of points each time. Puncture using the even method until a needling sensation is achieved; then connect the needles to an electric stimulator. Apply moderate intermittent wave stimulation for 30 minutes for grand mal and petit mal epilepsy; apply mild intermittent wave stimulation for 30 minutes for localized and psychomotor epilepsy and during the resting stage. Treat once a day or every other day. Thirty treatments constitute one course.

Point implantation therapy

This method is used to treat epilepsy during the resting stage. Commonly used points are the points of the Du and Ren meridians listed above. Select two or three points each time. Using a triangular surgical needle, implant surgical catgut on each point. (See Appendix 9.) Treat once every 20–30 days. Three treatments constitute one course.

Because of the intense and long-term stimulation it provides, point implantation therapy is an ideal choice for the treatment of epilepsy.

Scalp acupuncture

Scalp lines:

Ezhongxian	(MS1)
Dingzhongxian	(MS5)
Affected areas	

Determine abnormal loci by electroencephalogram (EEG) examination. Puncture using strong manipulation for 5 minutes, then retain the needles for 30 minutes to 2 hours. Treat once every other day. Ten treatments constitute one course.

Scalp acupuncture is usually used during the resting stage of epilepsy. It has been proven that scalp acupuncture can inhibit the abnormal firing of the brain cells that occurs in epilepsy and is therefore an effective treatment.

Auricular therapy

Auricular points:

Subcortex, Temple, Forehead, Occiput: correspond to the affected areas of the body. Locate positive points; tape both frontal and dorsal surfaces to increase stimulation.

Liver, Kidney: reinforce the liver and kidney.

Spleen, Abdomen: strengthen the spleen to remove phlegm.

Chest: widens the chest and regulates the flow of *qi*.

Heart, Ear Shenmen: calm the mind.

Apex of Ear: blood-letting puncturing of this point with a three-edged needle calms the mind and restores consciousness.

Use auricular taping with strong manipulation and blood-letting puncturing where indicated, twice a week. Ten treatments constitute one course.

Remarks

☯ Traditional therapies are very effective in relieving epileptic attack and may even provide a cure in some cases. However, extended treatment should be given to consolidate the results. Body acupuncture is the method used most often during epileptic attack; during the resting stage two or more methods are usually combined, for instance body acupuncture and scalp acupuncture, body acupuncture and electroacupuncture, or point implantation and scalp acupuncture.

☯ Patients who are currently taking antiepileptic drugs must not be suddenly withdrawn during treatment with traditional therapies. Drugs should be gradually reduced only after it is certain that the traditional treatment is playing a role in inhibiting epileptic attack.

☯ It cannot be emphasized strongly enough that great care must be taken when puncturing Dazhui (Du14) and Fengfu (Du16). The puncturing method used is very important. With the patient's head lowered, puncture Dazhui (Du14) obliquely upward to a depth of 0.5–0.8 *cun*; puncture Fengfu (Du16) toward the base of the lower jaw to a depth of 0.5–0.8 *cun*.

Manipulate both points using the even method for 3 to 5 minutes and then withdraw the needles.

Some experienced practitioners assert that better therapeutic results may be attained by inserting the needle into the vertebral canal, even touching the spinal cord, to cause the patient to experience a sensation of electric shock. However, this method is extremely dangerous and cannot be advocated. If the needle should accidentally enter the vertebral canal, producing sensations of shock or even paralysis, it must be withdrawn immediately. Paralysis may recover spontaneously within several hours in mild cases. Proper treatment should be given in severe cases to aid the recovery process. However, damage to the spinal cord may be irreversible.

☯ Additional modern methods should be combined with TCM when treating epilepticism.

49   Epistaxis

Epistaxis, or nosebleed, is a common symptom of various diseases and disorders. It may arise from either local or systemic problems. Local diseases and disorders include trauma of the nose, deviated septum, foreign bodies in the nose and inflammation or tumor of the nose or nasal sinuses. Systemic diseases and disorders include acute febrile infectious diseases, hypertension, haematopathy, dystrophia and vitamin deficiency. There are usually no general symptoms in cases of minor or occasional nasal haemorrhage, but anemia or shock may occur if nasal haemorrage is major or recurrent. Immediate and appropriate treatment is essential in these cases.

Aetiology

According to traditional Chinese medicine, epistaxis is classified into excessive and deficient types. The excessive type is caused either by invasion of the lungs by wind-heat, or by hyperactivity of the stomach fire due to overindulgence in spicy or greasy foods. Both of these conditions

may cause injury to the meridians and resultant nasal bleeding. The deficient type may occur when deficient fire caused by *yin* deficiency of the liver and kidneys rises up and damages the meridians, or when deficiency of the spleen *qi* results in loss of control of the blood.

Differentiation of syndromes

● Epistaxis due to invasion of the lungs by windheat.
  Characterized by profuse bright red nasal bleeding; accompanied by fever, headache, dry mouth, red tongue and rapid superficial pulse.
● Epistaxis due to hyperactivity of the stomach fire.
  Characterized by profuse bright red nasal bleeding; accompanied by dry mouth, constipation, red tongue with yellowish coating and rapid pulse.
● Epistaxis due to rising of deficient fire caused by *yin* deficiency of the liver and kidneys.
  Characterized by intermittent dark red nasal

bleeding; accompanied by dizziness, tinnitus, insomnia, dry mouth, red tongue with little coating and rapid thready pulse.

● Epistaxis due to deficiency of the spleen *qi*. Characterized by frequent scanty or profuse reddish nasal bleeding; accompanied by pale complexion, shortness of breath, lassitude, poor appetite, loose stool, pale tongue with thin whitish coating and weak pulse.

Treatment

Body acupuncture

Main acupuncture points:

Yingxiang	(LI20)
Hegu	(LI4)
Shangxing	(Du23)
Fengchi	(G20)

The Du and Large Intestine meridians are closely connected with the nose, so main points for stopping nasal bleeding are selected from these meridians. Yingxiang (LI20) is punctured obliquely upward towards Bitong (Ex32) for 0.5–1.0 *cun*. Hegu (LI4), the *yuan* (source) point of the Large Intestine meridian, functions to expel wind and dispel heat. Shangxing (Du23) is a local point proven through clinical experience to be effective for treating various nasal problems. Fengchi (G20), an important point of the Gallbladder meridian located at the base of the skull, functions to expel wind and dispel heat and is a main point for treating problems of the sensory organs.

Auxiliary points and appropriate manipulation are chosen according to differentiation of syndromes.

● For epistaxis due to invasion of the lungs by wind-heat, Shaoshang (L11) and Shangyang (LI1) are added and pricked with a three-edged needle to dispel heat.

● For epistaxis due to hyperactivity of the stomach fire, Lidui (S45) and Shaoshang (L11) are added and pricked with a three-edged needle to extinguish stomach fire.

● For epistaxis due to rising of deficient fire caused by *yin* deficiency of the liver and kidneys, Baihui (Du20) and Sanyinjiao (Sp6) are added and punctured using the even method to strengthen the liver and kidneys.

● For epistaxis due to deficiency of the spleen *qi*, antipathogenic *qi* is strengthened by puncturing

all main points using the reinforcing method and applying moxibustion to Shangxing (Du23).

Moxibustion

Points:

Xinhui	(Du22)
Shangxing	(Du23)
Fengfu	(Du16)
Yongquan	(K1)

Only one point is selected in each case. Apply moxa roll moxibustion for 20–30 minutes.

Auricular therapy

Auricular points:

Internal Nose: corresponds to the affected region.

Adrenal Gland: contracts the capillary vessels to stop bleeding.

Spleen: strengthens the spleen to control blood in the meridians.

Lung, Stomach: the lungs open into the nose and the Stomach meridian stems from the bilateral sides of the nose, so Lung and Stomach are treated to activate the meridians and arrest nasal bleeding.

Centre of Ear, Midpoint of Rim: clinically effective points for arresting bleeding.

Upper Ear Root: clinically effective points for arresting nasal haemorrhage. An old folk cure is to press this point with a stone or pencil point to stop nosebleeds.

Use auricular taping with strong manipulation.

Remarks

☙ The simplicity and effectiveness of traditional therapies make them ideal for treating nosebleeds. However, it is essential to diagnose the cause of epistaxis as soon as nasal bleeding has been arrested in order to treat it completely.

☙ For cases without obvious general symptoms and signs, acupuncture, moxibustion, or auricular therapy should be used only on the main points.

☙ There are two practical methods for stopping nosebleeds at home. One is press Upper Ear

Root with a stone or pencil point; the other is to apply a coating of pounded garlic to bilateral Yongquan (K1), located at the centres of the soles of the feet.

  It is recorded in *The Discussion on Febrile Diseases* by Zhang Zhongjing (150–219 A.D.) that onset of nasal bleeding may bring about an immediate cure of febrile diseases. This is referred to as 'red sweating' and works on the same principle as blood-letting puncturing.

  Additional treatments such as application of cold wet compresses and nasal packing may be undertaken concurrently with the above methods.

50 Erythromelalgia

Erythromelalgia is a disorder of the capillary tips caused by vagotonia. It occurs mainly in winter and more often in females than in males. It is marked by paroxysmal burning or stabbing pain and redness of the extremities and is aggravated at night, by walking, or by exposure to heat. There may be mild numbness and pain during the remission stage. The feet are affected much more often than the hands.

Aetiology and differentiation of syndromes

Traditional Chinese medicine classifies erythromelalgia as a *bi* syndrome. It is considered to be caused by invasion of the meridians by exogenous cold with resulting stagnation of the *qi* and blood, which are then transformed into heat. Primarily affected are the Yang meridians of the hands and feet, since they are rich in *qi* and blood which may be transformed into heat when invaded by exogenous cold. Erythromelalgia is marked by red tongue and wiry pulse.

Treatment

Body acupuncture

Acupuncture points:

Group 1:

Quchi	(LI11)
Waiguan	(SJ5)
Hegu	(LI4)
Baxie	(Ex6)
Shixuan	(Ex1)

Group 2:

Zusanli	(S36)
Jiexi	(S41)
Bafeng	(Ex23)
Taichong	(Liv3)

Main points for dredging the meridians, dispelling heat and relieving pain are selected from the Hand and Foot Yang meridians. Group 1 is used to treat erythromelalgia of the upper limbs. Shixuan (Ex1) is pricked with a three-edged needle to draw several drops of blood; for severe cases, Dazhui (Du14) is added and pricked with a three-edged needle and then cupped for 10 minutes to draw blood and dispel heat. Group 2 is used to treat erythromelalgia of the lower limbs. Taichong (Liv3), the *yuan* (source) point of the Liver meridian, is included to promote the flow of *qi* and blood and relieve pain.

Puncture using the reducing method and blood-letting acupuncture where indicated, once a day or once every other day. Five treatments constitute one course.

Auricular therapy

Auricular points:

Areas corresponding to the affected regions of the body: locate positive points; tape both frontal and dorsal surfaces to increase stimulation.

Heart, Liver, Lung: improve the circulation of *qi* and blood.

Sympathesis, Subcortex: regulate the function of the autonomic nervous system to harmonize vasomotoricity.

Ear Shenmen, Occiput: tranquillize the mind and relieve pain.

Apex of Ear: blood-letting puncturing of this point with a three-edged needle dispels heat and relieves pain.

Use auricular taping with strong manipulation and blood-letting puncturing where indicated, twice a week. Five treatments constitute one course.

Remarks

☙ The above therapies can effectively relieve the symptoms of erythromelalgia, as well as treat the cause.
☙ The hands and feet should be kept warm and alcohol avoided in order to avoid relapse.

51 External humeral epicondylitis

External humeral epicondylitis, commonly called tennis elbow, is caused by strain or sprain at the base of the carpal extensor muscle. It occurs primarily in adults; carpenters and tennis players are at especially high risk. External humeral epicondylitis is marked by pain on the lateral side of the elbow joint, usually radiating to the lateral side of the forearm or shoulder and aggravated when making a fist or wringing motion. There is severe tenderness on the external humeral epicondyle, but no swelling or impairment of joint movement.

Aetiology

According to traditional Chinese medicine, external humeral epicondylitis is caused by strain of the elbow leading to localized obstruction of the *qi* and blood. Primarily affected is the Large Intestine meridian. There are usually no general symptoms.

Treatment

Body acupuncture

Main acupuncture point:

Ashi (tender) point

Auxiliary acupuncture points:

Shousanli	(LI10)
Quchi	(LI11)
Zhouliao	(LI12)
Hegu	(LI4)

Have the patient sit with the elbow on a table, make a loose fist and flex the arm to 90°. Locate

the *ashi*, or tender point, on the external humeral epicondyle. Insert the needle between Quchi (LI11) and the tender point and puncture obliquely towards the base of the tender point. Manipulate using the reducing method until a needling sensation is felt in the local area and radiating to the forearm. Shousanli (LI10), Quchi (LI11), Zhouliao (LI12) and Hegu (LI4) may be added to increase stimulation.

Treat once a day or once every other day. Five treatments constitute one course.

Moxibustion

Acupuncture point:

Ashi (tender) point

Locate tender point. Apply moxa roll moxibustion for 10 minutes, or three to five medium-sized moxa rolls, once a day or once every other day. Five treatments constitute one course.

Point injection therapy

Acupuncture point:

Ashi (tender) point

Locate tender point. Insert syringe needle at the periosteum and inject with 2–4 ml of procaine, vitamin B_{12}, or hydroprednisone. Treat once every three days. Five treatments constitute one course.

Electroacupuncture

Points used are the same as for body acupuncture. Treat the *ashi* point and one auxiliary point each time. Puncture the points until a needling sensation is achieved, then connect the needles to an electrical stimulator. Apply continuous wave stimulation of the strongest bearable intensity for 30 minutes. Treat once a day or once every other day. Five treatments constitute one course.

Blood-letting puncturing and cupping

Acupuncture point:

Ashi (tender) point

Locate tender point. Prick with a three-edged needle or tap with a plum blossom needle to cause mild bleeding, then cup for 10–15 minutes. Treat once a week. Five treatments constitute one course.

Auricular therapy

Auricular points:

Elbow: corresponds to the affected area of the body. Locate posititve points; tape both frontal and dorsal surfaces to increase stimulation.

Large Intestine: the Large Intestine meridian distributes to the lateral humeral epicondyle, so Large Intestine is taped to clear and activate the meridians and collaterals.

Liver: the liver nourishes the tendons, so Liver is taped to strengthen them.

Ear Shenmen: relieves pain.

Use auricular taping with strong manipulation, twice a week. Five treatments constitute one course.

Remarks

☯ The above therapies are very effective for treating external humeral epicondylitis. They can be used singly or in combination.

☯ It is necessary to minimize movement of the affected limb and keep it warm during the course of treatment.

☯ Five to seven additional treatments must be given after the symptoms disappear in order to consolidate effects and prevent relapse.

52 Facial spasm

Facial spasm is an involuntary, paroxysmal spasm of the unilateral facial muscles. Some cases are sequelae of facial paralysis, but most do not have a clear and definite cause. The spasm usually originates in the orbicular muscle of the eye and gradually spreads to the homolateral facial muscles. Spasm of the angle of the mouth is most apparent. The spasm may stop spontaneously after sleep, but in some cases is persistent.

Aetiology

According to traditional Chinese medicine, facial spasm has three primary causes: exogenous wind-cold may affect the Stomach and Large Intestine meridians and obstruct the flow of *qi* and blood; *yin* deficiency of the liver and kidney may produce

endogenous wind; or mental injury may disturb the flow of *qi* in the meridians.

Differentiation of syndromes

● Facial spasm due to hyperactivity of the liver fire.
  Characterized by headache, vertigo, tinnitus, bitter taste in the mouth, restlessness, irritability, constipation, scanty yellowish urine, red tongue with yellowish coating and rapid wiry pulse.

● Facial spasm due to *yin* deficiency of the liver and kidneys.
  Characterized by dizziness, tinnitus, blurred vision, insomnia, bad dreams, poor memory, sore and weak back and knees, thin tongue with little coating and wiry thready pulse.

● Facial spasm due to deficiency of the heart and spleen.
Characterized by palpitation, shortness of breath, restlessness, insomnia, pale complexion, lassitude, poor appetite, loose stool, pale tongue with thin whitish coating and weak thready pulse.

Treatment

Body acupuncture

Main acupuncture points:

Fengchi	(G20)
Yifeng	(SJ17)
Hegu	(LI4)
Zusanli	(S36)
Baihui	(Du20)

Main points are chosen according to meridian theory. The Yangming and Shaoyang meridians of the hands and feet distribute to the face, therefore Fengchi (G20), Yifeng (SJ17), Hegu (LI4) and Zusanli (S36) are punctured to harmonize the flow of *qi* and blood and relieve spasm. Baihui (Du20), the meeting point of the Du, Liver and Hand and Foot Yang meridians, is an important point for tranquillizing the mind.

Auxiliary points and appropriate methods of manipulation are chosen according to differentiation of syndromes.

● For facial spasm due to hyperactivity of the liver fire, Taichong (Liv3) and Neiguan (P6) are added and punctured using the even method to eliminate hyperactive liver fire.
● For facial spasm due to *yin* deficiency of the liver and kidneys, Taixi (K3), Sanyinjiao (Sp6) and Shenshu (B23) are added and punctured using the reinforcing method to strengthen the liver and kidneys.
● For facial spasm due to deficiency of the heart and spleen, Shenmen (H7), Neiguan (P6) and Sanyinjiao (Sp6) are added and punctured using the reinforcing method to tranquillize mind and strengthen the spleen.

Treat once a day or once every other day. Ten treatments constitute one course.

Electroacupuncture

Points used are the same as for body acupuncture. Select one or two pairs of points each time.

Puncture the points until a needling sensation is achieved, then connect the needles to an electrical stimulator. Apply moderate intermittent wave stimulation for 30 minutes. Treat once a day or once every other day. Ten treatments constitute one course.

Auricular therapy

Main auricular points:

Cheek, Eye, Mouth: correspond to the affected areas of the body. Tape both frontal and dorsal surfaces to increase stimulation.

Large Intestine, Stomach: both the Large Intestine and Stomach meridians distribute to the face, so these points are taped to activate the meridians to expel wind and arrest spasm.

Spleen: nourishes the facial muscles to arrest spasm.

San Jiao: the mixed branches of the glossopharyngeal, vagus and facial nerves pass through this auricular area, so taping San Jiao can arrest spasm.

Subcortex, Ear Shenmen, Occiput: tranquillize the mind.

Auxiliary auricular points:

For facial spasm due to mental injury, Liver and Pancreas & Gallbladder are added.

For facial spasm due to *yin* deficiency of the liver and kidney, Liver and Kidney are added.

For facial spasm due to deficiency of the heart and spleen, Heart and Spleen are added.

Use auricular taping, concentrating on the affected side, twice a week. Five treatments constitute one course.

Remarks

☺ Traditional therapies are effective for treating facial spasm. Body acupuncture and auricular therapy are usually used in combination to increase stimulation and improve effect.
☺ Local points should not be punctured in order to avoid increasing nervous excitation and aggravating the condition.

53 Female infertility

Pregnancy will normally occur within six months in heterosexually active women of childbearing age who are not using contraceptive measures. Absence of conception may occur due to reproductive disorders of either the male or female partner. The possibility of infertility of the male partner must be considered before arriving at a diagnosis of female infertility.

Female infertility is classified clinically into primary and secondary types. Primary female infertility refers to absence of conception after three years by nullipara women of child-bearing age who are sexually active with fertile men and who are using no contraceptive measures. Secondary female infertility refers to absence of conception after two years in previously pregnant women of child-bearing age who are sexually active with fertile men and who are using no contraceptive measures. The causes of female infertility are various, including ovulatory dysfunction, hypoplasia of the uterus, inflammation or tumours of the genitals, problems of the immune system, psychological factors, or malnutrition. In some cases, failure to conceive may be due to simple ignorance of sexual function resulting in incomplete, insufficient or mistimed sexual intercourse.

Aetiology

According to traditional Chinese medicine, the female reproductive system is closely related to the kidneys and the Ren and Chong meridians. Development and maturation of the reproductive system and the ability to reproduce depend on an abundant supply of kidney essence, and conception and fetal development depend on normal and sufficient flow of *qi* and blood in the Ren and Chong meridians. The spleen functions to transform food into blood to supply the Ren and Chong meridians with *qi* and blood, and the liver promotes and regulates the flow of *qi* and blood in these meridians. Therefore, any factors which damage the kidneys, spleen or liver, or affect the normal flow of sufficient *qi* and blood in the Chong and Ren meridians, may result in female infertility.

Differentiation of syndromes

● Female infertility due to deficiency of the kidneys.
  Characterized by scanty red menstrual blood, dizziness, tinnitus, sore and weak back and knees, emaciation, pale tongue and deep, thready, weak pulse.
● Female infertility due to deficiency of *yin*.
  Characterized by scanty purple menstrual blood, dry mouth, restlessness, insomnia, sensation of heat in the palms and soles, mild fever, emaciation, red tongue and rapid thready pulse.
● Female infertility due to deficiency of *qi* and blood.
  Characterized by irregular menstruation, scanty red menstrual blood, dull pain in the lower abdomen and lumbosacral region during menstruation, pale complexion, palpitation, shortness of breath, lassitude, pale tongue with thin whitish coating and weak thready pulse.
● Female infertility due to coldness in the uterus.
  Characterized by delayed menstruation, scanty dark purple or clotted menstrual blood, pain or sensation of cold in the lower abdomen and lumbosacral region, aversion to cold, sensation of cold in the extremities, poor appetite, purple tongue with whitish coating and tense thready pulse.
● Female infertility due to stagnation of the liver *qi*.
  Characterized by long menstrual cycle, scanty purple menstrual blood; distending pain in the chest, lower abdomen and hypochondriac region; restlessness, thin whitish tongue coating and deep wiry pulse.
● Female infertility of the blood-heat type.
  Characterized by short menstrual cycle, profuse dark purple or clotted menstrual blood, restlessness, dry mouth, flushed face, red tongue and rapid slippery pulse.
● Female infertility due to accumulation of damp-heat in the Lower Jiao.
  Characterized by profuse, yellowish, strong-smelling leucorrhoea; pain in the lower abdomen and lumbosacral region, headache, dizziness, nausea, sensation of heat in the palms and

soles, frequent dripping urination, dark red tongue with greasy yellowish coating and rapid slippery pulse.

Treatment

Body acupuncture

Main acupuncture points:

Guanyuan	(Ren4)
Sanyinjiao	(Sp6)
Yinjiao	(Ren7)
Zigongxue	(Ex45)

Guanyuan (Ren4), the meeting point of the Ren and three Foot Yin meridians located on the lower abdomen, and Sanyinjiao (Sp6), the meeting point of the three Foot Yin meridians, are the main points for treating gynaecological and obstetrical problems. They are usually treated in combination. Yinjiao (Ren7), the meeting point of the Ren and Chong meridians, is punctured to regulate the Ren and Chong meridians. Zigongxue (Ex45) is a clinically effective point for treating infertility.

Auxiliary points and appropriate manipulation are chosen according to differentiation of syndromes.

- For female infertility due to deficiency of the kidneys, Shenshu (B23), Qixue (K13) and Taixi (K3) are added and punctured using the reinforcing method to strengthen the kidneys.
- For female infertility due to deficiency of *yin*, Taixi (K3) and Xuehai (Sp10) are added and punctured using the even method to nourish *yin*.
- For female infertility due to deficiency of *qi* and blood, Qihai (Ren6) and Zusanli (S36) are added and punctured using the reinforcing method to strengthen *qi* and blood.
- For female infertility due to coldness in the uterus, the uterus is warmed and cold expelled by adding and puncturing Mingmen (Du4) and Shenque (Ren8) using the reinforcing method and applying moxibustion as needed.
- For female infertility due to stagnation of the liver *qi*, Taichong (Liv3) and Neiguan (P6) are added and punctured using the reducing

method to promote the flow of the liver *qi*.
- For female infertility of the blood-heat type, Xuehai (Sp10) and Zhongji (Ren3) are added and punctured using the reducing method to dispel heat.
- For female infertility due to accumulation of damp-heat in the Lower Jiao, Qugu (Ren2), Guilai (S29) and Ciliao (B32) are added and punctured using the reducing method to remove damp-heat.

Treat once a day or once every other day. Ten treatments constitute one course.

Moxibustion

Points used are the same as for body acupuncture. Apply moxa roll moxibustion for 15–20 minutes to two or three points, once or twice a day. Ten treatments constitute one course.

Moxibustion functions to strengthen the antipathogenic *qi* and warm the meridians, so it is suitable for treating infertility due to deficiency of the kidneys or *qi* and blood, or coldness in the uterus.

Electroacupuncture

Points used are the same as for body acupuncture. Select one or two pairs of points each time. Puncture until a needling sensation is achieved, then connect the needles to an electrical stimulator. Apply moderate continuous wave stimulation for 30 minutes, once a day or once every other day. Ten treatments constitute one course.

Remarks

- Traditional therapies are effective for treating female infertility, with a high rate of cure for infertility due to anovulatory menstruation, tubal obstruction and hypoplasia of the uterus.
- Two or more therapies are usually used in combination to increase stimulation and raise effectiveness.

54 Flat wart

Flat wart is a viral skin problem which occurs primarily in adolescents. It is marked by flat circular or elliptical papules ranging from the size of a pinhead to that of a grain of rice, with a smooth surface, clearly defined border and brownish or normal colour. The papules may occur separately or in groups, usually on the face, back of the hands, or forearms. There are usually no subjective symptoms.

Aetiology and differentiation of syndrome

According to traditional Chinese medicine, flat wart is caused either by exogenous wind-heat attacking the meridians, or by stagnation of the liver *qi* which affects the flow of *qi* and blood. The papules occur primarily along the courses of the three Hand Yang meridians.

Treatment

Body acupuncture

Acupuncture points:

Hegu	(LI4)
Zhongzhu	(SJ3)
Zhizheng	(SI7)
Local points	

Points are selected according to meridian theory. Hegu (LI4) is the *yuan* (source) point of the Large Intestine meridian, Zhongzhu (SJ3) is the *shu* (stream) point of the San Jiao meridian and Zhizheng (SI7) is the *luo* (collateral) point of the Small Intestine meridian. These three points of the Hand Yang meridians are punctured to activate the meridians and clear the collaterals. Local points are selected according to the location of the papules. For example, Baxie (Ex6) is chosen for treating papules on the back of the hands; Sibai (S2), Jiache (S6) and Quanliao (SI18) are used to treat for papules on the face.

Puncture using the reducing method, once a day or once every other day. Local points are punctured obliquely towards the papules. Five treatments constitute one course.

Electroacupuncture

Points used are the same as for body acupuncture. Select one or two pairs of points each time. Puncture the points until a needling sensation is achieved, then connect the needles with an electrical stimulator. Apply continuous wave stimulation of the highest bearable intensity for 20–30 minutes. Treat once a day or once every other day. Five treatments constitute one course.

Auricular therapy

Auricular points:

Corresponding areas: tap with a plum blossom needle or prick with a three-edged needle to induce mild bleeding, expel wind and dispel heat.

Lung, Large Intestine: the lungs nourish the skin and the large intestine is connected internally and externally with the lungs, so Lung and Large Intestine are treated to improve the metabolism.

Liver: the liver regulates the flow of *qi* and blood, so Liver is treated to promote their flow.

Wind Stream, Adrenal Gland, Endocrine: relieve infection.

Apex of Ear: blood-letting puncturing of this point with a three-edged needle activates the meridians and clears the collaterals.

Use auricular taping with strong manipulation and blood-letting puncturing where indicated. Treat twice a week. Five treatments constitute one course.

Remarks

- Traditional therapies are effective for treating flat wart and may be used singly or in combination.
- If during the course of treatment the papules suddenly increase or become red and itchy, this indicates that they will disappear.

55 Furunculosis

Furuncle is an acute purulent inflammation of the hair follicle and its peripheral sebaceous glands caused by the *Staphylococcus aureus* bacteria. Cases of multiple or recurring furuncle are referred to as furunculosis. People with diabetes mellitus, chronic nephritis, malnutrition, eczema, prickly heat or pediculosis are at particularly high risk for this disorder. Furunculosis is marked in the initial stage by bright red conical papular eruptions which gradually enlarge and turn into extremely painful scleromata. The scleromata eventually suppurate, sometimes leaving a slough embolus in the centre of the lesion. When the embolus drops off pus is discharged and the pain is alleviated. A scar often remains after healing. General symptoms in the acute stage include chills, fever, headache, poor appetite or even haematosepsis. The furuncles usually occur on the face, back of the neck, back and buttocks.

Aetiology

According to traditional Chinese medicine, furunculosis is caused either by exogenous toxic heat which invades the body and accumulates in the skin, or by overindulgence in spicy or greasy foods resulting in endogenous toxic heat which accumulates in the skin. In both cases, the flow of *qi* and blood is obstructed, with furuncles forming due to the combination of stagnant blood and accumulated toxic heat. As the condition develops, *qi* and blood may be consumed.

Differentiation of syndromes

- Furunculosis due to excessive heat.
  Characterized by short course with redness, swelling, sensation of heat and severe pain in the affected region; accompanied by chills, fever, headache, red tongue with yellowish coating and rapid pulse.
- Furunculosis due to deficiency of *qi* and blood.
  Characterized by long course with frequently recurring painless furuncle with discharge of

pus; accompanied by lassitude, pale complexion, emaciation, poor appetite, pale tongue with thin white coating and weak thready pulse.

Treatment

Body acupuncture

Main acupuncture points:

Dazhui	(Du14)
Shenzhu	(Du12)
Lingtai	(Du10)
Weizhong	(B40)
Quchi	(LI11)

Main points are selected from the Yang meridians to activate the meridians and dispel heat and toxic pathogens. Dazhui (Du14), Shenzhu (Du12) and Lingtai (Du10) are selected from the Du meridian, the sea of all the Yang meridians. According to Five Element theory (see Glossary), the heart is governed by fire. Furuncles and other skin infections are due primarily to hyperactivity of the heart fire which obstructs the flow of *qi* and blood. Lingtai (Du10) (Seat of the Soul in Chinese) corresponds to the inner heart and therefore functions to dispel the heart fire and relieve the pain, swelling and redness of furuncles. It is an especially important point for treating furunculosis and other skin infections.

Weizhong (B40), the *he* (sea) and lower *he* (confluent) point of the Urinary Bladder meridian, is also an important point for dispelling heat and toxic pathogens. Quchi (LI11), the *he* (sea) point of the Large Intestine meridian, functions to activate the meridians and dispel heat.

Auxiliary points are chosen according to meridian theory.

- For furuncle on the face, Hegu (LI4) and Neiting (S44) are added.
- For furuncle on the back of the neck, Fengchi (G20) and Kunlun (B60) are added.
- For furuncle on the back, Feishu (B13), Jianjing (G21) and Xinshu (B15) are added.
- For furuncle on the buttocks, Zhiyin (B67) and Kunlun (B60) are added.

Appropriate manipulation is determined by differentiation of syndromes.

- For furunculosis due to excessive heat, heat and toxic pathogens are dispelled by pricking two or three main points with a three-edged needle and then cupping for 10–15 minutes to draw blood. Auxiliary points are punctured using the reducing method.
- For furunculosis due to deficiency of *qi* and blood, antipathogenic *qi* is strengthened and pathogens expelled by puncturing all points using the even method and applying moxibustion to the affected areas.

Treat excessive type furunculosis once a day. Five treatments consititute one course. Treat deficient type furunculosis once a day or once every other day. Ten treatments constitute one course.

Blood-letting puncturing

Points used are the same as for body acupuncture. Select two or three points each time. Prick with a three-edged needle to draw several drops of blood, then cup for 10–15 minutes to draw blood and increase stimulation.

This method functions to dispel heat and toxic pathogens, so it is an ideal therapy for treating furunculosis and other skin infections. Treat once a day or every other day. Five treatments constitute one course.

Auricular therapy

Auricular points:

Areas corresponding to the affected regions: locate positive points; tape both frontal and dorsal surfaces to increase stimulation.

Lung: the lungs nourish the skin, so Lung is treated to dispel toxic heat from the skin.

Heart: according to Five Element theory (see Glossary), the heart is governed by fire, so Heart is treated to dispel toxic heat.

Endocrine, Adrenal Gland, Wind Stream: relieve inflammation.

Ear Shenmen: relieves inflammation and pain.

Apex of Ear: blood-letting puncturing of this point with a three-edged needle dispels toxic heat.

Auxiliary points are added according to meridian theory.

For furuncle on the face, Large Intestine and Stomach are added.

For furuncle on the back of the neck, Urinary Bladder and Pancreas & Gallbladder are added.

Use auricular taping with strong manipulation and blood-letting puncturing where indicated, once every other day. Five treatments constitute one course.

Remarks

- Traditional therapies are very effective for treating furunculosis; in many cases there will be great improvement after two to three treatments.
- In cases with severe general symptoms, additional treatment should be undertaken concurrently.
- These methods are also suitable for treating carbuncle, impetigo herpetiformis, erysipelas, chronic folliculitis and various other skin infections. Additional points should be selected according to meridian theory.

56 Gastritis

Gastritis is an inflammatory condition of the gastric mucosa. It is classified into acute and chronic types. Acute gastritis includes acute simple gastritis, acute corrosive gastritis, acute erosive gastritis and acute purulent gastritis. Chronic gastritis includes chronic superficial gastritis, chronic atrophic gastritis, chronic hypertrophic gastritis. Most commonly seen in clinical practice is acute simple gastritis, characterized by distension and pain in the epigastric region, usually accompanied by poor appetite, nausea, vomiting, belching and acid regurgitation.

Aetiology

Traditional Chinese medicine refers to gastritis as epigastric pain and classifies it into excessive and deficient types. Excessive type gastritis is considered to be caused by invasion of the stomach by cold, irregular diet, or attack on the stomach by hyperactive liver *qi*; deficient type gastritis may either develop from the excessive type, or be caused by injury of the spleen and stomach arising from prolonged illness. Excessive type gastritis is marked by distending pain in the epigastric region aggravated by pressure. It is a relatively mild condition of short duration with a good prognosis. Deficient type gastritis is marked by dull pain in the epigastric region relieved by pressure. It is a relatively severe condition of long duration and correspondingly difficult to treat.

Differentiation of syndromes

- Gastritis due to attack on the stomach by exogenous cold.
  Characterized by sudden onset of severe stomach ache aggravated by cold and relieved by heat, aversion to cold drinks and preference for hot drinks, whitish tongue coating and tense wiry pulse.
- Gastritis due to retention of food in the stomach.
  Characterized by distension and pain in the epigastric region aggravated by pressure, eructation with fetid odor, acid regurgitation or vomiting of undigested food, anorexia, thick greasy tongue coating and slippery pulse.
- Gastritis due to attack on the stomach by hyperactive liver *qi*.
  Characterized by epigastric distension and pain radiating to the hypochondriac region, induced or aggravated by mental injury; feeling of fullness in the chest, sighing, depression or anxiety, thin whitish tongue coating and wiry pulse.
- Gastritis due to invasion of the stomach by liver fire.
  Characterized by severe epigastric pain radiating to the hypochondriac region, induced or aggravated by mental injury; restlessness or irritability, acid regurgitation, dry mouth with bitter taste, red tongue with yellowish coating and rapid wiry pulse.
- Gastritis due to *yang* deficiency of the spleen and stomach.

Characterized by intermittent dull epigastric pain alleviated by heat or pressure, vomiting of watery fluid, poor appetite, lassitude, emaciation, pale complexion, cold sensation of the hands and feet, loose stool, pale tongue with slimy whitish coating and weak thready pulse.
- Gastritis due to deficiency of the stomach *yin*.
  Characterized by dull burning pain in the epigastric region, anorexia, emaciation, sallow complexion, dry mouth and throat, thirst, constipation, red tongue with little coating and rapid thready pulse.

Treatment

Body acupuncture

Main acupuncture points:

Zusanli	(S36)
Zhongwan	(Ren12)
Weishu	(B21)
Neiguan	(P6)

Zusanli (S36), the *he* (sea) and lower *he* (confluent) point of the Stomach meridian, functions to strengthen the stomach and spleen. It is the first point chosen for all stomach and intestinal problems. Zhongwan (Ren12) and Weishu (B21), the front-*mu* and back-*shu* points respectively of the stomach, are treated in combination to strengthen the stomach and spleen. Neiguan (P6), the *luo* (collateral) point of the Pericardium meridian and one of the eight confluence points connecting with the Yinwei meridian, functions to regulate the flow of *qi* and relieve gastric pain.

Auxiliary points and appropriate manipulation are chosen according to differentiation of syndromes

- For gastritis due to attack on the stomach by exogenous cold, the stomach is warmed and cold dispelled by adding and puncturing Liangqiu (S34) using the reducing method and applying moxibustion to Zhongwan (Ren12).
- For gastritis due to retention of food in the stomach, Tianshu (S25) and Xiawan (Ren10) are added and punctured using the reducing method to activate the functions of transportation and transformation.
- For gastritis due to attack on the stomach by hyperactive liver *qi*, Taichong (Liv3), Sanyinjiao (Sp6) and Yanglingquan (G34) are added and punctured using the reducing method to soothe the liver and regulate the flow of *qi*.

- For gastritis due to invasion of the stomach by liver fire, liver fire is dispelled by combining two treatments: Xingjian (Liv2), Taichong (Liv3) and Yanglingquan (G34) are added and punctured using the reducing method, and Zhongwan (Ren12) is pricked with a three-edged needle to draw blood and then cupped for 10–15 minutes.
- For gastritis due to *yang* deficiency of the spleen and stomach, the spleen and stomach are warmed by adding and puncturing Pishu (B20) and Guanyuan (Ren4) using the reinforcing method and applying moxibustion to Shenque (Ren8), Zhongwan (Ren12) and Weishu (B21).
- For gastritis due to deficiency of the stomach *yin*, Pishu (B20), Sanyinjiao (Sp6) and Taixi (K3) are added and punctured using the even method to nourish the stomach *yin*.

Treat once a day or once every other day. Ten treatments constitute one course.

Electroacupuncture

Points used are the same as for body acupuncture. Select one or two pairs of points each time. Puncture until a needling sensation is achieved, then connect the needles to an electrical stimulator. Apply moderate intermittent wave stimulation for 20–30 minutes, once a day or once every other day. Ten treatments constitute one course.

Hot salt compress therapy

Acupuncture points:

Shenque	(Ren8)
Zhongwan	(Ren12)
Weishu	(B21)

Heat 500–1000 grams of salt in a dry pan over moderate heat until very hot. Fill a cloth bag with half of the hot salt and secure the mouth of the bag. Apply the compress to one point each time; replace with the second bag filled with the remaining hot salt when the first one has cooled off. Protect the skin from burns by applying a towel between the skin and the compress; as the compress cools down the towel can be removed and the bag applied directly to the skin. Apply to one point for 30–60 minutes, once or twice a day. Ten treatments constitute one course.

This method can effectively warm the spleen and stomach to dispel pathogenic cold and is therefore very effective for treating gastritis due to

yang deficiency of the stomach and spleen, as well as gastritis due to attack on the stomach by exogenous cold.

Point implantation therapy

Points used are the same as for body acupuncture. Select one or two points each time. Use a triangular needle to implant surgical catgut on each point. (See Appendix 9.) Treat once every 20–30 days. Three treatments constitute one course.

This method is especially suitable for treating chronic gastritis due to the long-term strong stimulation it provides.

Auricular therapy

Auricular points:

Stomach: corresponds to the affected region of the body.

Spleen: the spleen is connected both internally and externally with the stomach, so Spleen is treated to strengthen the spleen and stomach.

Liver: regulates the flow of *qi* to relieve pain and alleviate distension.

Subcortex, Endocrine: regulate the digestive function.

San Jiao, Abdomen, Middle of Superior Concha: regulate the flow of *qi* in the Middle Jiao to alleviate distension.

Apex of Ear: blood-letting puncturing of this point with a three-edged needle relieves inflammation and pain.

For acute gastritis use auricular taping and blood-letting puncturing where indicated, twice a week. Five treatments constitute one course. For chronic gastritis use auricular taping and blood-letting puncturing where indicated, twice a week, or auricular self-massage twice a day. Ten treatments constitute one course.

Remarks

- Traditional therapies are effective for treating gastritis, especially the acute type.
- Either body acupuncture or auricular therapy applied singly is sufficient to treat acute gastritis. However, two, three or more methods must be combined in order to provide stimulation sufficient to treat chronic gastritis effectively.

57 Gastrointestinal neurosis

Gastrointestinal neurosis is a functional disturbance of gastrointestinal secretion and movement caused by psychological factors. It occurs mainly in adults and more often in females than in males. Manifestations include anorexia, eructation, acid regurgitation, hiccups, nausea, vomiting, burning sensation in the epigastric region and abdominal distension or pain. Different types of gastrointestinal neurosis are characterized by typical primary symptoms. For example, nervous anorexia is marked by anorexia accompanied by emaciation and amenorrhoea; nervous vomiting is marked by vomiting without nausea and with no difficulty in eating immediately afterwards; nervous eructation is marked by repeated continuous belching; globus hystericus is marked by the sensation of a foreign body blocking the throat which cannot be swallowed or spat out, but with no accompanying functional difficulty in swallowing. Intestinal neurosis is marked by abdominal pain, discomfort, or distension; diarrhoea or constipation; and borborygmi. Nervous diarrhoea is marked by watery diarrhoea induced by mental injury; irritable colon syndrome is marked by paroxysmal intestinal colic in the left inferior abdomen, abdominal distension and constipation or diarrhoea.

Aetiology and differentiation of syndromes

Traditional Chinese medicine classifies gastrointestinal neurosis as stomach ache, diarrhoea, constipation, vomiting or hiccups, depending on the primary symptoms. It is considered to be caused primarily by mental injury which results in stagnation of the liver *qi*; the hyperactive liver *qi* thus produced then attacks the spleen and stomach. Besides gastrointestinal symptoms, additional manifestations include insomnia, bad dreams, depression or restlessness, feeling of fullness in the chest and hypochondriac region, sighing and lassitude. All of these symptoms may be induced or aggravated by mental injury.

Treatment

Body acupuncture

Main acupuncture points:

Neiguan	(P6)
Sanyinjiao	(Sp6)
Taichong	(Liv3)
Zusanli	(S36)
Zhongwan	(Ren12)

The *ben* (origin) of gastrointestinal neurosis is stagnation of the liver *qi*; the *biao* (expression) is disturbance of the gastrointestinal system. Therefore, soothing the liver *qi* and harmonizing the stomach and spleen are the basic principles for treating this disorder. Neiguan (P6), the *luo* (collateral) point of the Pericardium meridian and one of the eight confluence points connecting with the Yinwei meridian, functions both to soothe the liver *qi* and to harmonize the stomach and spleen. This point can thus concurrently treat both the *ben* (origin) and *biao* (expression) of gastrointestinal neurosis. Sanyinjiao (Sp6), the meeting point of the three Foot Yin meridians, also functions to regulate both the spleen and the liver. Taichong (Liv3), the *yuan* (source) point of the Liver meridian, soothes the liver and regulates the flow of *qi*. Zusanli (S36), the *he* (sea) point of the Stomach meridian and Zhongwan (Ren12), the front-*mu* point of the stomach and the *hui* (influential) point of the six *Fu* organs, are treated in combination to strengthen the stomach and spleen.

Auxiliary points and appropriate manipulation are chosen according to symptoms.

- For anorexia, Weishu (B21), Ganshu (B18), Pishu (B20) and Danshu (B19) are added and punctured using the reinforcing method to strengthen the spleen and stomach's functions of transportation and transformation.
- For nausea and vomiting, Danzhong (Ren17) and Geshu (B17) are added and punctured using the reducing method to subdue rebellious rising of the stomach *qi*.
- For abdominal disorders such as abdominal pain, constipation, or diarrhoea, Tianshu (S25) and Shangjuxu (S37) are added and punctured

using the even method to regulate the intestines.

● For globus hystericus, Taixi (K3) and Fenglong (S40) are added and punctured using the even method to strengthen the kidneys and dispel phlegm.

Treat once a day or once every other day. Ten treatments constitute one course.

Electroacupuncture

Points used are the same as for body acupuncture. Select one or two pairs of points each time. Puncture until a needling sensation is achieved, then connect the needles to an electrical stimulator. Apply moderate intermittent wave stimulation for 20–30 minutes, once a day or once every other day. Ten treatments constitute one course.

Hot salt compress therapy

Acupuncture point:

Shenque   (Ren8)

Heat 500–1000 grams of salt in a dry pan over moderate heat until very hot. Fill a cloth bag with half of the hot salt and secure the mouth of the bag. Apply the compress to Shenque (Ren8); replace with the second bag filled with the remaining hot salt when the first one has cooled off. Protect the skin from burns by applying a towel between the skin and the compress; as the compress cools down the towel can be removed and the bag applied directly to the skin. Apply for 30–60 minutes, once or twice a day. Ten treatments constitute one course.

This method not only effectively strengthens the spleen and stomach, but also reinforces the antipathogenic *qi*. It is therefore especially suitable for treating gastrointestinal neurosis marked by anorexia, abdominal pain, borborygmi or diarrhoea.

Auricular therapy

Auricular points:

Stomach, Small Intestine, Large Intestine, Abdomen: correspond to the affected area of the body; regulate the stomach and intestines.

Spleen: stengthens the spleen and regulates the stomach.

Liver: regulates the flow of the liver *qi*.

Subcortex: regulates the central nervous system.

Endocrine: regulates the gastrointestinal endocrine function.

Auxiliary auricular points.

For vomiting, Cardia is added.

For hiccups, Centre of Ear is added.

For acid regurgitation, Sympathesis is added.

For abdominal distension, Middle of Superior Concha is added.

For gastric or abdominal pain, Ear Shenmen and Sympathesis are added.

For diarrhoea, Ear Shenmen and Middle of Superior Concha are added.

For constipation, Rectum is added.

For globus hystericus, Throat and Oesophagus are added.

Use auricular taping, twice a week. Ten treatments constitute one course. Auricular massage may also be practised twice a day.

Remarks

● Traditional remedies are very effective for treating gastrointestinal neurosis.
● Because modern medicine still has no effective cure for gastrointestinal neurosis, many people with this disorder have been ill for a long time. They may have seen many doctors with no improvement, or even worsening of the condition. It is common for patients to be very worried about their condition and even suspect that they may have cancer. This pyschological influence aggravates the condition even more. Therefore, it is essential for patients to have a thorough understanding of gastrointestinal neurosis in order to dispel their misgivings and increase the effectiveness of traditional treatment.

58 Gastroptosis

Gastroptosis refers to abnormal position of the stomach, i.e. the lower notch of the lesser curvature of the stomach falls below the line of the interiliac crest when the torso is erect. It is caused primarily by weakness of the ligaments surrounding the stomach, and/or decreased abdominal pressure, which is insufficient to support the stomach in its normal position. There are no subjective symptoms or only mild discomfort in the initial stage; with development of the condition, digestive symptoms may occur, including distension or pain in the epigastric and abdominal regions, aggravated by eating; eructation, vomiting, acid regurgitation, poor appetite; and diarrhoea or constipation. Other manifestations may include emaciation, lassitude, dizziness, palpitation, or anaemia.

Aetiology

Traditional Chinese medicine refers to gastroptosis as *weihuan*, or flaccidity of the stomach. It is considered to be caused either by a congenitally weak constitution resulting in deficiency of the spleen and stomach, or by lack of proper care in infancy and childhood which results in injury to the stomach and spleen. Either circumstance can lead to deficiency of *qi* in the Middle Jiao with resulting flaccidity of the tissues and dropping of the stomach out of its normal position.

Differentiation of syndromes

- Gastroptosis due to sinking of *qi* in the Middle Jiao.
  Characterized by abdominal distension worsening after eating, anorexia, lassitude, emaciation, eructation or vomiting, sallow complexion, pale tongue with whitish coating and loose weak pulse.
- Gastroptosis due to deficient cold of the spleen and stomach.
  Characterized by distension or dull pain in the abdominal region aggravated by eating cold food and alleviated by pressure and warmth, vomiting of thin liquid, anorexia, pale complex-

ion, feeling of cold in the limbs, loose stool, pale tongue with whitish coating and slow deep pulse.
- Gastroptosis due to deficiency of the stomach *yin*.
  Characterized by distension or dull pain in the abdominal region worsening after eating, emaciation, eructation, acid regurgitation, vomiting, flushed cheeks, bad breath, constipation, red tongue with little coating and rapid thready pulse.

Treatment

Body acupuncture

Main acupuncture points:

Group 1:
Zhongwan (Ren12)   through Xiawan   (Ren10)
Tianshu   (S25) (left) through Wailing   (S26) (left)
Qihai   (Ren6)   through Guanyuan   (Ren4)
Zusanli   (S36)

Group 2:
Liangmen   (S21) (left) through Guanmen   (S22) (left)
Weishang   (Ex52)   through Shenque   (Ren8)
Huatuojiaji (Ex46) (T8-T12)
Zusanli   (S36)

Main points to strengthen *qi* and elevate the stomach are selected from the Stomach and Ren meridians. Two adjoining points are usually punctured simultaneously in one insertion in order to increase stimulation.

Puncture Group 1 and Group 2 alternately. Auxiliary points and appropriate methods of manipulation are chosen according to symptoms and differentiation of syndromes.

- For gastroptosis due to sinking of *qi* in the Middle Jiao or deficient cold of the spleen and stomach, the stomach and spleen are strengthened and sinking *qi* raised by adding and puncturing Baihui (Du20) and Shenque (Ren8) using the reinforcing method and applying moxibustion as needed.
- For gastroptosis due to deficiency of the stomach *yin*, Sanyinjiao (Sp6), Neiguan (P6) and Taixi (K3) are added and punctured using the even method to nourish the stomach *yin*.

- For cases with severe vomiting, Neiguan (P6) is added to subdue the rebellious stomach *qi*.
- For cases with severe acid regurgitation, Liang-qiu (S34), the *xi* (cleft) point of the Stomach meridian, is punctured to decrease gastric acid.

Treat once a day or once every other day. Ten treatments constitute one course.

Electroacupuncture

Points used are the same as for body acupuncture. Select two or three pairs of points each time. Puncture the points until a needling sensation is achieved, then connect the needles to an electrical stimulator. Apply moderate continuous wave stimulation for 30 minutes. Treat once a day or once every other day. Ten treatments constitute one course.

Point implantation therapy

Points used are the same as for body acupuncture. Using a triangular surgical needle, implant surgical catgut on two or three points each time. (See Appendix 9.) Treat once every 20–30 days. Three treatments constitute one course.

Auricular therapy

Main auricular points:

Stomach and Abdomen: correspond to the affected areas of the body. Locate positive points; tape both frontal and dorsal surfaces to increase stimulation.

Spleen: the spleen is internally and externally linked with the stomach, so Spleen is taped to strengthen the spleen and stomach and lift the sinking *qi* in the Middle Jiao.

Middle Superior Concha and San Jiao: relieve abdominal distension.

Subcortex: harmonizes the function of the digestive system.

Auxiliary auricular points:

For cases with constipation, Large Intestine and Rectum are added.

For cases with severe vomiting, Cardia is added.

Use auricular taping with strong manipulation, twice a week. Ten treatments constitute one course.

Remarks

☯ The stomach should be empty when receiving acupuncture treatment. Lying down for 15 minutes following treatment and after meals will assist recovery.
☯ Exercising the abdominal muscles and wearing an abdominal support belt can improve the results of treatment with traditional methods.

59 Habitual miscarriage

Miscarriage refers to spontaneous termination of pregnancy within the first seven months. Habitual miscarriage refers to three or more consecutive miscarriages, which usually occur at the same point in the pregnancy for each individual. The causes of habitual miscarriage are various. They include abnormality of the fertilized egg or placenta, chromosomal abnormalities, genital problems, endocrine dysfunction, severe acute or chronic disease in the pregnant woman, malnutrition or drug side effects.

Aetiology and differentiation of syndromes

According to traditional Chinese medicine, habitual miscarriage is due primarily to *qi* deficiency of the kidneys or spleen and stomach, resulting in insufficiency of the Chong and Ren meridians and insufficient nutrition for the fetus. General symptoms may include dizziness, lassitude, pale complexion, sore and weak back and knees and poor appetite.

Treatment

Moxibustion

Points:

Shenque	(Ren8)
Qihai	(Ren6)
Guanyuan	(Ren4)
Sanyinjiao	(Sp6)
Zusanli	(S36)
Zigongxue	(Ex45)

The Chong meridian, known as the Sea of Blood and the Ren meridian, which nourishes the fetus, both stem from the uterus. Therefore, main points to protect the fetus are chosen from the Ren meridian. Sanyinjiao (Sp6), the meeting point of the three Foot Yin meridians, is treated to strengthen the spleen and kidneys, the acquired and congenital foundations of life. Zusanli (S36), the *he* (sea) and lower *he* (confluent) point of the Stomach meridian, is an important tonification point for protecting the health. Zigongxue (Ex45) is a clinically effective point for treating gynaecological and obstetric problems.

Apply moxa roll moxibustion for 15–20 minutes to two or three points, once a day. Ten treatments constitute one course. Allow three to five days between courses. Treatment should be started immediately following conception and can be self-applied at home.

Remarks

- Moxibustion is effective for treating habitual miscarriage, but prolonged treatment should be given in order to achieve the greatest effect.
- It is reported that moxibustion is most effective in cases of habitual miscarriage occurring within the first trimester of pregnancy.
- It is important to undertake comprehensive measures for prevention of habitual miscarriage, including avoiding overstrain, regulating sexual activity, improving nutrition and maintaining a good psychological state.
- The causes of habitual miscarriage are various. It is important to determine the cause in each case in order to determine appropriate treatment and achieve the best results.

60 Headache

Headache is a very common symptom of numerous diseases and disorders. It is classified into two types according to pathogenesis. Functional headache has no clear cause, for instance, migraine or headache occurring during neurosism or menstruation. Organic headache is usually caused by inflammation or pressure on the meninges, cerebral blood vessels, or cranial nerves, for instance headache due to meningitis, hypertension, trigeminal neuralgia or intracranial space-occupying lesion.

Aetiology

According to traditional Chinese medicine, headache may be caused either by invasion of exogenous pathogens, or by endogenous factors such as mental injury, improper diet or excessive sexual activity. It is classified according to meridian theory. The Yangming meridian distributes to the forehead, so frontal headache is called Yangming headache. The Shaoyang meridian distributes to the bilateral sides of the head, so headache in the temporal region is called Shaoyang headache. The Taiyang meridian distributes to the occipital region, so headache in the occiput is called Taiyang headache. The Jueyin meridian distributes to the vertex, so headache in the vertex is called Jueyin headache.

Differentiation of syndromes

- Wind-cold type headache.
  Characterized by headache usually radiating to the neck and back; accompanied by chills, aversion to wind, thin whitish tongue coating and tense superficial pulse.

- Wind-heat type headache.
  Characterized by severe headache, fever, flushed face, pink eyes, thirst with desire for cold drinks, constipation or difficult defecation, yellowish urine, red tongue tip with thin yellowish tongue coating and rapid superficial pulse.
- Wind-damp type headache.
  Characterized by dull muffled pain in the head, heavy sensation in the body, feeling of fullness in the chest, poor appetite, nausea, greasy whitish tongue coating and soft pulse.
- Headache due to flaring up of the stomach fire.
  Characterized by severe frontal headache, flushed face, pink eyes, dry mouth, thirst with desire for cold drinks, constipation, scanty yellowish urine, dry or greasy yellowish tongue coating and rapid pulse.
- Headache due to stagnation of the liver *qi*.
  Characterized by distending pain in the vertex of the head, aggravated by mental injury; accompanied by feeling of fullness in the chest and hypochondriac region, sighing, depression or irritability, poor appetite, thin greasy tongue coating and wiry pulse.
- Headache due to flaring up of the liver and gallbladder fire.
  Characterized by severe unilateral or bilateral headache; accompanied by restlessness or irritability, bitter taste in the mouth, red or painful eyes, tinnitus or pain in the ears, red edges of the tongue with yellowish tongue coating and rapid wiry pulse.
- Headache due to hyperactivity of the liver *yang*.
  Characterized by headache and vertigo, aggravated by mental injury; accompanied by restlessness or irritability, flushed face, blurred vision, chirping tinnitus, insomnia, poor memory, sore and weak back and knees, dry red tongue with little coating and rapid wiry or thready pulse.
- Headache due to accumulation of turbid phlegm.
  Characterized by dull muffled pain in the entire head; accompanied by feeling of fullness in the chest and abdomen, nausea or vomiting, anorexia, greasy whitish tongue coating and slippery pulse.
- Headache due to stagnation of blood in the collaterals.
  Characterized by refractory fixed stabbing pain occurring on the unilateral or bilateral sides of the head or in areas which have suffered traumatic injury; accompanied by dark complexion, thirst, purple or purple-spotted tongue and uneven thready pulse.
- Headache due to deficiency of *qi* and blood.
  Characterized by dull pain in the head aggravated by overstrain; accompanied by dizziness, pale complexion, palpitation, lassitude, pale tongue with thin coating and weak thready pulse.
- Headache due to deficiency of the kidney essence.
  Characterized by dull headache, usually accompanied by vertigo; chirping tinnitus, sore and weak back and knees, seminal emission, sexual dysfunction, poor memory, pale tongue with thin coating and deep, thready, weak pulse.
- Headache due to deficient cold.
  Characterized by cold pain in the head, aggravated by cold and alleviated by warmth; accompanied by cold feeling in the extremities, pale complexion, spontaneous sweating, sore and weak back and knees, pale tongue with thin whitish coating and slow deep pulse.

Treatment

Body acupuncture

Main acupuncture points:

Fengchi	(G20)
Baihui	(Du20)
Taiyang	(Ex30)

Fengchi (G20), an important point of the Gallbladder meridian located on the base of the skull, functions to expel wind, tranquillize the mind and relieve pain. Baihui (Du20), the meeting point of the Du, Liver and Hand and Foot Yang meridians located on the top of the head, is treated to tranquillize the mind and relieve pain. Taiyang (Ex30) is a clinically effective point for relieving headache.

Auxiliary points may be selected according to either meridian theory or differentiation of syndromes. Either or both methods may be used according to condition.

Auxiliary points selected according to meridian theory:

- For Yangming (frontal) headache

Touwei	(S8)
Zanzhu	(B2)
Yintang	(Ex27)

Shenting	(Du24)
Hegu	(LI4)
Neiting	(S44)

● For Shaoyang (temporal) headache

Hanyan	(G4)
Shuaigu	(G8)
Jiaosun	(SJ20)
Zulinqi	(G41)

● For Taiyang (occipital) headache

Naohu	(Du17)
Tianzhu	(B10)
Houxi	(SI3)
Shenmai	(B62)

● For Jueyin (vertex) headache

Sishencong	(Ex26)
Taichong	(Liv3)

Auxiliary points and appropriate methods of manipulation selected according to differentiation of syndromes:

● For wind-cold type headache, wind-cold is dispelled by adding Dazhui (Du14) and puncturing using the reducing method and then cupping for 10–15 minutes.
● For wind-heat type headache, wind-heat is dispelled by adding and pricking Dazhui (Du14) using a three-edged needle, then cupping for 10–15 minutes.
● For wind-damp type headache, Sanyinjiao (Sp6), Zusanli (S36) and Zhongwan (Ren12) are added and punctured using the reducing method to remove dampness.
● For headache due to flaring-up of the stomach fire, Tianshu (S25) and Shangjuxu (S37) are added and punctured using the reducing method to purge excess heat. (This method is similar to stopping water from boiling by removing fuel from the fire.)
● For headache due to stagnation of the liver *qi*, Taichong (Liv3), Neiguan (P6) and Yanglingquan (G34) are added and punctured using the reducing method to promote flow of the liver *qi* and relieve pain.
● For headache due to flaring up of the liver and gallbladder fire, Xingjian (Liv2) and Xiaxi (G43) are added and punctured using the reducing method to clear away pathogenic fire.
● For headache due to hyperactivity of the liver *yang*, Taichong (Liv3), Taixi (K3) and Sanyinjiao (Sp6) are added and punctured using the even method to reinforce the kidney *yin* and subdue the liver *yang*.

● For headache due to accumulation of turbid phlegm, Fenglong (S40), Zhongwan (Ren12) and Sanyinjiao (Sp6) are added and punctured using the even method to strengthen the spleen and remove phlegm.
● For headache due to stagnation of blood in the collaterals, *ashi* points and Taiyang (Ex30) are pricked with a three-edged needle to dredge the collaterals and relieve pain.
● For headache due to deficiency of *qi* and blood, Zusanli (S36), Qihai (Ren6) and Sanyinjiao (Sp6) are added and punctured using the reinforcing method to strengthen the spleen and stomach.
● For headache due to deficiency of the kidney essence, the kidney essence is tonified by adding and puncturing Taixi (K3), Shenshu (B23) and Guanyuan (Ren4) using the reinforcing method and adding moxibustion as needed.
● For headache due to deficient cold, Shenshu (B23), Mingmen (Du4) and Dazhui (Du14) are added and punctured using the reinforcing method and moxibustion is added to strengthen the body's *yang*.

Select all main points and two to four auxiliary points each time. Treat acute cases once a day; five treatments constitute one course. Treat chronic cases once a day or once every other day; ten treatments constitute one course.

Electroacupuncture

Points used are the same as for body acupuncture. Select one or two pairs of points each time. Puncture the points until a needling sensation is achieved, then connect the needles to an electrical stimulator. Apply continuous wave stimulation of the highest bearable intensity for 20–30 minutes. Treat acute cases once a day; five treatments constitute one course. Treat chronic cases once a day or once every other day; ten treatments constitute one course.

Auricular therapy

Main auricular points:

Ear Shenmen, Subcortex: tranquillize the mind and relieve pain.

Apex of Ear: blood-letting puncturing of this point with a three-edged needle tranquillizes the mind, clears the brain and relieves pain.

Auxiliary auricular points:

For frontal headache, Forehead and Stomach are added.

For bilateral or unilateral headache, Temple and Pancreas & Gallbladder are added.

For occipital headache, Occiput and Urinary Bladder are added.

For vertex headache, Liver and positive points on the lateral side of the antitragus are added.

Use auricular taping and blood-letting puncturing where indicated, twice a week. Five treatments constitute one course. For chronic headache, auricular self-massage may also be practised twice a day.

Remarks

☯ Both body acupuncture and auricular therapy are effective for treating headache and may be used either singly or in combination. Cupping, blood-letting puncturing and moxibustion may be used as auxiliary measures according to specific conditions.

☯ Acupuncture points are selected according to either meridian theory or differentiation of syndromes. The two methods of selection may be used singly, alternately, or in combination in clinical practice. In cases of localized headache, points are usually chosen according to meridian theory; in cases of headache with no clear position, points are generally selected according to differentiation of syndromes.

☯ Traditional therapies are very effective for treating all types of functional headache and some types of organic headache, but are ineffective in cases caused by intracranial space-occupying lesion.

61 Haemorrhoids

Haemorrhoids are venous masses which are formed when backflow obstruction of the haemorrhoidal veins causes dilatation and varicosity of the submucosal venous plexus of the blind end of the rectum and the subcutaneous venous plexus of the anal canal.

Haemorrhoids are classified into three types according to location of the venous masses. Internal haemorrhoids are marked by bleeding during defecation, prolapse of the haemorrhoids, or severe pain when complicated by infection. External haemorrhoids are marked by the sensation of a foreign body in the anus and severe pain aggravated by defecation, walking, or sitting, any of which may cause thrombosis or splitting of the haemorrhoidal veins to occur. Mixed haemorrhoids have characteristics of both internal and external haemorrhoids, but the condition is more severe than either alone.

Aetiology

According to traditional Chinese medicine, haemorrhoids are caused primarily by overindulgence in spicy or greasy food, or protracted diarrhoea or constipation. These conditions result in stagnation of *qi* and blood and subsequent injury to the collaterals of the anus.

Differentiation of syndromes

● Haemorrhoids due to injury of the collaterals by excessive heat.
   Characterized by bright red bleeding during defecation and severe pain in the anus; accompanied by thirst, constipation, red tongue with yellowish coating and strong rapid pulse.
● Haemorrhoids due to deficiency of *qi* and blood.

Characterized by copious pale bleeding during defecation and prolapse of the haemorrhoids, the rectal mucosa, or even the entire rectum, aggravated by defecation, coughing, sneezing, or walking; accompanied by dizziness, palpitation, sallow complexion, lassitude, poor appetite, pale or purple-spotted tongue and weak thready pulse.

Treatment

Body acupuncture

Main acupuncture points:

Changqiang	(Du1)
Chengshan	(B57)
Dachangshu	(B25)
Erbai	(Ex11)

Both the Du and Urinary Bladder meridians connect with the anus; therefore Changqiang (Du1), the local point of the Du meridian and Chengshan (B57), the distal point of the Urinary Bladder meridian, are punctured to activate the meridians and promote the flow of blood. Dachangshu (B25), the back-*shu* point of the large intestine, is punctured to strengthen the functioning of the large intestine. Erbai (Ex11) is a clinically effective point for treating haemorrhoids.

Auxiliary points and appropriate methods of manipulation are chosen according to differentiation of syndromes.

- For haemorrhoids due to injury of the collaterals by excessive heat, Zhiyin (B67) and Xialiao (B34) are added and pricked with a three-edged needle, then cupped for 10–15 minutes to draw blood and clear away heat.
- For haemorrhoids due to deficiency of *qi* and blood, *qi* and blood are tonified by adding and puncturing Baihui (Du20), Zusanli (S36), Sanyinjiao (Sp6) and Qihai (Ren6) using the reinforcing method, or adding moxibustion as needed.

Treat once a day or once every other day. Ten treatments constitute one course.

Electroacupuncture

Points used are the same as for body acupuncture. Select one or two pairs of points each time. Puncture the points until a needling sensation is achieved, then connect the needles to an electrical stimulator. Apply continuous wave stimulation of the strongest bearable intensity for 30 minutes. Treat once a day or once every other day. Ten treatments constitute one course.

Blood-letting puncturing

Acupuncture points:

Yinjiao	(Du28)
Baliao	(B31-B34)
Dachangshu	(B25)
Positive points in the lumbosacral region.	

Yinjiao (Du28) and Dachangshu (B25) are pricked with a three-edged needle and the other points tapped with a plum blossom needle. Any whitish papuloid matter often found on Yinjiao (Du28) must first be excised and some bleeding induced to achieve good results. Dachangshu (B25) is cupped after being pricked to increase stimulation. The points may be treated sequentially or alternately.

Treat once every two days. Five treatments constitute one course. Blood-letting puncturing functions to clear away heat and stimulate the blood circulation. It is therefore especially suitable for treating haemorrhoids due to injury of the collaterals by excessive heat. Many cases will show improvement in symptoms such as pain and bleeding after only one or two treatments.

Auricular therapy

Auricular points:

Anus, Rectum: correspond to the affected areas of the body. Locate positive points; tape both frontal and dorsal surfaces to increase stimulation.

Large Intestine: improves transportation in the large intestine.

Liver: regulates the flow of *qi* and blood and relieves pain.

Spleen: controls the flow of blood in the meridians and collaterals to arrest bleeding.

Urinary Bladder: the Urinary Bladder meridian connects with the anus, so Urinary Bladder is taped to activate the meridan *qi* and improve blood circulation to relieve pain.

Endocrine, Adrenal Gland: relieve inflammation.

Subcortex: regulates the nervous and circulatory functions.

Ear Shenmen: relieves inflammation and pain.

Apex of Ear: blood-letting puncturing of this point with a three-edged needle activates the meridians to relieve pain.

Use auricular taping with strong manipulation and blood-letting puncturing where indicated, twice a week. Five treatments constitute one course.

Remarks

☯ The above therapies can effectively relieve the symptoms of haemorrhoids, including bleeding and pain.
☯ Changqiang (Du1) is punctured with the patient in a knee-chest position. Strong manipulation should be used to cause the needling sensation to spread to the peripheral area of the anus.
☯ These methods are also suitable for treating anal fissure, eczema of the anus, postoperative pain of anal fistula and prolapse of the anus.

62 Herpes zoster

Herpes zoster is an acute herpetic skin disease caused by the neurotropic herpes virus, which distributes along the peripheral nerves causing skin lesions. Primarily affected are the intercostal nerves; lesions are usually unilateral. Premonitory symptoms, or prodrome, include mild fever, general malaise and pain in the affected region. Two or three days after the onset of prodrome, a band of lesions appears as the herpes virus distributes along the affected nerve pathways. The course of the disease generally lasts two or three weeks. Children may experience little or no pain, but severe pain persisting even after disappearance of the lesions may occur in the elderly. Specific immunity is usually developed after the first attack, so recurrence is rare.

Aetiology and differentiation of syndromes

According to traditional Chinese medicine, herpes zoster is caused primarily by damp-heat and toxic pathogens affecting the meridians. Usually affected are the Liver and Gallbladder meridians. Local manifestations may be accompanied by restlessness, thirst, bitter taste in the mouth, poor appetite, scanty urine and rapid, wiry, thready pulse.

Treatment

Body acupuncture

Main acupucnture points:

　　Areas of skin lesions

Two methods are used to puncture the areas of the skin lesions. First, several needles may be used simultaneously to puncture the area surrounding the lesions from different directions. The needles are positioned approximately 0.5–1.0 *cun* away from the border of the affected area and inserted obliquely towards the centre of the area to a depth of 1.5–2.0 *cun*. The number of needles used depends on the size of the affected area; generally four to eight needles are applied. Second, the affected area and surrounding region may be moderately to heavily tapped with a plum blossom needle to induce bleeding. The blood is then absorbed with dry cotton.

Auxiliary points are added according to the location of the skin lesions:

● For lesions on the head and face, Hegu (LI4) and Neiting (S44) are added.
● For lesions on the chest and hypochondriac region, Zhigou (SJ6), Yanglingquan (G34) and corresponding Huatuojiaji (Ex46) are added.

● For lesions on the lower back and abdomen, Weizhong (B40), Zusanli (S36), Sanyinjiao (Sp6) and Taichong (Liv3) are added.

All points are punctured using the reducing method, once a day. Five treatments constitute one course.

Electroacupuncture

Points used are the same as for body acupuncture. Select one or two pairs of points each time. Puncture until a needling sensation is achieved; then connect the needles to an electrical stimulator. Apply intermittent wave stimulation of the highest bearable intensity for 30 minutes, once a day. Five treatments constitute one course.

Blood-letting puncturing

Acupuncture points:

Areas of skin lesions

Strictly sterilize the affected areas. Tap heavily several times with a plum blossom needle, then cup for 10–15 minutes to draw blood.

Because of the strong stimulation this method provides, it is especially suitable for treating refractory cases and the elderly. Treat once every two or three days. Three treatments constitute one course.

Auricular therapy

Auricular points:

Areas corresponding to the location of the skin lesions: locate tender points; tape both frontal and dorsal surfaces to increase stimulation.

San Jiao: drains water to dispel damp-heat and toxic pathogens.

Endocrine, Adrenal Gland: relieve infection.

Apex of Ear: blood-letting puncturing of this point with a three-edged needle dispels heat and pathogens and relieves pain.

Ear Shenmen, Occiput: calm the mind and relieve pain.

Auxiliary auricular points:

For herpes zoster of the intercostal nerve, Liver and Pancreas & Gallbladder are added.

For herpes zoster of the trigeminal nerve, Stomach and Large Intestine are added.

Use auricular taping with strong manipulation and blood-letting puncturing where indicated, concentrating on the affected side, once every other day. Five treatments constitute one course.

Remarks

๑ Traditional therapies can effectively relieve the pain and shorten the course of herpes zoster.
๑ These therapies may be used singly or in combination.
๑ These methods are also suitable for treating residual neuralgia of herpes zoster.

63 Hiccups

Hiccups are a common symptom of various diseases and disorders including phrenospasm, gastrointestinal neurosis, gastritis and hepatic conditions. They are caused primarily by spasm of the diaphragm.

Aetiology

Traditional Chinese medicine classifies hiccups into excessive and deficient types. The excessive type is caused by exogenous wind-cold, improper diet or mental injury, any of which can result in rebellious rising of the stomach *qi*. The deficient type is caused by either febrile disease which consumes the stomach *yin*, or by chronic disease which consumes the stomach and spleen *yang*, resulting in either rebellious rising of the stomach *qi* or failure of the stomach *qi* to descend.

Differentiation of syndromes

- Hiccups caused by attack on the stomach by pathogenic cold.
  Characterized by hiccups aggravated by cold and relieved by warmth, discomfort in the epigastric region, poor appetite, no thirst, whitish tongue coating and tense pulse.
- Hiccups caused by attack on the stomach by hyperactive liver *qi*.
  Characterized by hiccups induced and aggravated by mental injury, distension in the chest and hypochondriac region, sighing, depression or restlessness, thin greasy tongue coating and wiry pulse.
- Hiccups caused by deficiency of the stomach *yin*.
  Characterized by intermittent hiccups, sensation of heat in the palms and soles, insomnia, dry mouth and tongue, red tongue with little coating and rapid thready pulse.
- Hiccups caused by attack on the stomach by *yang* deficiency of the spleen and kidneys.
  Characterized by onset of hiccups following protracted illness, abdominal discomfort alleviated by heat or pressure, anorexia, lassitude, pale complexion, loose stool or diarrhoea, weak and sore back and knees, sensation of cold in the hands and feet, pale tongue with thin whitish coating and deep thready pulse.

Treatment

Body acupuncture

Main acupuncture points:

Neiguan	(P6)
Geshu	(B17)

Neiguan (P6), the *luo* (collateral) point of the Pericardium meridian and one of the eight confluence points connecting with the Yinwei meridian, relieves hiccups by subduing rebellious rising of the stomach *qi*. It is punctured obliquely upwards until the needling sensation ascends to the epigastric region. For patients who cannot accept acupuncture, or in cases when acupuncture proves ineffective, pressure may be applied to this point with the thumb instead of puncturing with a needle. Geshu (B17), the *hui* (influential) point of the blood, is located at the level of the diaphragm and can effectively relieve hiccups by alleviating spasm of the diaphragm.

Auxiliary points and appropriate manipulation are chosen according to syndromes.

- For hiccups caused by attack on the stomach by pathogenic cold, cold is expelled by adding and puncturing Zhongwan (Ren12) using the reducing method, or applying moxibustion as needed.
- For hiccups caused by attack on the stomach by hyperactive liver *qi*, Taichong (Liv3), Gongsun (Sp4), Yanglingquan (G34) and Zusanli (S36) are added and punctured using the reducing method to regulate the flow of the liver *qi*.
- For hiccups caused by deficiency of the stomach *yin*, Pishu (B20), Weishu (B21), Sanyinjiao (Sp6) and Zusanli (S36) are added and punctured using the even method to nourish the stomach *yin*.
- For hiccups caused by attack on the stomach by *yang* deficiency of the spleen and kidneys, the spleen and kidneys are warmed by adding and puncturing Pishu (B20), Shenshu (B23), Zhongwan (Ren12) and Zusanli (S36) using the reinforcing method, or applying moxibustion as needed.

Treat once a day. Five treatments constitute one course for the excessive type; ten treatments constitute one course for the deficient type.

Point injection therapy

Acupuncture points:

Danzhong	(Ren17)
Zhongwan	(Ren12)
Neiguan	(P6)
Geshu	(B17)

Select two or three points each time. Inject each point with 1–2 ml of procaine, vitamins B_1 or B_6, or atropine. Treat once every other day. Five treatments constitute one course.

Auricular therapy

Auricular points:

Centre of Ear: corresponds to the diaphragm; relieves spasm of the diaphragm.

Stomach, Spleen: regulate the stomach *qi* to suppress its adverse rising.

Liver: soothes the liver *qi* and regulates the stomach *qi*.

Sympathesis: alleviates spasm of the diaphragm.

Subcortex: regulates the digestive and nervous functions.

Ear Shenmen, Occiput: tranquillize the mind.

Use auricular taping or pressure. Auricular therapy is very effective for treating hiccups; in most cases the hiccups will have stopped by the end of the treatment session. For deficient type hiccups, auricular therapy can temporarily stop spasm of the diaphragm to relieve symptoms.

Remarks

◐ Excessive type hiccups are relatively mild, of short duration and easily cured. Deficient type hiccups are relatively severe, of longer duration and more difficult to treat.
◐ Point injection therapy may be utilized in cases which do not respond to body acupuncture or auricular therapy.

64 High fever

High fever refers to body temperature in the human over 39 °C. It is a common manifestation of various diseases and disorders, including acute infectious or communicable diseases, sunstroke or rheumatic fever.

Aetiology and differentiation of syndromes

According to traditional Chinese medicine, fever results from the struggle between the body's antipathogenic *qi* and pathogenic factors. It is classified into exogenous and endogenous types. The exogenous type is caused by exogenous pathogens or epidemic factors which invade the body. The resulting fever is usually high, marked by sudden onset and short course and accompanied by additional exterior symptoms and signs. The endogenous type is caused by dysfunction of the internal *zangfu* organs, resulting in deficiency of the *qi*, blood, *yin* or *yang*. The fever is usually intermittent and relatively low, marked by slow onset and long course and accompanied by additional interior symptoms and signs. Generally speaking, exogenous fever is excessive; endogenous fever may be either deficient, or deficient in origin (*ben*) and excessive in expression (*biao*). The following treatments are for exogenous fever. For treatment of endogenous fever, refer to the related disease or disorder of which the fever is a symptom.

Treatment

Body acupuncture

Acupuncture points:

Dazhui	(Du14)
Quchi	(LI11)
Hegu	(LI4)
Fengchi	(G20)
Shixuan	(Ex1)

Main points are chosen from the Yang meridians. The following points are punctured in combination using the reducing method to activate the meridians and dispel heat: Dazhui (Du14), the meeting point of the Du and the six Hand and Foot Yang meridians; Quchi (LI11) and Hegu (LI4), the *he* (sea) and *yuan* (source) points respectively of the Large Intestine meridian; and Fengchi (G20), an important point of the Gallbladder meridian located at the base of the skull.

Shixuan (Ex1), an extraordinary point for dispelling heat, is pricked with a three-edged needle to let several drops of blood. Bilateral Shixuan (Ex1) points located on the right and left hands may be treated either alternately or simultaneously.

Treat once or twice a day.

Blood-letting puncturing

Acupuncture points:

Shixuan   (Ex1)
Jing (well) points of the Hand meridians

Auricular point:

Apex of Ear

Prick each point with a three-edged needle to let several drops of blood. Shixuan (Ex1) and the twelve *jing* (well) points are punctured alternately; points of the hands are punctured unilaterally or bilaterally. Treat once or twice a day.

This method functions to expel wind and dispel heat. It is an ideal method for treating high fever caused by invasion of the body by exogenous pathogens.

Cupping therapy

Acupuncture points:

Dazhui   (Du14)
Feishu   (B13)

Dazhui (Du14) is the meeting point of the Du meridian and the six Hand and Foot Yang meridians; Feishu (B13), the back-*shu* point of the lungs, nourishes the skin to defend against invasion by exogenous pathogens. The two points may be treated either alternately or simultaneously. First prick using a three-edged needle and then cup for 10–15 minutes to draw blood.

Treat once or twice a day.

Remarks

☯ Traditional therapies are among the most important measures available for lowering high fever. In many cases, fever may be greatly reduced or even become normal after just one treatment. Fever may begin to go down approximately 15 minutes after treatment.

☯ High fever is an acute disorder commonly seen in clinical practice. It is essential to establish the cause of the fever when determining treatment. Additional measures should be concurrently undertaken in severe cases.

☯ All therapies may be used singly, or may be combined in order to increase stimulation and improve effect.

65 Hypertension

Hypertension, a commonly seen complaint in clinical practice, is characterized by high arterial blood pressure. It is classified into primary and secondary types according to aetiology and pathogenesis. Primary hypertension is an independent disease with no clear cause. It is marked by high arterial blood pressure; additional manifestations include headache, dizziness, tinnitus, flushed face, insomnia and irritability. In severe cases, blurred vision, palpitation, shortness of breath, poor memory, numbness of the fingers or even stroke may occur. There is often a family history of hypertension. The primary pathogenesis of primary hypertension is disorder of the central nervous system.

Secondary hypertension occurs secondary to organic problems such as nephric, cardiac or endocrine disorder. In these cases, hypertension is a symptom of the disease and is therefore also referred to as symptomatic hypertension.

Aetiology

Traditional Chinese medicine classifies hypertension as headache or vertigo. It has three primary causes: mental injury, which results in stagnation of the liver *qi* and subsequent flaring up of the liver fire; improper diet, which causes deficiency of the spleen and accumulation of phlegm in the interior; and wasting diseases, which damage the kidney *yin*, causing hyperactivity of the liver *yang*.

Differentiation of syndromes

- Hypertension due to flaring up of the liver fire.
  Characterized by headache, dizziness, flushed face, pink eyes, rumbling tinnitus, dry mouth with bitter taste, restlessness, irritability, constipation, yellowish urine, red tongue with yellowish coating and rapid wiry pulse.
- Hypertension due to hyperactivity of the liver *yang*.
  Characterized by dizziness, headache, flushed face, blurred vision, chirping tinnitus, insomnia, poor memory, restlessness, sore and weak back and knees, dry red tongue with little coating and rapid thready or wiry pulse.
- Hypertension due to *yin* deficiency of the liver and kidneys.
  Characterized by dizziness, palpitation, blurred vision, dry eyes, chirping tinnitus or even deafness, sore and weak back and knees, pain in the heels, frequent urination at night, sensation of heat in the palms and soles, night sweating, dry reddish tongue with no coating and deep thready or weak pulse.
- Hypertension due to accumulation of phlegm in the Middle Jiao.
  Characterized by vertigo, heavy muffled feeling in the head, feeling of fullness in the chest, drowsiness, pale swollen tongue with tooth marks and greasy whitish coating and slippery or wiry pulse.

Treatment

Body acupuncture

Main acupuncture points:

Baihui	(Du20)
Fengchi	(G20)
Taichong	(Liv3)
Renying	(S9)
Taiyang	(Ex30)

Baihui (Du20), the meeting point of the Du, Liver and six Hand and Foot Yang meridians, is treated to subdue endogenous wind and calm the mind. Fengchi (G20), an important point of the Gallbladder meridian, functions to tranquillize the mind. Taichong (Liv3), the *yuan* (source) point of the Liver meridian, calms the liver and arrests endogenous wind. Taiyang (Ex30) is a clinically effective point for treating hypertension.

Renying (S9) is located close to the carotid sinus and functions to lower blood pressure by stimulating the carotid sinus pressoreceptor. With the patient lying supine with no pillow, use a one inch needle to puncture Renying (S9) perpendicularly for 0.3–0.5 *cun* until the handle of the needle quivers in time with the beating of the carotid. The needle should be retained for 5 minutes. Manipulate using the even method to avoid overreaction.

Auxiliary points and appropriate methods of manipulation are chosen according to differentiation of syndromes:

- For hypertension due to flaring up of the liver fire, pathogenic fire is dispelled by adding and puncturing Xingjian (Liv2), Quchi (LI11) and Zulinqi (G41) using the reducing method; and pricking Taiyang (Ex30) with a three-edged needle to draw several drops of blood and then cupping for 10–15 minutes.
- For hypertension due to hyperactivity of the liver *yang*, Taixi (K3), Yongquan (K1) and Sanyinjiao (Sp6) are added and punctured using the even method to strengthen the kidney *yin* in order to subdue hyperactive liver *yang*.
- For hypertension due to *yin* deficiency of the liver and kidneys, Taixi (K3), Sanyinjiao (Sp6), Yanglingquan (G34), Ganshu (B18) and Shenshu (B23) are added and punctured using the reinforcing method to strengthen the liver and kidneys.
- For hypertension due to accumulation of phlegm in the Middle Jiao, Zhongwan (Ren12), Fenglong (S40), Zusanli (S36) and Neiguan (P6) are added and punctured using the even method to strengthen the spleen and eliminate phlegm.

Treat once a day or once every other day. Ten treatments constitute one course.

Blood-letting puncturing

Acupuncture points:

Taiyang	(Ex30)
Quchi	(LI11)
Dazhui	(Du14)

Select one or two points each time. Prick with a three-edged needle and then cup for 10–15 minutes to extract 3–5 ml of stagnant blood. Treat once a week. Five treatments constitute one course. Blood-letting puncturing functions to clear away fire and tranquillize the mind and is therefore especially suitable for treating hypertension due to flaring-up of the liver fire and hyperactivity of the liver *yang*.

Auricular therapy

Main auricular points:

Subcortex, Sympathesis: regulate vasomotoricity to alleviate spasm of the blood vessels.

Superior Triangular Fossa: clinically effective point for treating hypertension, also called Blood Pressure Lowering point.

Ear Shenmen, Occiput: tranquillize the mind.

Apex of Ear, Groove of Dorsal Surface: bloodletting puncturing of these two points in turn with a three-edged needle lowers the blood pressure.

Auxiliary auricular points:

For hypertension caused by hyperactivity of the liver *yang*, Liver, Kidney and Heart are added.

For hypertension caused by accumulation of phlegm in the interior, Spleen and Stomach are added.

Use auricular taping and blood-letting puncturing where indicated, twice a week. Ten treatments constitute one course.

Remarks

☯ Traditional therapies are effective for treating hypertension, especially primary hypertension during the first and second stages. They can provide immediate relief of the symptoms of hypertension, including headache, dizziness and blurred vision, but a radical cure is difficult to achieve.

☯ Experimental studies indicate that acupuncture can lower vasotonia of the brain and relieve peripheral vasospasm, with resulting lowering of the blood pressure.

66 Hyperthyroidism

Hyperthyroidism is caused by autoimmunity or mental injury resulting in thyroid enlargement and hypersecretion of thyroxin. It is marked by hyperexcitation of the sympathetic nervous system and hypermetabolism. It occurs primarily in adult females. Manifestations include irritability, trembling of the fingers and tongue, lassitude, polyphagia, emaciation, frequent defecation, aversion to heat and profuse perspiration. Signs include mild to moderate diffuse thyroid enlargement, tremor and vascular murmur, premature heartbeat, paroxysmal tachycardia, auricular fibrillation and exophthalmos. In some cases there may be additional atypical symptoms such as listlessness, dry or cold skin, poor appetite and bradycardia.

Aetiology

According to traditional Chinese medicine, hyperthyroidism is caused primarily by mental injury or improper diet which leads to stagnation of the liver *qi* and accumulation of phlegm in the interior. The prolonged combination of stagnant *qi* and accumulated phlegm results in the formation of pathogenic fire which consumes the body's *yin*; the *yin* deficiency then causes deficient fire.

Differentiation of syndromes

● Hyperthyroidism due to stagnation of the liver *qi* and accumulation of phlegm.
  Characterized by thyroid enlargement, depression or irritability, feeling of fullness in the chest and hypochondriac region, frequent sighing, bad dreams, frequent defecation, whitish greasy tongue coating and slippery wiry pulse.
● Hyperthyroidism due to hyperactivity of the liver fire.
  Characterized by thyroid enlargement, restlessness, palpitation, insomnia, bad dreams,

exophthalmos, flushed face, aversion to heat, profuse sweating, dry mouth with bitter taste, polyphagia, red tongue with yellowish coating and rapid wiry pulse.

- Hyperthyroidism due to deficient fire.
  Characterized by thyroid enlargement, exophthalmos, restlessness, palpitation, insomnia, bad dreams, dizziness, blurred vision, lassitude, emaciation, sensation of heat in the palms and soles, night sweating, polyphagia, thin red tongue with little coating and rapid thready pulse.

Treatment

Body acupuncture

Main acupuncture points:

Renying	(S9)
Shuitu	(S10)
Tianding	(LI17)
Futu	(LI18)
Hegu	(LI4)
Fenglong	(S40)
Neiguan	(P6)

The pathogenesis of hyperthyroidism has its origin in stagnation of the liver-*qi* and accumulated phlegm which obstruct the Large Intestine and Stomach meridians. Accordingly, both local and distal points of the Large Intestine and Stomach meridians are selected as main points to clear the meridians and soften hardened glands. Neiguan (P6), the *luo* (collateral) point of the Pericardium meridian, is effective for improving the flow of *qi* and tranquillizing the mind.

Ashi points may be chosen as an alternative to puncturing the local points. Use three or four needles to puncture the mass from the border to the centre. Manipulate 30–50 times using the even lifting and thrusting method, then withdraw the needles for mild cases or retain for 20 minutes for severe cases.

Auxiliary points and appropriate manipulation are selected according to symptoms and differentiation of syndromes:

- For hyperthyroidism due to stagnation of the liver *qi* and accumulation of phlegm, Taichong (Liv3), Zusanli (S36), Zhongwan (Ren12) and Danzhong (Ren17) are added and punctured using the reducing method to improve the flow of *qi* and remove phlegm.

- For hyperthyroidism due to hyperactivity of the liver fire, Fengchi (G20), Xingjian (Liv2) and Zulinqi (G41) are added and punctured using the reducing method to dispel liver fire.
- For hyperthyroidism due to deficient fire, Sanyinjiao (Sp6), Taixi (K3) and Shenmen (H7) are added and punctured using the even method to reinforce *yin* and subdue deficient fire.
- For cases involving exophthalmos, Fengchi (G20), Taiyang (Ex30), Zanzhu (B2) and Tongziliao (G1) are added to benefit the eyes.
- For cases involving profuse sweating, Yinxi (H6) and Fuliu (K7) are added and punctured using the reinforcing method to arrest perspiration.

Auricular therapy

Main auricular points:

Neck: corresponds to affected area of the body.

Liver: soothes the liver to regulate the flow of *qi*.

Spleen: strengthens the spleen to remove phlegm.

Kidney: nourishes *yin* to reduce pathogenic fire.

Endocrine, Midpoint of Rim: regulate endocrine function.

Subcortex: regulates nervous and endocrine functions.

Auxiliary auricular points:

For aversion to heat and profuse sweating, Sympathesis is added.

For cardiac problems, Heart is added.

For sexual dysfunction or irregular menstruation, Internal Genitals is added.

For exophthalmos, Eye is added.

Use auricular taping, twice a week. Ten treatments constitute one course.

Remarks

- Acupuncture can effectively improve the symptoms and signs of hyperthyroidism, but long-term treatment should be given to consolidate the results. Therapeutic results are closely related to the course and state of the disease, i.e., the earlier it is treated and the milder it is, the better the results will be.

☯ The occurrence and development of hyperthyroidism is closely related to psychological factors. It is therefore important to help patients maintain a positive outlook and avoid

harmful emotions during treatment in order to increase the therapy's effectiveness.

☯ When puncturing local points, care should be taken to avoid injuring the trachea and large blood vessels.

☯ In cases of emergency hyperthyroid crisis, additional modern treatment should be given.

67 Hysteria

Hysteria is a functional disorder caused by mental injury, occurring primarily in adults and more often in females than in males. The first hysterical attack is usually related to psychological trauma. Hysteria may manifest in mental disorders, including emotional outbursts of irrational laughing or crying, hysterical syncope, or mutism; physical problems, including hysterical paralysis, aphonia, spasm, blindness, deafness and globus hystericus; and internal disorders, including nervous vomiting, anorexia, hiccups and frequent urination.

Aetiology and differentiation of syndromes

Hysteria is classified by traditional Chinese medicine into *jue*, *yu*, *zangzao*, *meiheqi* and *bentunqi* syndromes. Although manifestations are various, the main pathogenesis for all syndromes is abnormal flow of *qi* due to mental injury. For example, anger results in adverse flow of the liver *qi*, which may either rise abnormally and draw up blood causing headache, syncope, blindness, deafness or aphonia; or disturb the mind leading to irrational laughing or crying. Brooding may result in stagnation of *qi* and subsequent accumulation of stagnant phlegm, leading to either aphonia or the subjective sensation of a foreign object stuck in the throat (referred to as globus hystericus in modern medicine or *meiheqi* syndrome in TCM). If the abnormal flow of *qi* disturbs the internal organs, symptoms such as vomiting, hiccups, anorexia, abdominal pain, tachycardia or shortness of breath may occur. Insufficient nourishment of the muscles and tendons due to stagnation of *qi* may cause hemiplegia, paralysis or convulsions.

Treatment
Body acupuncture

Main acupuncture points:

Taichong	(Liv3)
Hegu	(LI4)

The liver governs the normal flow of *qi* and the Large Intestine meridian of Hand Yangming is rich in both *qi* and blood. Therefore Taichong (Liv3) and Hegu (LI4), the *yuan* (source) points of the Liver and Large Intestine meridians respectively and located symmetrically on the hands and feet, are the main points selected for treating hysteria. Treated in combination (known as 'opening the four passes'), these points soothe the flow of *qi* and tranquillize the mind.

Although manifestations of hysteria are various, clinically each individual only exhibits one or two symptoms which generally remain consistent throughout the course of the attack. Accordingly, auxiliary points are selected according to individual manifestations.

● For hysterical syncope, Renzhong (Du26) and Yongquan (K1) are added and punctured using the reducing method to restore consciousness and refresh the spirit.
● For emotional outburst, Baihui (Du20), Fengchi (G20) and Neiguan (P6) are added and punctured using the reducing method to tranquillize the mind.
● For hemiplegia, Waiguan (SJ5), Houxi (SI3), Quchi (LI11), Huantiao (G30), Yanglingquan (G34) and Zusanli (S36) are added and punctured using the reducing method to promote the flow of *qi* and blood.
● For paralysis of the lower limbs, Huantiao (G30), Yanglingquan (G34), Zusanli (S36)

and Xuanzhong (G39) are punctured using the reducing method. Electroacupuncture may be used to increase the stimulation. Alternatively, Yongquan (K1) may be punctured using strong manipulation for 3–5 minutes. The patient should be encouraged to walk and move about immediately following treatment.

- For spasm, Waiguan (SJ5), Quchi (LI11), Fengchi (G20), Yanglingquan (G34) and Sanyinjiao (Sp6) are added and punctured using the even method to tranquillize endogenous wind and relax spasticity.
- For aphonia, Lianquan (Ren23) and Tongli (H5) are added and punctured using the reducing method to soothe the flow of *qi* and recover use of the voice.
- For deafness, Tinghui (G2), Yifeng (SJ17) and Fengshi (G31) are added and punctured using the reducing method to soothe the flow of *qi* and improve hearing.
- For blindness, Fengchi (G20), Taiyang (Ex30) and Guangming (G37) are added and punctured using the reducing method to soothe the flow of *qi* and brighten the eyes.
- For vomiting and hiccups, Neiguan (P6), Zhongwan (Ren12) and Zusanli (S36) are added and punctured using the reducing method to harmonize the stomach *qi* and arrest vomiting and hiccups.
- For anorexia, Zusanli (S36), Zhongwan (Ren12) and Sanyinjiao (Sp6) are added and punctured using the even method to strengthen the spleen and stomach.
- For abdominal pain, Tianshu (S25), Liangqiu (S34) and Zusanli (S36) are added and punctured using the reducing method to regulate the flow of *qi* and relieve pain.
- For frequent urination, Guanyuan (Ren4) and Sanyinjiao (Sp6) are added and punctured using the even method to reinforce the kidneys and control urination. Moxibustion may also be applied to Guanyuan (Ren4).
- For retention of urine, Zhongji (Ren3) and Sanyinjiao (Sp6) are added and punctured using the reducing method to promote urination.
- For palpitation and shortness of breath, Neiguan (P6) and Danzhong (Ren17) are added and punctured using the reducing method to open the chest and tranquillize the mind.
- For globus hystericus, Lianquan (Ren23), Tiantu (Ren22) and Fenglong (S40) are added and punctured using the reducing method to open the flow of *qi* and reduce phlegm.

Electroacupuncture

Commonly used points are the same as for body acupuncture. Choose one or two pairs of points each time; puncture using the reducing method until a needling sensation is achieved, then connect with electrical stimulator. Apply moderate intermittent stimulation for 30 minutes.

Auricular therapy

Main auricular points:

Liver: soothes the liver *qi* to relieve mental depression.

Chest: opens the chest to regulate the flow of *qi*.

Heart: nourishes the heart to calm the mind.

Spleen: strengthens the spleen and stomach to remove phlegm.

Subcortex: regulates the central nervous function.

Ear Shenmen, Occiput: tranquillize the mind.

Apex of Ear: blood-letting puncturing of this point with a three-edged needle calms the mind and dispels heat.

Auxiliary points are added according to symptoms, for example:

For globus hystericus, Throat is added.

For nervous vomiting, Cardia is added.

For hysterical blindness, Eye is added.

Use auricular taping with strong stimulation and blood-letting pucturing where indicated, twice a week. Ten treatments constitute one course.

Remarks

- Traditional Chinese therapies, especially body acupuncture and electroacupuncture, are excellent for treating all types of hysteria. In many cases the attack is relieved as soon as the needles are inserted and a needling sensation achieved.
- It is essential to relieve patients' anxiety before treatment by encouraging a positive attitude and confidence that traditional therapies can cure their disorder.
- Select a minimum of points, correctly located. Use strong stimulation and try to achieve therapeutic results at the first treatment.

68 Impotence

Impotence is a common male sexual dysfunction caused by functional disturbance of the central nervous system or organic disease. It is marked by inability to achieve or maintain an erection, making sexual intercourse problematic. Other manifestations may include dizziness, blurred vision, lassitude, listlessness, insomnia and night or spontaneous sweating.

Aetiology

According to traditional Chinese medicine, impotence has several primary causes. Either protracted illness or excessive sexual activity may result in decline of fire from Mingmen, the Gate of Life; mental injury may damage the heart and spleen or affect the liver *qi*; or overindulgence in fatty foods or alcohol may damage the spleen's functions of transportation and transformation, resulting in accumulation of damp-heat which flows downward to create impotence.

Differentiation of syndromes

- Impotence due to decline of fire from the Gate of Life.
  Characterized by dizziness, tinnitus, listlessness, pale complexion, sore and weak back and knees, sensation of cold in the extemities, frequent urination, pale tongue with whitish coating and deep thready pulse.
- Impotence due to deficiency of the heart and spleen.
  Characterized by lassitude, sallow complexion, insomnia, bad dreams, susceptibility to fright, palpitation, poor appetite, loose stool, pale tongue with thin greasy coating and weak thready pulse.
- Impotence due to stagnation of the liver *qi*.
  Characterized by feeling of fullness in the chest and hypochondriac region, frequent sighing, depression, anxiety, poor appetite, abdominal distension, thin tongue coating and wiry thready pulse.
- Impotence due to downward flow of damp-heat.
  Characterized by dampness and fetid odor in the scrotal region, soreness and heaviness of the

body, scanty yellowish urine, greasy yellowish tongue coating and soft rapid pulse.

Treatment

Body acupuncture

Main acupuncture points:

Guanyuan	(Ren4)
Sanyinjiao	(Sp6)

Guanyuan (Ren4), the meeting point of the Ren and three Foot Yin meridians, is punctured to reinforce *yuan* (original) *qi*. Sanyinjiao (Sp6), the meeting point of the three Foot Yin meridians, is an important point for treating urogenital problems.

Auxiliary points and proper manipulation are chosen according to differentiation of syndromes:

- For impotence due to decline of fire from the Gate of Life, the kidney *yang* is tonified by adding and puncturing Mingmen (Du4), Shenshu (B23) and Taixi (K3) using the reinforcing method, or applying moxibustion as needed.
- For impotence due to deficiency of the heart and spleen, Shenmen (H7), Zusanli (S36) and Zhongwan (Ren12) are added and punctured using the reinforcing method to tonify the heart and spleen.
- For impotence due to stagnation of the liver *qi*, Neiguan (P6), Taichong (Liv3), Sishencong (Ex26) and Zusanli (S36) are added and punctured using the even method to promote the flow of the liver *qi* and calm the mind.
- For impotence due to downward flow of damp-heat, damp-heat is removed by adding and puncturing Zhongji (Ren3), Yinlingquan (Sp9) and Ligou (Liv5) using the reducing method, or pricking Dadun (Liv1) with a three-edged needle to draw several drops of blood.

Treat once a day or once every other day. Ten treatments constitute one course.

Moxibustion/hot salt compress therapy

Points:

Guanyuan	(Ren4)
Shenque	(Ren8)
Mingmen	(Du4)

Apply moxa roll or moxa cone moxibustion, or hot salt compress. Use only one method for each course. Moxa roll moxibustion is applied to all three points for 20–30 minutes, once a day. Ten treatments constitute one course. When using moxa cone moxibustion, 100–200 small cones (0.5 cm diameter and height) are applied to one point each time, once a week. Three treatments constitute one course. Hot salt compress is applied only to Shenque (Ren8), every other day. Ten treatments constitute one course. (See Appendix 8.)

Moxibustion is suitable for treating all types of impotence with the exception of impotence due to downward flow of damp-heat.

Electroacupuncture

Points used are the same as for body acupuncture. Select two or three pairs of points each time. Puncture until a needling sensation is achieved, then connect the needles to an electrical stimulator. Apply moderate intermittent wave stimulation for 30 minutes. Treat once a day or once every other day. Ten treatments constitute one course.

Point injection therapy

Points:

Guanyuan	(Ren4)
Sanyinjiao	(Sp6)
Baliao	(B31-B34)
Qugu	(Ren2)

Select two or three points each time. Inject each point with 2–4 ml of 5% glucose solution containing either 1 mg strychnine, 50 mg vitamin B_{12}, or 5 mg of testosterone propionate. Treat once every two or three days. Five treatments constitute one course. The same two or three points may be chosen for each course, or four to five points may be treated in turn.

Auricular therapy

Main auricular points:

Internal Genitals, External Genitals: correspond to the affected region of the body.

Kidney: the kidneys open into the external genitals and dominate reproduction, so Kidney is taped to activate the Kidney *yang*.

Liver: the Liver meridian connects with the external genitals, so Liver is taped to activate the Liver meridian and regulate the flow of *qi* and blood.

Heart, Spleen: strengthen the spleen and nourish the heart to calm the mind.

Midpoint of Rim, Endocrine: regulate endocrine function.

Subcortex, Forehead: harmonize excitement and inhibition of the central nervous system.

Ear Shenmen, Occiput: tranquillize the mind.

Use auricular taping, twice a week. Five treatments constitute one course. Auricular self-massage and pressure may also be practised twice a day.

Remarks

- Traditional therapies are effective for treating impotence because of their ability to regulate functional disturbance of the central nervous system.
- Points on the lower abdomen must be punctured obliquely downward so a needling sensation is felt in the external genitals.
- Masturbation and other sexual activity should be avoided during the course of treatment.
- Most cases of impotence are due to functional rather than organic problems and can be cured using the above methods. Functional impotence is closely related to psychological factors; it is therefore essential to encourage a positive attitude and confidence in a cure in order to maximize the effectiveness of traditional therapies.
- Self-massage of the testes is helpful for curing impotence. Hold the left testis in the left hand and massage it with the right hand one hundred times; repeat the process with the right testis. Massage twice a day, before going to sleep at night and before getting up in the morning. Massage must be given over an extended period of time to be effective.
- The above methods are also suitable for treating premature ejaculation, absence of ejaculation and spermatopathy.

69 Influenza

Influenza is an acute communicable disease of the respiratory tract caused by the influenza virus, usually occurring epidemically in the winter and spring. It is marked by sudden onset of high fever, chills, headache, soreness of the entire body, lassitude, poor appetite, nausea and vomiting, usually accompanied by nasal discharge, dry cough and sore throat.

Aetiology

According to traditional Chinese medicine, influenza is an exterior syndrome which primarily affects the lungs. The lungs nourish the skin and open into the nose, so exogenous pathogens such as wind-cold, wind-heat or summer heat and dampness can invade the lungs through the skin and nose, with resulting inability of the lungs to perform their normal function of dispersal and descent.

Differentiation of syndromes

- Influenza due to wind-cold.
  Characterized by severe chills, mild fever, anhidrosis, nasal obstruction with dilute discharge, sneezing, itching of the throat, cough with dilute whitish sputum, headache, soreness of the entire body, thin whitish tongue coating and tense superficial pulse.
- Influenza due to wind-heat.
  Characterized by high fever, mild chills, hidrosis, nasal obstruction with thick discharge, swollen and painful throat, cough with sticky yellowish sputum, headache, thirst with preference for cold drinks, thin yellowish tongue coating and rapid superficial pulse.
- Influenza due to summer heat and dampness.
  Characterized by mild fever and chills, pain and heavy muffled sensation in the head, soreness and heaviness of the entire body, cough with sticky sputum, feeling of fullness in the chest, abdominal distension, nausea, vomiting, scanty urine, loose stool, poor appetite, greasy yellowish tongue coating and soft rapid pulse.

Treatment

Body acupuncture

Main points:

Dazhui	(Du14)
Fengchi	(G20)
Hegu	(LI4)
Feishu	(B13)

Main points are selected from the Yang meridians to activate the meridians and expel exogenous pathogens. The Du meridian is the sea of all the Yang meridians, so Dazhui (Du14), the meeting point of the Du meridian and six Hand and Foot Yang meridians, is punctured to activate the flow of *qi* and expel exogenous pathogens. Fengchi (G20) (Wind Pool in Chinese) functions to expel wind. Hegu (LI4), the *yuan* (source) point of the Large Intestine meridian, functions to strengthen antipathogenic *qi* and expel exogenous pathogens. The lungs open into the nose and nourish the skin, so Feishu (B13), the back-*shu* point of the lungs, is punctured to strengthen the function of the lungs.

Auxiliary points and appropriate manipulation are chosen according to differentiation of syndromes and symptoms.

- For influenza due to wind-cold, wind-cold is expelled by adding and puncturing Yingxiang (LI20) and Taiyang (Ex30) using the reducing method, or by cupping Dazhui (Du14) for 10–15 minutes.
- For influenza due to wind-heat, wind-heat is dispelled by letting several drops of blood; Shaoshang (L11) is added and pricked with a three-edged needle; and Dazhui (Du14) and Feishu (B13) are pricked with a three-edged needle and then cupped for 10–15 minutes.
- For influenza due to summer heat and dampness, Neiguan (P6), Zhongwan (Ren12) and Zusanli (S36) are added and punctured using the reducing method to regulate the stomach and spleen.
- For high fever, heat is dispelled by adding and pricking Shixuan (Ex1) with a three-edged needle to let several drops of blood.
- For severe headache, Taiyang (Ex30) and Baihui (Du20) are added.

● For severe vomiting, Neiguan (P6) and Yanglingquan (G34) are added.

Treat once a day. Five treatments constitute one course.

Blood-letting puncturing

Main points:

Dazhui	(Du14)
Feishu	(B13)
Shixuan	(Ex1)

Dazhui (Du14) and Feishu (B13) are pricked simultaneously using a three-edged needle and then cupped for 10–15 minutes to draw blood. Sixuan (Ex1) is pricked with a three-edged needle to let several drops of blood. Dazhui (Du14) and Feishu (B13) are treated alternately with Shixuan (Ex1). Treat once a day. Five treatments constitute one course. This method functions to dispel heat and is suitable for treating influenza due to wind-heat.

Cupping therapy

Main acupuncture points:

Dazhui	(Du14)
Feishu	(B13)

Cup one point for 10–15 minutes, once a day. Five treatments constitute one course. Treat the two points alternately. This method functions to expel cold and is suitable for treating influenza due to wind-cold.

Auricular therapy

Main auricular points:

Lung, Internal Nose, External Nose, Throat: the lungs open into the nose and relate to the throat, so these points are chosen to facilitate the flow of lung *qi*, expel wind and dispel heat.

Auxiliary auricular points:

For high fever, Apex of Ear and Apex of Tragus are pricked with a three-edged needle to let several drops of blood.

For frontal headache, Forehead is added.

For bilateral headache, Temple is added.

For occipital headache, Occiput is added.

For cough, Trachea and Mouth are added.

For poor appetite, nausea and vomiting, Stomach and Cardia are added.

Use auricular taping and blood-letting puncturing where indicated, twice a week.

Remarks

☻ Traditional therapies are very effective for treating influenza; there will often be great improvement in all symptoms after only one treatment.
☻ All therapies can be used singly or in combination.
☻ These methods are also effective for treating the common cold.

70 Insufficient lactation

Insufficient lactation refers to lack or absence of milk secretion following parturition, or sudden decrease or cessation of previously normal milk secretion. Causes may include malnutrition, or psychological or physical factors.

Aetiology

According to traditional Chinese medicine, insufficient lactation has two causes. A weak constitution or excessive blood loss during delivery may result in deficiency of *qi* and blood and insufficient nutrients for production of milk; or mental injury may result in stagnation of the liver *qi*, affecting the production and transportation of milk.

Differentiation of syndromes

● Insufficient lactation due to deficiency of *qi* and blood.

Characterized by thin, scanty, or no milk and soft breasts with no distending pain; accompanied by dizziness, pale complexion, lassitude, palpitation, shortness of breath, pale tongue and weak thready pulse.

● Insufficient lactation due to stagnation of the liver *qi*.
Characterized by scanty or no milk following parturition, or sudden decrease or cessation of previously normal milk secretion due to anger or anxiety; hard breasts with distending pain; accompanied by feeling of fullness in the chest and hypochondriac region, depression or restlessness, frequent sighing, poor appetite, insomnia, whitish tongue coating and wiry pulse.

Treatment

Body acupuncture

Main acupuncture points:

Danzhong	(Ren17)
Shaoze	(SI1)
Yingchuang	(S16)
Rugen	(S18)

Danzhong (Ren17), the *hui* (influential) point of *qi*, functions to tonify *qi* and open the chest. It is punctured horizontally towards both breasts for 1.5–2.0 *cun*.

The heart controls the flow of blood in the blood vessels and the small intestine functions to digest food and separate nutrients from waste; therefore Shaoze (SI1), the *jing* (well) point of the Small Intestine meridian and the meeting point of the Heart and Small Intestine meridians, is chosen to strengthen the heart and small intestines and promote the transformation and transportation of milk.

Yingchuang (S16) and Rugen (S18), two points of the Stomach meridian located above and below the nipple respectively, are rich in blood and *qi*.

They are treated to strengthen the blood and *qi* and promote the transformation and transportation of milk. Yingchuang (S16) is punctured downward and Rugen (S18) upward.

Auxiliary points and appropriate methods of manipulation are chosen according to differentiation of syndromes.

● For insufficient lactation due to deficiency of *qi* and blood, Zusanli (S36), Zhongwan (Ren12), Qihai (Ren6) and Sanyinjiao (Sp6) are added and punctured using the reinforcing method to tonify the *qi* and blood.
● For insufficient lactation due to stagnation of the liver *qi*, Taichong (Liv3), Neiguan (P6) and Qimen (Liv14) are added and punctured using the even method to stimulate the flow of the liver *qi* and promote transportation of milk.

Treat once a day. Five treatments constitute one course.

Moxibustion

Points used are the same as for body acupuncture. Local points and Shaoze (SI1) are most commonly used. Apply moxa roll moxibustion for 15–20 minutes to two or three points, once or twice a day. Five treatments constitute one course.

Remarks

☯ Both acupuncture and moxibustion are very effective for treating insufficient lactation. In many cases, two or three treatments are sufficient to improve the condition. However, these methods are ineffective for treating insufficient lactation due to mammary aplasia.
☯ Improving nutrition and maintaining a good psychological state are helpful for promoting lactation.

71 Intercostal neuralgia

Intercostal neuralgia refers to pain in one or more intercostal spaces due to inflammation of the intercostal nerves. It is caused mainly by pleuritis, pneumonia, costal chondritis, herpes zoster or chest trauma such as heart surgery. It is marked by persistent stabbing pain along the pathway of the affected intercostal nerves, radiating to the lumbar region of the affected side and aggravated by coughing or deep breathing, localized hyper-aesthesia and tenderness.

Aetiology and differentiation of syndromes

Traditional Chinese medicine classifies intercostal neuralgia as hypochondriac pain and considers it to be caused by stress, trauma or exogenous pathogens which lead to stagnation of *qi* and blood in the chest and hypochondriac region. Mainly affected is the Gallbladder meridian. It is characterized by purple-spotted tongue and wiry pulse.

Treatment

Body acupuncture

Acupuncture points:

Yanglingquan	(G34)
Zhigou	(SJ6)
Huatuojiaji	(Ex46)

The Gallbladder meridian passes through the hypochondriac region, therefore Yanglingquan (G34), the *he* (sea) point of the Gallbladder meridian, is punctured to activate the meridian and relieve pain. Zhigou (SJ6) is an important point for treating all problems of the hypochondriac region. Huatuojiaji (Ex46) points which correspond to the affected intercostal nerves are selected to relieve pain.

Puncture using strong manipulation. A needling sensation should be felt in the affected area. Treat once a day or once every other day. Five treatments constitute one course.

Electroacupuncture

Points used are the same as for body acupuncture. Select one or two pairs of points each time. Puncture the points until a needling sensation is achieved, then connect the needles to an electric stimulator. Apply intermittent wave stimulation of the strongest bearable intensity for 30 minutes. Treat once a day. Five treatments constitute one course.

Auricular therapy

Auricular points:

Chest, Thoracic Vertebrae: correspond to the affected areas of the body. Locate positive points; tape both frontal and dorsal surfaces to increase stimulation.

Liver, Pancreas & Gallbladder: the Liver and Gallbladder meridians pass through the chest and hypochondriac region, so these points are taped to clear and activate the meridians and collaterals.

Ear Shenmen, Subcortex: tranquillize the mind and relieve pain.

Apex of Ear: blood-letting puncturing of this point with a three-edged needle dispels heat and relieves pain.

Use auricular taping with strong manipulation and blood-letting puncturing where indicated, twice a week. Five treatments constitute one course.

Remarks

☯ The above therapies can immediately relieve the pain of intercostal neuralgia; however, it is necessary to treat the underlying disease concurrently.

72 *Jue* syndrome

Jue syndrome refers to sudden fainting and loss of consciousness. There are ususally no post-recovery sequelae, although some cases may be marked by cold limbs. *Jue* syndrome is a common manifestation of various diseases and disorders including shock, sunstroke, hypoglycaemic coma and hysterical syncope.

Aetiology

According to traditional Chinese medicine, the main pathogenesis of *jue* syndrome is disorder in the flow of *qi*, resulting in disruption of the linkage of *yin* and *yang*. The causes are various, including overindulgence in food, alcohol, or sexual activity;

exogenous pathogens, mental injury; loss of blood or body fluid, severe pain, pathogenic phlegm or stagnant blood.

Differentiation of syndromes

- *Qi jue* syndrome of the excessive type.
  Characterized by sudden fainting and loss of consciousness following mental injury such as extreme anger; accompanied by lockjaw, clenched fists, rapid respiration, cold limbs, thin whitish tongue coating and deep or deep and wiry pulse.
- *Qi jue* syndrome of the deficient type.
  Characterized by sudden dizziness and fainting following overstrain or mental injury such as extreme fear; accompanied by pale complexion, weak respiration, profuse sweating, cold limbs, pale tongue with whitish coating and deep thready weak pulse.
- Blood *jue* syndrome of the excessive type.
  Characterized by sudden fainting and loss of consciousness following extreme anger; accompanied by trismus, clenched fists, flushed complexion and purple lips, red tongue and deep wiry pulse.
- Blood *jue* syndrome of the deficient type.
  Characterized by sudden fainting and loss of consciousness following major loss of blood; accompanied by pale complexion and lips, trembling of the extremities, profuse sweating, weak respiration, pale tongue and weak thready pulse.
- Cold *jue* syndrome.
  Characterized by grey complexion, lying in flexed position, cold sensation in the entire body, especially the limbs; diarrhoea containing undigested food, pale tongue with thin whitish coating and deep thready, slow pulse.
- Heat *jue* syndrome.
  Characterized in the initial stage by fever, headache, burning sensation in the chest and abdomen, thirst with a preference for cold drinks, constipation, yellowish urine and restlessness; followed by cold limbs, mental confusion or even loss of consciousness, red tongue with dry yellowish coating and deep rapid pulse.
- Phlegm *jue* syndrome.
  Characterized by sudden fainting and loss of consciousness; accompanied by wheezing, excessive salivation, feeling of fullness in the chest, greasy whitish tongue coating and deep slippery pulse.
- Food *jue* syndrome.
  Characterized by sudden fainting and loss of consciousness following overindulgence in food or alcohol; accompanied by abdominal distension, vomiting, thick greasy tongue coating and forceful slippery pulse.
- Sexual *jue* syndrome.
  Characterized by sudden fainting and loss of consciousness during or following sexual activity; accompanied by profuse sweating, cold limbs, weak respiration, pale tongue and deep thready, weak pulse.

Treatment

Body acupuncture

Main acupuncture points:

Shuigou	(Du26)
Baihui	(Du20)
Zhongchong	(P9)

The Du meridian is the sea of all Yang meridians and connects with the brain; the pericardium covers and protects the heart. Therefore, points of the Du and Pericardium meridians are chosen as main points to restore consciousness.

Shuigou (Du26) lies in the nasolabial groove between the nose and mouth. The nose receives *qi* from the sky and the mouth receives nourishment from the earth, so this point is also called Renzhong, the centre or midpoint of the human being, just as the human being is located between sky and earth. Shuigou (Du26) is also the meeting point of the Du meridian and the Hand and Foot Yangming meridians, which are rich in both *qi* and blood. This point is therefore very effective for harmonizing the flow of *qi* and blood and is the most important point for restoring consciousness.

Baihui (Du20), the meeting point of the Du, Liver and six Hand and Foot meridians, functions to induce resuscitation. Zhongchong (P9), the *jing* (well) point of the Pericardium meridian and one of the Shixuan (Ex1) points, functions to restore consciousness.

Shuigou (Du26) is punctured obliquely upward to a depth of 0.3–0.5 *cun*. For deficient type *jue* syndromes, Zhongchong (P9) is punctured to a depth of 0.2–0.3 *cun*; for excessive type *jue* syndromes, it is pricked with a three-edged needle to let several drops of blood. The needles should be retained and manipulated every 5 minutes until consciousness returns and all other signs and symptoms improve.

Auxiliary points and appropriate manipulation are chosen according to differentiation of syndromes:

- For *qi jue* syndrome of the excessive type, Hegu (LI4) and Taichong (Liv3) are added and punctured using the reducing method to regulate the flow of *qi* and blood. This is known as 'opening the four passes'.
- For *qi jue* syndrome of the deficient type, *qi* is tonified by either adding and puncturing Guanyuan (Ren4), Qihai (Ren6) and Zusanli (S36) using the reinforcing method, or applying moxibustion to Baihui (Du20), Qihai (Ren6) and Guanyuan (Ren4).
- For blood *jue* syndrome of the excessive type, Yongquan (K1) and Xingjian (Liv2) are added and punctured using the reducing method to regulate the flow of *qi* and blood.
- For blood *jue* syndrome of the deficient type, the blood is supplemented and consciousness restored by adding and puncturing Guanyuan (Ren4), Qihai (Ren6) and Sanyinjiao (Sp6) using the reinforcing method, and/or applying moxibustion to these points.
- For cold *jue* syndrome, Shenque (Ren8) and Guanyuan (Ren4) are added and punctured using the reinforcing method to restore *yang* and expel cold. Moxibustion may also be applied to Baihui (Du20), Shenque (Ren8) and Guanyuan (Ren4) to increase the effect.
- For heat *jue* syndrome, Shixuan (Ex1) is added and pricked with a three-edged needle to induce mild bleeding in order to dispel heat and restore consciousness.
- For phlegm *jue* syndrome, Neiguan (P6), Fenglong (S40), Danzhong (Ren17) and Hegu (LI4) are added and punctured using the reducing method to clear phlegm and induce resuscitation.
- For food *jue* syndrome, Zhongwan (Ren12), Neiguan (P6) and Zusanli (S36) are added and punctured using the reducing method to relieve retention of food and widen the chest.
- For sexual *jue* syndrome, Shenque (Ren8) and Guanyuan (Ren4) are added and punctured using the reinforcing method to supplement *yuan* (primal) *qi* and restore consciousness. Moxibustion may also be applied to Baihui (Du20), Shenque (Ren8) and Guanyuan (Ren4) to improve effectiveness.

Electroacupuncture

Points used are the same as for body acupuncture. Choose one to three pairs of points each time. Puncture the points until a needling sensation is achieved, then connect the needles with an electrical stimulator. Apply moderate continuous or intermittent wave stimulation until consciousness returns and all other signs and symptoms improve.

Moxibustion

Acupuncture points:

Baihui	(Du20)
Shenque	(Ren8)
Guanyuan	(Ren4)
Qihai	(Ren6)
Danzhong	(Ren17)
Zhongwan	(Ren12)
Zusanli	(S36)

Points of the Du and Ren meridians are selected to regulate the flow of *qi* and restore consciouness. Moxa roll or moxa cone moxibustion is applied simultaneously to four or five points until consciousness returns and there is improvement in all other signs and symptoms.

Moxibustion functions to supplement *qi* and arrest *yang*, so it is an ideal therapy for treating *jue* syndromes of the deficient and cold types.

Auricular Therapy

Main auricular points:

Heart: the heart functions to circulate blood throughout the meridians and is the storehouse of the mind, so Heart is stimulated to promote the flow of blood and restore consciousness.

Subcortex, Sympathesis: regulate the neurovascular function to promote the flow of blood.

Endocrine, Adrenal Gland: strengthen endocrine function to raise the blood pressure.

Teeth (also called Blood Pressure Raising Point): clinically effective point for raising the blood pressure.

Auxiliary auricular points are added according to differentiation of syndromes:

- For *qi* or blood *jue* syndrome of the excessive type, Liver is added to promote the flow of *qi* and blood.

- For heat *jue* syndrome, Apex of Ear is added and pricked with a three-edged needle to let several drops of blood in order to dispel pathogenic heat.
- For phlegm or food *jue* syndrome, Stomach and Abdomen are added to regulate the flow of *qi* in the Middle Jiao.

Use auricular taping with strong manipulation and blood-letting puncturing where indicated, or apply auricular puncturing using the reducing method. Press or manipulate every five minutes during treatment to increase stimulation.

Remarks

☯ The treatment of *jue* syndrome with traditional therapies has a very long history. Numerous contemporary clinical reports also indicate that

traditional therapies are both reliable and effective for treating *jue* syndrome. Immediate and appropriate treatment is usually extremely successful.

☯ There are specific advantages in using traditional therapies to treat *jue* syndrome. *Jue* syndrome usually occurs in an emergency situation and treatment should be given as soon as possible. When needles or moxa are not available, Shuigou (Du26) and Zhongchong (P9) may be pressed with the thumbnail; other points may be pressed with the balls of the thumbs.

☯ Modern research indicates that traditional therapies can prevent and to some extent cure shock; when used in combination with other anti-shock measures, traditional therapies can increase the body's receptivity to those measures and raise their effectiveness.

73 Leukorrhagia

Leukorrhagia refers to abnormal changes in the vaginal secretions. It is a common symptom of various diseases and disorders of both the internal and external female genitals. Simple leukorrhagia is marked by profuse, thin, whitish vaginal discharge. It may occur either during the preovulatory phase, before or after the menstrual period, during pregnancy, or after administration of oestrogens. Sticky, yellowish, strong-smelling vaginal discharge occurs primarily in the presence of inflammation of either the internal or external genitals; bloody vaginal discharge occurs primarily in the presence of senile vaginitis, cervical polyps, or tumours.

Aetiology

Traditional Chinese medicine classifies leukorrhagia into excessive and deficient types. The excessive type is caused primarily by downward flow of damp-heat in the Liver meridian, or by invasion of damp-heat or toxic pathogens. The deficient type is caused primarily by deficiency of the spleen or kidneys, resulting in accumulation of dampness in the interior and its subsequent down-

ward flow. Primarily affected in both types are the spleen, liver and kidneys.

Differentiation of syndromes

- Leukorrhagia of the damp-cold type.
  Characterized by profuse, thin, whitish vaginal discharge; accompanied by pain and sensation of cold in the lower abdomen, sore and weak back, lassitude, poor appetite, loose stool, whitish tongue coating and soft weak pulse.
- Leukorrhagia of the damp-heat type.
  Characterized by sticky, yellowish, strong-smelling vaginal discharge; accompanied by abdominal distension, nausea or vomiting, poor appetite, yellowish urine, greasy yellowish tongue coating and slippery or wiry pulse.
- Leukorrhagia of the damp-toxic type.
  Characterized by strong-smelling vaginal discharge which may be cheesy whitish, purulent yellow, or contain blood; accompanied by abdominal distension, itching of the vulva, bitter taste in the mouth, dry throat, scanty yellowish urine, red tongue with yellowish coating and rapid slippery pulse.

Treatment

Body acupuncture

Main acupuncture points:

Zhongji	(Ren3)
Sanyinjiao	(Sp6)
Ciliao	(B32)
Daimai	(G26)

The main pathogenesis of leukorrhagia is accumulation of dampness in the Lower Jiao. Zhongji (Ren3), the front-*mu* point of the urinary bladder and the meeting point of the Ren and three Foot Yin meridians; and Ciliao (B32), a point of the Urinary Bladder meridian located in the sacral region, both function to expel dampness. Sanyinjiao (Sp6), the meeting point of the three Foot Yin meridians, is an important point for treating gynaecological and genital problems. Daimai (G26), the meeting point of the Gallbladder and Dai meridians, is usually quite tender in people with leukorrhagia. Reports indicate that moxibustion applied to Daimai (G26) alone can cure leukorrhagia.

Auxiliary points and proper manipulation are chosen according to differentiation of syndromes:

● For leukorrhagia of the damp-cold type, cold and dampness are dispelled by adding and puncturing Baihuanshu (B30) and Zusanli (S36) using the reinforcing method and applying moxibustion as needed.
● For leukorrhagia of the damp-heat type, Ligou (Liv5), Yinlingquan (Sp9) and Xialiao (B34) are added and punctured using the reducing method to expel heat and remove dampness.
● For leukorrhagia of the damp-toxic type, Ligou (Liv5), Qugu (Ren2) and Yaoshu (Du2) are added and punctured using the reducing method to expel damp-toxic pathogens.

Treat once a day or once every other day. Ten treatments constitute one course.

Moxibustion

Points used are the same as for body acupuncture. Apply moxa roll moxibustion for 15–20 minutes, or three to five medium-sized moxa cones, to two or three points each time. Treat once a day or once every other day. Ten treatments constitute one course.

Moxibustion functions to dispel cold and remove dampness and is therefore especially suitable for treating leukorrhagia of the damp-cold type.

Electroacupuncture

Points used are the same as for body acupuncture. Select one or two pairs of points each time. Puncture until a needling sensation is achieved, then connect the needles to an electrical stimulator. Apply moderate continuous wave stimulation for 30 minutes, once a day or once every other day. Ten treatments constitute one course.

Auricular therapy

Main auricular points:

Internal Genitals, External Genitals, Pelvis, Abdomen: correspond to the affected regions. Locate positive points; tape both frontal and dorsal surfaces to increase stimulation.

San Jiao: dispels dampness.
Endocrine, Midpoint of Rim, Subcortex: regulate endocrine function.

Adrenal Gland, Wind Stream: relieve inflammation.

Auxiliary auricular points:

For damp-heat leukorrhagia, Liver is added and Apex of Ear is punctured with a three-edged needle to draw blood.

For damp-cold leukorrhagia, Spleen and Kidney are added.

Use auricular taping and blood-letting puncturing where indicated, twice a week. Five treatments constitute one course.

Remarks

☙ Leukorrhagia is a common symptom of many gynaecological problems. It is essential to establish a diagnosis prior to treatment in order to avoid overlooking conditions such as tumours, especially in women over 40 years old or when bloody or strong-smelling vaginal discharge is present.
☙ Traditional therapies are effective for treating leukorrhagia. Two or more treatments are usually used in combination in order to increase stimulation and improve effectiveness.

74 Lochiorrhagia

Lochia is a type of normal vaginal discharge occurring for up to two weeks following parturition. However, lochia that persists for more than two weeks may be caused by subinvolution of the uterus and is called lochiorrhagia.

Aetiology

Traditional Chinese medicine classifies lochiorrhagia into excessive and deficient types. The excessive type is caused either by invasion of the uterus by exogenous cold following parturition with resulting stagnation of blood in the uterus, or by mental injury leading to stagnation of the liver *qi* and its subsequent transformation into pathogenic fire. The deficient type is caused by general weakness or overstrain immediately following parturition which damages the *qi*, with subsequent loss of control of the blood.

Differentiation of syndromes

- Lochiorrhagia due to stagnation of blood in the uterus.
  Characterized by scanty, purple, clotted lochia; accompanied by severe pain in the lower abdomen aggravated by pressure, purple or spotted tongue and deep uneven pulse.
- Lochiorrhagia due to overflow of blood caused by pathogenic fire.
  Characterized by profuse, sticky, strong-smelling, red lochia; accompanied by restlessness, insomnia, dry mouth and throat, red tongue and rapid thready pulse.
- Lochiorrhagia due to deficiency of *qi*.
  Characterized by profuse, thin, red lochia; accompanied by lassitude, pale complexion, dizziness, poor appetite, pale tongue and weak thready pulse.

Treatment

Body acupuncture

Main acupuncture points:

| Guanyuan | (Ren4) |
| Sanyinjiao | (Sp6) |

Guanyuan (Ren4), the meeting point of the Ren and three Foot Yin meridians located on the lower abdomen and Sanyinjiao (Sp6), the meeting point of the three Foot Yin meridians, are treated in combination. They are the main pair of points used for treating gynaecological and obstetric problems.

Auxiliary points and proper manipulation are chosen according to differentiation of syndromes.

- For lochiorrhagia due to stagnation of blood in the uterus, the flow of blood is promoted by adding and puncturing Diji (Sp8) and Xuehai (Sp10) using the reducing method, and applying moxibustion as needed.
- For lochiorrhagia due to overflow of blood caused by pathogenic fire, Xingjian (Liv2) and Xuehai (Sp10) are added and punctured using the reducing method to dispel heat and arrest bleeding.
- For lochiorrhagia due to deficiency of *qi*, *qi* is strengthened and blood controlled by adding and puncturing Qihai (Ren6) and Zusanli (S36) using the reinforcing method, and applying moxibustion as needed.

Treat once a day. Five treatments constitute one course.

Moxibustion

Points:

Guanyuan	(Ren4)
Qihai	(Ren6)
Shenque	(Ren8)
Sanyinjiao	(Sp6)

Select one or two points each time. Apply moxa roll moxibustion to each point for 15–20 minutes. Treat once or twice a day. Five treatments constitute one course.

Moxibustion is suitable for treating lochiorrhagia due to stagnation of blood in the uterus and lochiorrhagia due to deficiency of *qi*. It can be self-applied at home.

Remarks

- Both body acupuncture and moxibustion are effective for treating lochiorrhagia.
- Lochiorrhagia due to stagnation of blood in the uterus is the condition most commonly seen in clinical practice.

75 Lumbar muscle strain

Lumbar muscle strain refers to chronic lower back pain. It is marked by intermittent or persistent soreness, pain and heaviness in the lumbar region, alleviated by proper exercise and aggravated by extended sitting or standing or cold and rainy weather. There is usually a history of acute lumbar strain, work involving excessive bending or standing, or invasion by wind-cold or damp-cold.

Aetiology and differentiation of syndromes

According to traditional Chinese medicine, the lumbus is the storehouse of the kidneys. Excessive sexual activity or prolonged illness may damage the kidney essence and result in malnutrition of the muscles and tendons of the lumbar region. Malnourished lumbar muscles and tendons and subsequent persistent dull lumbar pain and soreness may also occur if cases of external trauma or invasion by wind-cold or damp-cold are not treated in a timely and proper manner. Additional manifestations include sore and weak back and knees, lassitude, feeling of cold in the extremities, pale tongue and deep thready pulse. Primarily affected are the Urinary Bladder and Du meridians.

Treatment

Body acupuncture

Acupuncture points:

> *Ashi* points
> Shenshu   (B23)
> Mingmen   (Du4)
> Weizhong   (B40)
> Kunlun   (B60)
> Taixi   (K3)

Shenshu (B23), the back-*shu* point of the kidneys, is punctured to tonify the kidneys. Mingmen (Du4), a local point of the Du meridian, is an important kidney-strengthening point. Weizhong (B40) and Kunlun (B60), the *he* (sea) and *jing* (river) points respectively of the Urinary Bladder meridian, are treated in combination to activate the

flow of *qi* and blood in the Urinary Bladder meridian. Taixi (K3), the *yuan* (source) point of the Kidney meridian, is punctured to strengthen the kidneys.

Puncture using the reinforcing method, once a day or once every other day. Ten treatments constitute one course.

Electroacupuncture

Points used are the same as for body acupuncture. Select one or two pairs of points each time. Puncture the points until a needling sensation is achieved, then connect the needles to an electrical stimulator. Apply moderate intermittent wave stimulation for 30 minutes. Treat once a day or once every other day. Ten treatments constitute one course.

Point injection therapy

Ashi and local points are injected with 2–4 ml of procaine, dexamethasone or vitamin B_{12} once every three days. Three treatments constitute one course.

Auricular therapy

Auricular points:

> Lumbosacral Vertebrae: locate tender points; tape both frontal and dorsal surfaces to increase stimulation. The most tender point is usually located between the crest of the antihelix and the scaphoid fossa.

> Kidney: the kidneys are connected to the lumbus, so Kidney is taped to strengthen the kidneys.

> Urinary Bladder: the Urinary Bladder meridian passes through the lumbus, so Urinary Bladder is taped to clear and activate the meridians and collaterals.

> Liver, Spleen: nourish and strengthen the tendons and muscles.

> Ear Shenmen: main point for relieving pain.

Use auricular taping, twice a week. Five treatments constitute one course. Auricular pressure and self-massage may be practised twice a day as well.

Remarks

◑ Traditional therapies are very effective for treating lumbar muscle strain; two or more methods are usually used in combination to increase stimulation and raise effect.

◑ Self-massage of the lumbar region during and after treatment is beneficial.

◑ It is essential to keep the back and lower extremities warm, avoid overstrain and regulate sexual activity in order to avoid relapse.

76 Malaria

Malaria is an infectious parasitic disease transmitted by the anopheline mosquito. It is marked by intermittent chills, high fever and sweating. Splenomegaly and anemia may also occur in some cases. Malaria is classified according to the interval between attacks, into quotidian, tertian, quartan, quintan and malignant (non-specific interval) types. Cerebral malaria refers to malignant malaria marked by loss of mental acuity, delirium, convulsion or amentia.

Aetiology

According to traditional Chinese medicine, malaria is caused by the malaria pathogen, which invades the body and hides in the area between interior and exterior, i.e. the Shaoyang meridians (including the Gallbladder and San Jiao meridians.) Chills occur when the pathogen penetrates the interior and struggles with the *yin qi*; high fever, headache and sweating occur when the pathogen emerges and struggles with the *yang qi*. Remission from alternating attacks of chills and high fever occurs when the pathogen evades the antipathogenic *qi* to hide once again in the area between interior and exterior. If the pathogen remains in the body for an extended time, damage may occur to the *qi* and blood, resulting in anaemia, or the stagnant pathogen may produce phlegm which accumulates in the hypochondriac region, resulting in splenomegaly.

Differentiation of syndromes

● Simple malaria.
  Characterized by chills and aversion to cold in the initial stage. This is followed by the fever stage, marked by high fever, headache, flushed face, thirst and restlessness which last for several hours until profuse sweating occurs, and then abate. The resting stage is marked by mild dizziness and lassitude. Tongue coating is thin and whitish or yellowish; pulse is tense and wiry during the initial stage and rapid and wiry during the fever stage. The attacks occur once a day in most cases, sometimes every other day or every two days.

● Heat-type malaria.
  Attacks are similar to those of simple malaria; marked by high fever, mild aversion to cold, shortness of breath, restlessness, sensation of heat in the hands and feet, headache, thirst with preference for cold drinks, pain in the chest and hypochondriac region, vomiting, jaundice and delirium; tongue is red with yellowish coating and pulse wiry and rapid.

● Cold-type malaria.
  Attacks are similar to those of simple malaria; marked by severe aversion to cold, chills, mild or no fever, no thirst or thirst with preference for hot drinks, feeling of stuffiness in the chest and hypochondriac region, lassitude, greasy whitish tongue coating and slow wiry pulse.

● Damp-type malaria.
  Attacks are similar to those of simple malaria; marked by chills and moderate fever, heavy sensation and pain in the entire body, distended chest and abdomen, vomiting, greasy tongue coating and slippery wiry pulse.

● Malignant-type malaria.
  Characterized by irregular attack of chills and fever or high fever with no chills, sweating, pantalgia, flushed face, pink eyes, thirst with a

preference for cold drinks, feeling of stuffiness in the chest, vomiting, constipation, scanty yellowish urine; possible delirium, convulsions, manic behaviour, or loss of mental acuity; dark red tongue with greasy black coating and wiry rapid or full pulse.

- Gastrointestinal-type malaria.
  Attacks are similar to those of simple malaria; marked by abdominal pain, diarrhoea with bloody pussy stool, tenesmus, emaciation, shortness of breath, greasy whitish tongue coating and wiry thready slippery pulse.
- Chronic malaria.
  Characterized by long-standing malaria or frequent relapse following overstrain; accompanied by pale complexion, listlessness, dizziness, mass in the hypochondriac region, pale or purple-spotted tongue and weak thready pulse.

Treatment

Body acupuncture

Main acupuncture points:

Dazhui	(Du14)
Houxi	(SI3)
Jianshi	(P5)

Dazhui (Du14), the meeting point of the Du and six Hand and Foot Yang meridians, is punctured to stimulate antipathogenic *qi* and expel exogenous pathogens. Houxi (SI3), one of the eight confluence points connecting with the Du meridian, is punctured to help Dazhui (Du14) expel exogenous pathogens. Jianshi (P5), the *jing* (river) point of the Pericardium meridian, is a clinically effective point for treating malaria.

Puncture the three main points using the even method every day two hours prior to expected onset to tonify antipathogenic *qi* and prevent regularly occurring malarial attack. Needles should be retained for 30 minutes.

Auxiliary points and appropriate methods of manipulation are chosen according to differentiation of syndromes:

- For heat-type malaria, heat is expelled by adding and puncturing Hegu (LI4) and Neiting (S44) using the reducing method and pricking Shixuan (Ex1) with a three-edged needle.

- For cold-type malaria, the meridians are warmed and cold expelled by adding and puncturing Zusanli (S36), Zhongwan (Ren12) and Taixi (K3) using the even method and applying moxibustion to Dazhui (Du14) and Zhongwan (Ren12).
- For damp-type malaria, Sanyinjiao (Sp6), Zusanli (S36) and Yinlingquan (Sp9) are added and punctured using the even method to remove dampness.
- For malignant-type malaria, Dazhui (Du14), Quze (P3), Weizhong (B40) and Shixuan (Ex1) are added and pricked with a three-edged needle to draw blood and dispel toxic heat.
- For gastrointestinal-type malaria. Tianshu (S25), Zusanli (S36) and Sanyinjiao (Sp6) are added and punctured using the even method to harmonize the stomach and spleen.
- For chronic malaria, Zhongwan (Ren12), Pishu (B20), Zusanli (S36) and Sanyinjiao (Sp6) are added and punctured using the reinforcing method to strengthen antipathogenic *qi* and expel pathogens.

Treat once a day or once every other day. Ten treatments constitute one course.

Electroacupuncture

Points used are the same as for body acupuncture. Select one or two pairs of points each time. Puncture until a needling sensation is achieved, then connect the needles to an electrical stimulator. Apply moderate intermittent wave stimulation for 30–40 minutes. Treat once each day two hours before the attack is expected. Ten treatments constitute one course.

Moxibustion

Points:

Dazhui	(Du14)
Taodao	(Du13)
Neiguan	(P6)
Shenque	(Ren8)

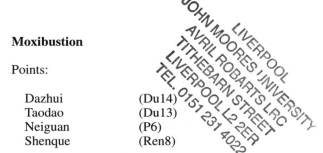

Apply moxa roll moxibustion for 10–15 minutes, or three to five medium-sized moxa cones to one or two points each time. Treat once a day two hours before the attack is expected. Ten treatments constitute one course. This method is very effective for treating tertian malaria.

Remarks

☯ Traditional therapies can not only immediately

relieve the symptoms of malaria, but also effect a radical cure, as proven by elimination of malarial parasites from the blood.
☯ Many reports indicate that applying acupuncture or moxibustion two hours prior to expected daily onset effectively prevents malarial attack.

77 Male infertility

Pregnancy will generally occur within six months in heterosexually active women of childbearing age who are not using contraceptive measures. Infertility, or absence of conception after two years, may occur due to reproductive disorders of either the male or female partner.

The causes of male infertility are complex. Clinically, male infertility is classified into three types: infertility due to sexual dysfunction, including impotence, seminal emission, premature ejaculation or absence of ejaculation; infertility due to spermatopathy, such as oligospermia, azoospermia, or cacospermia; and infertility due to congenital or acquired problems of the genitals, such as hypoplagia of the testis, undescended testis, obstruction of the spermatic duct, or hypospadia. In some cases, failure to conceive may be due to simple ignorance of sexual function resulting in incomplete, insufficient or mistimed sexual intercourse.

Acupuncture has been shown to be clinically effective for treating male infertility due to sexual dysfunction and spermatopathy.

Aetiology

According to traditional Chinese medicine, male infertility is related primarily to dysfunction of the kidneys and liver. The kidneys store essence, open into both the external genitals and the anus and dominate reproduction. If the *qi*, essence, *yin* or *yang* of the kidneys is consumed due to congenital insufficiency, early or excessive sexual activity, or prolonged illness, the kidneys will be weakened and infertility may result.

The liver governs the flow of *qi* and blood in the body. The Liver meridian and its collaterals,

divergent meridian and muscle region are all connected with the external genitals. Sexual function or sperm production may be affected if mental injury affects the ability of the liver to regulate the flow of *qi* and blood, or if damp-heat pathogens in the liver and gallbladder descend to the external genitals.

Differentiation of syndromes

● Male infertility due to unconsolidated kidney *qi*.
Characterized by premature ejaculation or waking spermatorrhoea; accompanied by dizziness, tinnitus, sore and weak back and knees, frequent urination or urinary incontinence, pale tongue with thin whitish coating and deep, thready pulse.
● Male infertility due to deficiency of the kidney essence.
Characterized by oligospermia, azoospermia, cacospermia, or impotence; accompanied by lassitude, dizziness, tinnitus, poor memory, sore and weak back and knees, pale tongue and deep thready weak pulse.
● Male infertility due to hyperactivity of deficient fire arising from insufficiency of the kidney *yin*.
Characterized by seminal emission while dreaming, priapism and absence of ejaculation; accompanied by dizziness, tinnitus, emaciation, restlessness, sensation of heat in the palms and soles, night sweating, dry red tongue with little coating and rapid thready pulse.
● Male infertility due to decline of fire from the Gate of Life.
Characterized by impotence, oligospermia and

hyposexuality; accompanied by dizziness, tinnitus, pale complexion, lassitude, sensation of cold in the hands and feet, aversion to cold, dilute and frequent urination, pale thin tongue and slow deep thready pulse.

● Male infertility due to stagnation of the liver *qi*.
Characterized by impotence, seminal emission, premature ejaculation hyposexuality; accompanied by depression, feeling of fullness in the chest and hypochondriac region, frequent sighing, thin whitish tongue coating and wiry pulse.

● Male infertility due to descent of damp-heat from the liver and gallbladder.
Characterized by swelling and pain of the testis, bloody semen and impotence or priapism; accompanied by bitter taste in the mouth, dry throat, restlessness, scanty yellowish urine, scrotal itching, red tongue with greasy yellowish coating and rapid wiry pulse.

● Male infertility due to stagnation of *qi* and blood.
Characterized by absence of ejaculation and priapism; accompanied by distension or pain in the lower abdomen and scrotal region, feeling of fullness in the chest, depression or restlessness, purple or purple-spotted tongue and deep uneven pulse.

Treatment

Body acupuncture

Main acupuncture points:

Shenshu	(B23)
Mingmen	(Du4)
Guanyuan	(Ren4)
Sanyinjiao	(Sp6)
Ciliao	(B32)

Shenshu (B23), the back-*shu* point of the kidneys, is punctured to strengthen the kidneys and restore fertility.

The *yin* and *yang* of the kidneys are the source of the entire body's *yin* and *yang*. The body's *yin* and *yang* are governed by the Du and Ren meridians respectively, so points of these two meridians are selected to rebalance the body's *yin* and *yang*. Mingmen (Du4) (Gate of Life in Chinese) is treated to warm the body's *yang*. Guanyuan (Ren4), the meeting point of the Ren and three Foot Yin meridians located on the lower abdomen, functions to tonify the primordial *qi*.

Sanyinjiao (Sp6), the meeting point of the three Foot Yin meridians, functions to strengthen the kidneys, liver and spleen and is an important point for treating urogenital problems. Ciliao (B32), a point of the Urinary Bladder meridian located in the second posterior sacral foramen, is a clinically effective point for treating problems of the genitals.

Auxiliary points and appropriate methods of manipulation are chosen according to differentiation of syndromes.

● For male infertility due to unconsolidated kidney *qi*, the kidney *qi* is strengthened by adding and puncturing Zhishi (B52) and Taixi (K3) using the reinforcing method, or adding moxibustion as needed.

● For male infertility due to deficiency of the kidney essence, the kidney essence is tonified by adding and puncturing Qihai (Ren6), Baihui (Du20), Taixi (K3) and Zusanli (S36) using the reinforcing method, or adding moxibustion as needed.

● For male infertility due to hyperactivity of deficient fire resulting from insufficiency of the kidney *yin*, Xinshu (B15), Shenmen (H7) and Taixi (K3) are added and punctured using the even method to inhibit the heart fire and tonify the kidney water.

● For male infertility due to decline of fire from the Gate of Life, the kidney *yang* is warmed by adding and puncturing Baihui (Du20) and Qihai (Ren6) using the reinforcing method and adding moxibustion on Mingmen (Du4) and Guanyuan (Ren4).

● For male infertility due to stagnation of the liver *qi*, Taichong (Liv3), Neiguan (P6) and Yanglingquan (G34) are added and punctured using the reducing method to soothe the liver *qi*.

● For male infertility due to descent of damp-heat from the liver and gallbladder, Zhongji (Ren3), Ligou (Liv5) and Yinlingquan (Sp9) are added and punctured using the reducing method to expel heat and dredge dampness.

● For male infertility due to stagnation of *qi* and blood, Taichong (Liv3), Qugu (Ren2) and Guilai (S29) are added and punctured using the reducing method to improve circulation of the *qi* and blood.

Treat once a day or once every other day. Ten treatments constitute one course.

Moxibustion

Acupuncture points:

Guanyuan	(Ren4)
Qihai	(Ren6)
Shenque	(Ren8)
Shenshu	(B23)
Mingmen	(Du4)
Yaoyangguan	(Du3)
Sanyinjiao	(Sp6)

Select two to four points each time. Apply moxa roll moxibustion to each point for 10–20 minutes. Treat once a day or once every other day. Ten treatments constitute one course.

Non-scarring moxa cone moxibustion is usually used on Guanyuan (Ren4). Apply 100–200 small moxa cones (0.5 cm height and diameter) once every other week. Three treatments constitute one course.

Moxa cone moxibustion on Shenque (Ren8) is usually used in combination with salt. Put a layer of fine salt on the umbilicus, then burn 10–30 small moxa cones on the salt. Treat once a day or once every other day. Ten treatments constitute one course.

Moxibustion functions to strengthen the kidneys, warm *yang* and improve the circulation of *qi* and blood, so it is suitable for treating male infertility due to unconsolidated kidney *qi*, deficiency of the kidney essence, decline of fire from the Gate of Life, stagnation of the liver *qi*, stagnation of *qi* and blood.

Electroacupuncture

Points used are the same as for body acupuncture. Select two or three pairs of points each time. Puncture the points until a needling sensation is achieved, then connect the needles to an electrical stimulator. Apply moderate intermittent wave stimulation for 15–20 minutes. Treat once a day or once every other day. Ten treatments constitute one course.

Remarks

- The causes of male infertility are complex. It is essential to establish a diagnosis prior to treatment. Acupuncture is not effective for male infertility due to congenital or acquired organic problems of the genitals.
- When puncturing points in the lower abdomen and lumbosacral region, a needling sensation should be felt in the scrotal region.
- Men with this condition are often anxious and disturbed; it is essential to encourage them to develop a positive attitude and confidence that traditional therapies can provide a cure in order to shorten the course and improve effectiveness of treatment.
- Spermacrasia may be due to excessive sexual activity. Regulation of sexual activity should be encouraged.
- For male infertility due to impotence or seminal emission, refer to sections on these conditions.

78 Meniere's disease

Meniere's disease is a type of auditory vertigo caused by hydrops in the labyrinth of the ear. It is marked by transient paroxysmal episodes of rotatory vertigo, aggravated by changes in body position and usually accompanied by tinnitus, hearing loss, parallel nystagmus, nausea, vomiting, perspiration and pale complexion. Spontaneous cure and repeated occurrence are often seen in clinical practice.

Aetiology

Traditional Chinese medicine classifies Meniere's disease as vertigo. It is considered to be caused either by rebellious rising of hyperactive liver *yang* which disturbs the ears, or by accumulation of turbid phlegm in the Middle Jiao which obstructs the rising of clear *qi* to the ears. Pathogenic factors include endogenous wind and phlegm; primarily affected are the liver, spleen and kidneys.

Differentiation of syndromes

- Meniere's disease caused by hyperactivity of the liver *yang*.
  Characterized by sudden onset of vertigo, tinnitus or deafness; accompanied by restlessness, irritability, bitter taste in the mouth, nausea, vomiting and wiry pulse.

- Meniere's disease caused by accumulation of turbid phlegm in the Middle Jiao.

  Characterized by paroxysmal vertigo and tinnitus; accompanied by heaviness and muffled sensation in the head, drowsiness, poor appetite, nausea, vomiting, pale complexion, greasy whitish tongue coating and slippery pulse.

Treatment

Body acupuncture

Main acupuncture points:

Fengchi	(G20)
Yifeng	(SJ17)
Baihui	(Du20)
Neiguan	(P6)
Taiyang	(Ex30)
Ermen	(SJ21)
Tinggong	(SI19)
Tinghui	(G2)

The San Jiao and Gallbladder meridians are closely connected with the ears, so main points are selected from these two meridians to activate the meridians and halt vertigo. Fengchi (G20), an important point of the Gallbladder meridian located at the base of the skull, functions to dispel wind and tranquillize the mind. Yifeng (SJ17), a meeting point of the San Jiao and Gallbladder meridians located close to the ears, functions to activate the meridians and halt vertigo.

Baihui (Du20), a meeting point of the Du, Liver and six Hand and Foot Yang meridians located on the top of the head, functions to dispel endogenous wind and tranquillize the mind. Neiguan (P6), the *luo* (collateral) point of the Pericardium meridian and one of the eight confluence points connecting with the Yinwei meridian, subdues rebellious rising of *qi* and arrests nausea and vomiting. Taiyang (Ex30) has been proven through clinical experience to be effective for treating head problems. Ermen (SJ21), Tinggong (SI19) and Tinghui (G2) are three local points effective for treating ear problems.

Four to five main points are selected each time. Auxiliary points and appropriate manipulation are chosen according to differentiation of syndromes.

- For Meniere's disease caused by hyperactivity of the liver *yang*, Taichong (Liv3), Taixi (K3) and Zulinqi (G41) are added and punctured using the even method to soothe the liver *yang*.

- For Meniere's disease caused by accumulation of turbid phlegm in the Middle Jiao, Zhongwan (Ren12), Zusanli (S36), Fenglong (S40) and Sanyinjiao (Sp6) are added and punctured using the reinforcing method to strengthen the spleen and eliminate phlegm.

Treat once a day or once every other day. Ten treatments constitute one course.

Electroacupuncture

Points used are the same as for body acupuncture. Select one or two pairs of points each time. Puncture until a needling sensation is achieved, then connect the needles to an electrical stimulator. Apply moderate intermittent wave stimulation for 20–30 minutes, once a day or once every other day. Ten treatments constitute one course.

Scalp acupuncture

Scalp lines:

Ezhongxian	(MS1)
Dingzhongxian	(MS5)
Niehouxian	(MS11)

Puncture the lines using the even method for 5 minutes, or connect the needles to an electrical stimulator and apply moderate continuous wave stimulation for 20–30 minutes, once a day or once every other day. Ten treatments constitute one course.

Auricular therapy

Auricular points:

Internal Ear, External Ear: correspond to the affected area.

San Jiao, Pancreas & Gallbaldder: the San Jiao and Gallbladder meridians distribute to the ear, so San Jiao and Pancreas & Gallbaldder are treated to activate the meridians and halt vertigo.

Subcortex: regulates the nervous and circulatory systems.

Ear Shenmen, Occiput: tranquillize the mind.

Apex of Ear: blood-letting puncturing of this point with a three-edged needle calms the mind and expels wind.

Use auricular taping with strong manipulation and blood-letting puncturing where indicated, twice a week. Five treatments constitute one course.

Remarks

☯ Traditional therapies are effective for treating Meniere's disease. They can not only prevent vertigo, but can also treat the cause of the condition by relieving hydrops in the labyrinth of the ear.

☯ Auricular therapy is a simple and effective method for treating Meniere's disease. One patient reported that she had been suffering from Meniere's disease for seven years; after starting to wear earrings positioned at Internal Ear, the condition quickly disappeared.

79 Menopausal syndrome

Menopausal syndrome refers to a series of symptoms occurring during the beginning of menopause. Menopause, or cessation of the menses, and the accompanying symptoms of menopausal syndrome, are caused by a relatively sudden decrease in the production of the female hormones oestrogen and progesterone by the ovaries, with resulting changes in the endocrine and autonomic nervous systems. Menopause generally occurs between the ages of 45 and 50, although women with anovarism due to trauma, surgery or pelvic radiotherapy may also experience it much earlier.

Manifestations of menopausal syndrome are various. Cardiovascular symptoms may include intermittent flushing and sensation of heat on the face (popularly known as 'hot flashes'), palpitation, discomfort or pain in the precardial region, formication and numbness or pain of the extremities. Mental symptoms such as insomnia and unexpected mood changes are common; if they are understood to be a normal part of menopause, accompanying anxiety and irritability can often be avoided. Symptoms of metabolic dysfunction, such as obesity or oedema, may sometimes occur.

Vaginal dryness due to the decrease of hormones which stimulate the production of natural lubricants may cause irritation and soreness during sexual activity; this can be relieved by the use of commercial water-based lubricants or natural vegetable oils. Osteoporosis, or thinning of the bones that begins with menopause, can be largely prevented by sufficient calcium in the diet (1200–1500 mg per day) and regular weight-bearing exercise.

Aetiology

According to traditional Chinese medicine, menopausal syndrome is caused by gradual decline of both the *yin* and *yang* of the kidneys due to ageing, leading to dysfunction of the *zangfu* organs. Usually affected are the liver, spleen and heart. According to Five Elements Theory (see Glossary), the kidneys (water) stimulate the liver (wood), which react with the heart (fire). If the kidney *yin* is insufficient, the liver *yang* will not be nourished and will become hyperactive, the heart fire will not be controlled and the heart blood will be consumed. The kidney *yang*, also called *yuan* (original) *yang*, is the motivating force for all physiological functions of the entire body. If the kidney *yang* is insufficient, the spleen *yang* will not be warmed and will fail to transport and transform nutrients and dampness.

Differentiation of syndromes

● Menopausal syndrome due to hyperactivity of the liver *yang*.
   Characterized by dizziness, restlessness, irritability, sensation of heat throughout the body, sweating, sore and weak back and knees, red tongue and rapid wiry thready pulse.
● Menopausal syndrome due to insufficiency of the heart blood.
   Characterized by palpitation, insomnia, bad dreams, restlessness, sensation of heat in the palms and soles, mood changes, red tongue with little coating and rapid thready pulse.

- Menopausal syndrome due to deficiency of the spleen.
  Characterized by lassitude, pale complexion, poor appetite, abdominal distension, loose stool, oedema, pale tongue with whitish coating and weak pulse.
- Menopausal syndrome due to accumulation of phlegm-damp arising from deficiency of the spleen.
  Characterized by obesity, feeling of fullness in the chest, vomiting of phlegm, abdominal distension, poor appetite, loose stool, oedema, greasy tongue coating and slippery pulse.

Treatment

Body acupuncture

Main acupuncture points:

Sanyinjiao	(Sp6)
Neiguan	(P6)
Baihui	(Du20)
Fengchi	(G20)

Sanyinjiao (Sp6), the meeting point of the three Foot Yin meridians, functions to strengthen the kidneys, liver and spleen. Neiguan (P6), the *luo* (collateral) point of the Pericardium meridian and one of the eight confluence points connecting with the Yinwei meridian, functions to open the chest and calm the mind. Baihui (Du20), the meeting point of the Du, Liver and six Hand and Foot Yang meridians, is punctured to tranquillize the mind. Fengchi (G20), an important point of the Gallbladder meridian, functions to tranquillize the mind.

Auxiliary points and proper manipulation are chosen according to differentiation of syndromes.

- For menopausal syndrome due to hyperactivity of the liver *yang*, Taichong (Liv3), Taixi (K3) and Taiyang (Ex30) are added and punctured using the even method to nourish the kidney *yin* and subdue the liver *yang*.
- For menopausal syndrome due to insufficiency of the heart blood, Shenmen (H7) and Taixi (K3) are added and punctured using the even method to strengthen the kidney *yin* and calm the mind.
- For menopausal syndrome due to deficiency of the spleen, the spleen and stomach are strengthened by adding and puncturing Zusanli (S36), Qihai (Ren6) and Zhongwan (Ren12) using the reinforcing method, or applying moxibustion as needed.

- For menopausal syndrome due to accumulation of phlegm-dampness arising from deficiency of the spleen, Fenglong (S40), Danzhong (Ren17), Zhongwan (Ren12) and Zusanli (S36) are added and punctured using the even method to strengthen the spleen and dispel phlegm-dampness.

Treat once a day or once every other day. Ten treatments constitute one course.

Electroacupuncture

Points used are the same as for body acupuncture. Select one or two pairs of points each time. Puncture until a needling sensation is achieved, then connect the needles to an electrical stimulator. Apply moderate continuous wave stimulation for 20–30 minutes. Treat once a day or once every other day. Ten treatments constitute one course.

Auricular therapy

Main auricular points:

Internal Genitals: correspond to the affected region.

Kidney: strengthens the congenital essence to regulate *yin* and *yang*.

Liver: soothes the liver *qi* and calms the mind.

Endocrine, Midpoint of Rim: regulate the endocrine function.

Ear Shenmen, Subcortex: regulate the nervous function.

Auxiliary auricular points:

For insomnia, Anterior Ear Lobe and Occiput are added.

For palpitation, Heart and Chest are added.

For oedema, Spleen and Middle Superior Concha are added.

For problems of the extremities, Sympathesis and points corresponding to the affected areas are added.

Use auricular taping, twice a week. Five treatments constitute one course. Auricular self-massage may also be practised twice a day.

Remarks

☯ Traditional therapies are effective for treating menopausal syndrome. The above therapies may be either used singly, or combined to increase stimulation and improve effectiveness.

☯ The onset and development of the symptoms of menopausal syndrome are closely related to psychological factors. It is essential that women entering menopause understand its causes and manifestations; this will encourage a positive attitude and confidence that traditional therapies can relieve the symptoms of menopausal syndrome.

80 Morning sickness

Morning sickness refers to varying degrees of nausea and vomiting experienced by some women during the first trimester of pregnancy. In mild cases, symptoms are limited to mild nausea and some vomiting, usually in the morning; hence the name. Additional manifestations may include poor appetite and unusual food preferences. Morning sickness usually ends with the first trimester and does not require treatment. However, severe cases, called hyperemesis gravidarum, should be treated. In these cases vomiting is frequent or persistent and the patient may be unable to keep down any liquids or solids. Vomit may contain gall bile and coffeeground-like substance, in addition to food and mucus. General manifestations include lassitude, emaciation, palpitation, shortness of breath and impairment of hepatic and renal function. The cause of morning sickness is still not clear, but it may be related to high levels of chorionic gonadotropin, nervous or psychological factors, or hypovitaminosis.

Aetiology

According to traditional Chinese medicine, the general pathogenesis of morning sickness is rebellious rising of the stomach *qi*. There are three major causes. The abundant *qi* which is present in the Chong meridian during pregnancy may ascend to attack and deplete the stomach *qi*; mental injury may result in stagnation of the liver *qi*, which then affects the stomach; or accumulation of phlegm-dampness in the Middle Jiao caused by deficiency of the spleen may block the normal ascent and descent of the stomach *qi*.

Differentiation of syndromes

● Morning sickness due to deficiency of the stomach *qi*.
Characterized by severe nausea and vomiting, or vomiting immediately following eating, during the first trimester of pregnancy; accompanied by lassitude, anorexia, distension of the epigastric region, pale tongue with whitish coating and soft weak pulse.

● Morning sickness due to lack of coordination between the stomach and liver.
Characterized by severe vomiting during the first trimester of pregnancy with bitter vomit; accompanied by dizziness, distending pain in the chest and hypochondriac region, frequent sighing, depression, whitish tongue coating and wiry slippery pulse.

● Morning sickness due to accumulation of phlegm-dampness in the Middle Jiao.
Characterized by severe vomiting during the first trimester of pregnancy with phlegmy vomit; accompanied by feeling of fullness or distension in the epigastric region, shortness of breath, poor appetite, dizziness, greasy whitish tongue coating and slippery pulse.

Treatment

Body acupuncture

Main acupuncture points:
Neiguan   (P6)
Zhongwan   (Ren12)
Zusanli   (S36)

Neiguan (P6), the *luo* (collateral) point of the Pericardium meridian and one of the eight confluence points connecting to the Yinwei meridian, functions to subdue the rebellious rising of the stomach *qi* and is one of the most important points for treating vomiting. Zhongwan (Ren12), the front-*mu* point of the stomach, functions to strengthen the stomach. Zusanli (S36), the *he* (sea) point and lower *he* (confluent) point of the Stomach meridian, is the most important point for treating stomach problems.

Auxiliary points and proper manipulation are chosen according to differentiation of syndromes.

- For morning sickness due to deficiency of the stomach *qi*, the spleen and stomach are strengthened to arrest vomiting by adding and puncturing Gongsun (Sp4) using the reinforcing method, and applying moxibustion as needed.
- For morning sickness due to lack of coordination between the stomach and liver, Taichong (Liv3) and Yanglingquan (G34) are added and punctured using the even method to harmonize the liver and stomach.
- For morning sickness due to accumulation of phlegm-dampness in the Middle Jiao, Dangzhong (Ren17), Shangwan (Ren13) and Yinlingquan (Sp9) are added and punctured using the even method to strengthen the spleen and remove phlegm-dampness.

Treat once a day. Five treatments constitute one course.

Moxibustion

Points used are the same as for body acupuncture. Select two to four points each time. Apply moxa roll moxibustion to each point for 15–20 minutes, two or three times a day. Five days constitute one course.

Auricular therapy

Auricular points:

Stomach, Cardia: harmonize the stomach and arrest vomiting.

Liver, Spleen: soothe the liver and strengthen the spleen.

Ear Shenmen, Subcortex: tranquillize the mind.

Endocrine: regulates endocrine function.

Use auricular therapy with moderate stimulation, once every other day. Five treatments constitute one course.

Remarks

- Many clinical reports indicate that traditional therapies are very safe and effective for treating nausea and vomiting during pregnancy. Many cases show great improvement after only one or two treatments.
- Moxibustion is an especially safe, simple and effective treatment for morning sickness and can be self-applied at home.
- For those unwilling to receive acupuncture, susceptible to fainting, or with a history of repeated miscarriage, bilateral Neiguan (P6) may be pressed with the thumbs.
- A minimum of points and mild to moderate stimulation should by used. Treating the main points is generally sufficient in most cases.
- For cases with severe acidosis, electrolyte disturbance, or impairment of hepatic or renal functions, appropriate additional measures should be concurrently undertaken.

81 Motion sickness

Motion sickness commonly occurs while travelling in buses, trains, cars, aeroplanes or boats. It is caused by motion which affects the semicircular canal of the inner ear. Primary manifestations include nausea, vomiting and headache; accompanied by pale complexion, cold sweat and exhaustion.

Aetiology and differentiation of syndromes

According to traditional Chinese medicine, motion sickness is caused internally by deficiency of the stomach and spleen and externally by irritation by noxious fumes or odours. The combination of internal and external factors results in rebellious rising of the stomach *qi*.

Treatment

Body acupuncture

Acupuncture points:

Neiguan   (P6)

The primary pathogenesis of motion sickness is rebellious rising of the stomach *qi*. Neiguan (P6), the *luo* (collateral) point of the Pericardium meridian and one of the eight confluence points connecting with the Yinwei meridian, is punctured to subdue rebellious rising of the stomach *qi*. The point is punctured obliquely upward to cause a needling sensation to ascend. If it is not possible to use needles during travel, pressing the point with the thumb is also effective.

Auricular therapy

Auricular points:

Internal Ear, External Ear: harmonize the function of the vestibular organ to relieve dysfunction of the semicircular canal caused by motion.

Cardia: main point for vomiting.

Occiput, Ear Shenmen, Liver: calm the mind.

Wind Stream: main anti-allergy point; relieves irritation caused by noxious fumes and odours.

Use auricular taping and pressure. Tape the point half an hour before boarding and press periodically during travel. Most cases of motion sickness can be prevented in this way.

Remarks

☻ Both body acupuncture and auricular therapy are very effective for treating and preventing motion sickness.

82 Mumps

Mumps is an acute communicable disease caused by the mumps virus. It occurs most commonly in children and is usually epidemic in the winter and spring. Symptoms include fever, aversion to cold, headache and pain and swelling of the parotid glands. The prognosis is generally good, but if appropriate and timely treatment is not given complications may arise, including testitis or ovaritis with possible subsequent sterility, or meningitis.

Aetiology and differentiation of syndrome

According to traditional Chinese medicine, mumps is caused by exogenous wind-heat and toxic pathogens which invade the San Jiao and Gallbladder meridians, leading to obstruction of *qi* and blood in the parotid glands. The Gallbladder meridian passes through the external genitals, so invasion of the Gallbladder meridian by exogenous pathogens may result in swelling and pain of the

testes or ovaries. Mumps is characterized by pain and swelling of the parotid glands; accompanied by fever, chills, headache, thirst, constipation, scanty urine, swelling and pain of the testes or ovaries, yellowish tongue coating and rapid pulse. Loss of consciousness may occur in some severe cases.

Treatment

Body acupuncture

Main acupuncture points:

Yifeng	(SJ17)
Waiguan	(SJ5)
Fengchi	(G20)
Guanchong	(SJ1)
Shaoshang	(L11)
Jiache	(S6)

Both the San Jiao and Gallbladder meridians distribute to the parotid glands, so points on these two meridians are treated to expel exogenous pathogens. Yifeng (SJ17), a meeting point of the

San Jiao and Gallbladder meridians, is a local point for treating mumps. Waiguan (SJ5), the *luo* (collateral) point of the San Jiao meridian and one of the eight confluence points connecting with the Yangwei meridian, functions to expel wind and dispel heat and toxic pathogens. Fengchi (G20), an important point of the Gallbladder meridian located at the base of the skull, functions to expel exogenous pathogens.

Guanchong (SJ1) and Shaoshang (L11), the *jing* (well) points of the San Jiao and Lung meridians respectively, are pricked with a three-edged needle to let several drops of blood in order to dispel heat and toxic pathogens. Jiache (S6) is a local point of the Stomach meridian for treating mumps.

Auxiliary points are selected according to symptoms.

- For high fever, Dazhui (Du14) is added and punctured with a three-edged needle and then cupped for 10–15 minutes to draw blood and lower fever.
- For swelling and pain of the testes or ovaries, Taichong (Liv3), Ligou (Liv5) and Qugu (Ren2) are added.
- For nausea and vomiting, Neiguan (P6) is added.
- For loss of consciousness, Renzhong (Du26) and Shixuan (Ex1) are added.

Puncture all points using the reducing method, once a day. Five treatments constitute one course.

Auricular therapy

Main auricular points:

Jaw, Neck: correspond to the affected region of the body. Locate positive points; tape both frontal and dorsal surfaces to increase stimulation.

San Jiao, Pancreas & Gallbladder: both the San Jiao and Gallbladder meridians pass through the parotid region, so San Jiao and Pancreas & Gallbladder are taped to activate the meridian *qi* and discharge exogenous pathogens.

Endocrine, Adrenal Gland, Wind Stream: relieve inflammation.

Apex of Ear, Apex of Antitragus: blood-letting puncturing of these points with a three-edged needle dispels heat and expels pathogens.

Auxiliary auricular points:

For complication by meningitis, Subcortex, Forehead, Temple and Occiput are added.

For complication by testitis or ovaritis, Internal Genitals and Liver are added.

Use auricular taping with strong manipulation and blood-letting puncturing where indicated, once every other day. Five treatments constitute one course.

Remarks

- Both body acupuncture and auricular therapy are very effective for treating mumps. In many cases great improvement will be seen after two or three treatments.
- Traditional therapies can be used as a preventative during the mumps season.
- Body acupuncture and auricular therapy can be used singly or in combination.

83 Myocarditis

Myocarditis refers to acute, subacute or chronic inflammation, or localized or diffuse lesion of the cardiac muscles. It is caused by various factors including biopathogens, physiochemical irritation, or allergic reaction. General manifestations include palpitation, feeling of fullness in the chest, shortness of breath or even loss of consciousness. Physical exam-ination may reveal abnormal ECG and cardiac dilatation.

Aetiology

Traditional Chinese medicine classifies myocarditis as palpitation and considers it to be caused primarily by exogenous toxic heat pathogens which attack the pericardium and consume the *qi*, blood, *yin* and *yang* of the heart.

Differentiation of syndromes

● Myocarditis due to deficiency of *qi* and heart *yin*.
  Characterized by palpitation, feeling of fullness in the chest, lassitude, sensation of heat in the palms and soles, night sweating, red tongue with little coating and rapid thready pulse.
● Myocarditis due to deficiency of the heart *yang*.
  Characterized by palpitation, feeling of fullness in the chest, pale complexion, spontaneous sweating, aversion to cold, loss of consciousness, pale or swollen tongue with teeth marks and whitish coating and knotty intermittent pulse.
● Myocarditis due to deficiency of the heart and spleen.
  Characterized by palpitation, shortness of breath, lassitude, poor appetite, abdominal distension, loose stool, pale and swollen tongue with whitish coating and weak thready pulse.

Treatment

Body acupuncture

Main acupuncture points:

Shenmen	(H7)
Tongli	(H5)
Neiguan	(P6)
Danzhong	(Ren17)
Xinshu	(B15)
Jueyinshu	(B14)

Points of the Heart and Pericardium meridians and their back-*shu* points are selected as main points to strengthen the heart and calm the mind. Shenmen (H7), the *yuan* (source) point and Tongli (H5), the *luo* (collateral) point respectively of the Heart meridian, are treated in combination to calm the mind and relieve palpitation. Neiguan (P6), the *luo* (collateral) point of the Pericardium meridian and one of the eight confluence points connecting with the Yinwei meridian, is an important point for treating all heart problems.
    Jueyinshu (B14) and Xinshu (B15), the back-*shu* points of the pericardium and heart respec-tively and Danzhong (Ren17), the front-*mu* point of the pericardium and the *hui* (influential) point of *qi*, are treated in combination to strengthen the heart and increase its supply of nutrients.
    Auxiliary points and appropriate methods of manipulation are chosen according to differentiation of syndromes:

● For myocarditis due to deficiency of *qi* and heart *yin*, Zusanli (S36), Sanyinjiao (Sp6) and Yinxi (H6) are added and punctured using the even method to tonify *qi* and nourish *yin*.
● For myocarditis due to deficiency of the heart *yang*, the heart is warmed by adding and puncturing Dazhui (Du14) and Mingmen (Du4) using the reinforcing method, or adding moxibustion as needed.
● For myocarditis due to deficiency of the heart and spleen, Zusanli (S36), Sanyinjiao (Sp6) and Zhongwan (Ren12) are added and punctured using the reinforcing method to strengthen the spleen and stomach.

Treat once a day or once every other day. Ten treatments constitute one course.

Auricular therapy

Auricular points:

Heart, Chest: correspond to the affected areas of the body. Locate positive points; tape both frontal and dorsal surfaces to increase stimulation.

Spleen, Stomach: strengthen the spleen and stomach.

Subcortex, Ear Shenmen, Occiput: tranquillize the mind.

Use auricular taping with moderate stimulation, twice a week. Ten treatments constitute one course.

Remarks

☙ Traditional therapies can effectively relieve the symptoms of myocarditis, shorten the duration of the disease and decrease the occurrence of chronic myocarditis and sequelae of myocarditis.
☙ Most cases of myocarditis can be cured if treated promptly and correctly. Patients should be educated concerning their condition in order to increase effectiveness of treatment.

84 Myopia

Myopia is a visual disorder caused by dysfunction of the optic dioptric system. The visual focus is formed in the front of the retina when light passes through the optic dioptric system; dysfunction of this system affects the ability to focus normally. Myopia is marked by poor distance vision and normal near-range vision. The more extreme the condition, the shorter the range of normal vision. A common cause of myopia is improper or overuse of the eyes, although severe myopia is usually related to heredity.

Aetiology

According to traditional Chinese medicine, myopia is caused either by congenital insufficiency or by acquired factors which damage the liver, kidneys and spleen, leading to insufficient nourishment of the eyes.

Differentiation of syndromes

- Myopia due to insufficiency of the liver and kidneys.
  Characterized by reduced or blurred vision; accompanied by dizziness, headache, poor memory, lassitude, thin pale tongue with thin whitish coating and deep thready pulse.
- Myopia due to deficiency of the spleen and stomach.
  Characterized by reduced vision; accompanied by lassitude, emaciation, sallow complexion, poor appetite, pale tongue with whitish coating and weak pulse.

Treatment

Body acupuncture

Main acupuncture points:

Taichong	(Liv3)
Fengchi	(G20)
Guangming	(G37)
Muchuang	(G16)
Zanzhu	(B2)
Sibai	(S2)
Taiyang	(Ex30)
Yuyao	(Ex28)

The liver opens into the eyes and the Liver and Gallbladder meridians connect with the eyes. The liver and gallbladder are connected both internally and externally. Therefore, main distal points are selected from the Liver and Gallbladder meridians to brighten the eyes. Taichong (Liv3), the *yuan* (source) point of the the Liver meridian, functions to activate the meridians and brighten the eyes. Fengchi (G20), an important point of the Gallbladder meridian located at the base of the skull, is treated to expel wind and brighten the eyes. It is a main point for treating various eye problems. Guangming (G37), (Brightness in Chinese), the *luo* (collateral) point of the Gallbladder meridian, strengthens both the liver and gallbladder and brightens the eyes. Muchuang (G16) (Window of the Eyes in Chinese) is effective for treating various eye problems.

Zanzhu (B2), Sibai (S2), Yuyao (Ex28) and Taiyang (Ex30) are local points for treating eye problems. Sibai (S2) is punctured obliquely towards Jingming (B1) for 1.0 *cun* until soreness, distension or tears occur.

Auxiliary points and appropriate manipulation are chosen according to diffentiation of syndromes:

- For myopia due to insufficiency of the liver and kidneys, Ganshu (B18), Shenshu (B23) and Taixi (K3) are added and punctured using the reinforcing method to strengthen the liver and kidneys.
- For myopia due to deficiency of the spleen and stomach, Zusanli (S36) and Sanyinjiao (Sp6) are added and punctured using the reinforcing method to strengthen the spleen and stomach.

Treat once a day or once every other day. Ten treatments constitute one course.

Auricular therapy

Auricular points:

Eye, Eye 2: correspond to the affected area. Locate positive points; tape both frontal and dorsal surfaces to increase stimulation.

Liver, Pancreas & Gallbladder: activate the meridians and brighten the eyes.

Spleen, Kidney: strengthens the spleen and kidneys.

Occiput, Subcortex: regulate the optic nerve function.

Apex of Ear: blood-letting puncturing of this point with a three-edged needle brightens the eyes.

Use auricular taping with strong manipulation and blood-letting puncturing where indicated, twice a week. Ten treatments constitute one course.

Remarks

- ☯ Traditional therapies are much more effective for treating pseudomyopia than genuine myopia. The earlier treatment is instituted, the better the results will be.
- ☯ Body acupuncture and auricular therapy can be either used singly or combined to increase effectiveness. Auricular therapy is more commonly used in clinical practice because of its effectiveness, simplicity and acceptability to patients.
- ☯ Avoidance of eye strain and daily practice of eye exercises will increase the effectiveness of traditional therapies.
- ☯ The following self-massage eye exercise based on meridian theory can prevent and treat myopia:
  - Step 1: With eyes closed, use the balls of the thumbs to press Jingming (B1) towards the root of the nose 32 times (Fig. 1).
  - Step 2: With the thumbs on Taiyang (Ex30), use the radial sides of the index fingers to massage the supraorbital and intraorbital margins 32 times; then use the thumbs to press Taiyang (Ex30) 32 times (Fig. 2).
  - Step 3: Use the index fingers to press Sibai (S2) 32 times (Fig. 3).
  - Step 4: Use the index and middle fingers to press Fengchi (G20) 32 times (Fig. 4).
  - Step 5: Holding the fingers together, massage along the nose to the forehead, to bilateral Taiyang (Ex30) and downward along the cheeks. Repeat eight times (Fig. 5). This motion resembles washing the face and is called 'dry face washing.'

Self-massage Eye Exercise (figs 1–5)

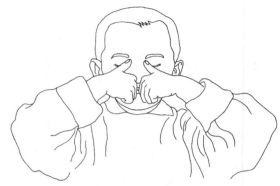

Fig. 1 Press Jingming (B1)

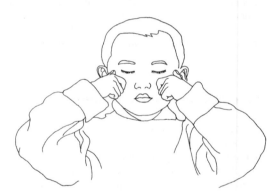

Fig. 2 Massage orbital margins and press Taiyang (Ex30)

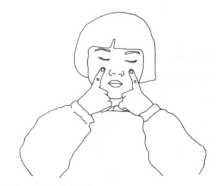

Fig. 3 Press Sibai (S2)

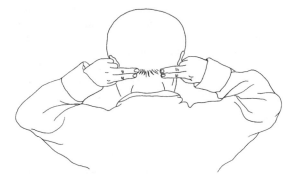

Fig. 4 Press Fengchi (G20)

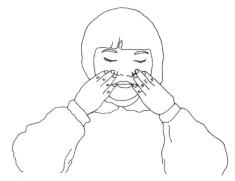

Fig. 5 Dry-wash face

85 Neurodermatitis

Neurodermatitis is a type of itching dermoneurosis usually induced by mental injury or localized physical irritation. It is marked by lichenoid skin lesions accompanied by paroxysmal itching. Localized itching occurs in the initial stage, with dense groups of circular or polygonal pimples appearing as the result of extensive scratching. As the condition develops, deep dermatoglyph, dermal ridging and brown pachyderma appear.

Neurodermatitis is classified into localized and disseminated types. The former is much more common and occurs primarily on the bilateral sides and back of the neck, the elbows, the extension aspect of the forearm, the sacral region, the medial sides of the thighs and the fibular aspect of the legs. The latter occurs mainly in the craniofacial region or on the shoulders, the extremities or the trunk.

Aetiology

According to traditional Chinese medicine, neurodermatitis is caused either by exogenous pathogens such as wind, dampness, or heat which obstruct the flow of *qi* and blood in the skin; or by deficiency of blood which produces endogenous wind and subsequent insufficient nourishment of the skin.

Differentiation of syndromes

● Neurodermatitis caused by obstruction of *qi* and blood by exogenous pathogens.

Characterized by short course, severe itching, dense groups of circular or polygonal pimples, oozing erosion and scabs; accompanied by restlessness, dryness of the mouth, greasy or thin yellowish tongue coating and rapid pulse.
● Neurodermatitis caused by endogenous wind resulting from blood deficiency.

Characterized by long course, severe itching, various skin lesions including deep dermatoglyph, dermal ridging and brown pachyderma; pale tongue with thin whitish coating and thready pulse.

Treatment

Body acupuncture

Main acupuncture points:

Quchi	(LI11)
Hegu	(LI4)
Xuehai	(Sp10)
Sanyinjiao	(Sp6)
Areas of skin lesions	

Quchi (LI11) and Hegu (LI4), the *he* (sea) and *yuan* (source) points respectively of the Large Intestine meridian, are treated in combination to activate the meridians and relieve itching. Xuehai (Sp10) (Sea of Blood in Chinese) functions to promote the flow of blood and is one of the most important points for treating skin conditions. Sanyinjiao (Sp6), the meeting point of the three Foot Yin meridians, functions to strengthen the liver and spleen and promote the flow of blood.

For localized neurodermatitis, either of two methods are used to puncture the areas of the skin lesions to promote the flow of blood and expel wind. First, several needles may be used simultaneously to puncture the area surrounding the lesions from different directions. The needles are positioned approximately 0.5–1.0 *cun* away from the border of the affected area and inserted subcutaneously towards the centre of the area to a length of 1.5–2.0 *cun*. The number of needles used depends on the size of the affected area; generally four to eight needles are applied. Second, the affected area and surrounding region may be moderately to heavily tapped with a plum blossom needle to induce bleeding. The blood is then absorbed with dry cotton.

Auxiliary points and appropriate manipulation are added according to differentiation of syndromes:

● For neurodermatitis caused by obstruction of *qi* and blood by exogenous pathogens, pathogens are expelled by adding and puncturing Fengchi (G20), Dazhui (Du14) and Weizhong (B40) using the reducing method; or pricking Dazhui (Du14) and Weizhong (B40) with a three-edged needle to let several drops of blood and then cupping for 10–15 minutes.
● For neurodermatitis caused by endogenous wind resulting from blood deficiency, *qi* is strengthened and endogenous wind extinguished by adding and puncturing Geshu (B17), Feishu (B13), Qihai (Ren6) and Zusanli (S36) using the reinforcing method and applying moxibustion to the affected areas.

Treat once a day or once every other day. Ten treatments constitute one course.

Moxibustion

Points:

   Areas of skin lesions

Two method of applying moxibustion may be used.

Moxa cone moxibustion

Make small moxa cones approximately the size of a match-head. Coat the affected area with garlic juice and apply moxa cones to the area, one to three cones to each point, spaced about 0.5 *cun* apart. Ignite the cones and allow them to burn freely. Remove the ashes and cover the area with

sterilized material. Treat once every ten days, choosing different points each time. There will generally be great improvement after two or three treatments. To alleviate pain during treatment, tap the area surrounding the affected region with the palms of the hands, or puncture with two needles on opposite sides of the affected area and connect with an electrical stimulator for an anaesthetic effect.

Herbal moxibustion, or medicinal vesiculation

Grind 12 g of Chinese blistering beetle and 4 g of realgar into a powder and mix with enough honey to make a thick paste. Apply a piece of paste the size of a small bean to the centre of the affected area for approximately 32 hours, then remove the paste. A yellowish blister the size of a small bean will be left. The blister will heal after about one week. Repeat the treatment, applying three or four additional bean-sized pieces of herbal paste to other parts of the affected area. This method is effective, painless and will not leave scars.

Both cone and herbal moxibustion are suitable for treating localized neurodermatitis.

Electroacupuncture

Points used are the same as for body acupuncture. Select one or two pairs of points each time. Puncture until a needling sensation is achieved; then connect the needles to an electrical stimulator. Apply intermittent wave stimulation of the highest bearable intensity for 20–30 minutes, once a day or once every other day. Ten treatments constitute one course.

Blood-letting puncturing

Points:

   Areas of skin lesions

Strictly sterilize the affected areas. Tap heavily several times with a plum blossom needle, then cup for 10–15 minutes to draw blood.

Treat once every two to three days. Five treatments constitute one course. This method is suitable for treating localized neurodermatitis.

Auricular therapy

Auricular points:

   Areas corresponding to location of the skin lesions: tap with a plum blossom needle to cause bleeding and expel wind, dispel damp-heat and relieve itching.

Lung: the lungs nourish the skin, so Lung is treated to dispel pathogens from the skin.

Liver: soothes the liver to regulate the flow of *qi* and blood.

Endocrine, Adrenal Gland, Wind Stream: relieve infection.

Apex of Ear: blood-letting puncturing of this point with a three-edged needle expels wind and dispels heat to relieve itching.

Heart, Ear Shenmen, Occiput, Subcortex: calm the mind and relieve itching.

Use auricular taping with strong manipulation and blood-letting puncturing where indicated, twice a week. Five treatments constitute one course.

Remarks

😊 Traditional remedies are effective for treating neurodermatitis, especially the localized type.

😊 Neurodermatitis is a chronic and refractory skin problem. Two or more therapies are usually used in combination to increase stimulation.

😊 Avoid scratching the affected areas.

86 Neurosism

Neurosism is one of the neuroses most commonly seen in clinical practice. It occurs primarily in adults and more often in women than in men. It is caused either by mental injury such as depression, anxiety, anger, or grief; or by inappropriate mental exertion during the weakened physical state following prolonged illness. These conditions result in imbalance between excitement and inhibition of the cerebral cortex. Symptoms include insomnia, bad dreams, dizziness, headache, palpitation, perspiration, depression, restlessness, irritability, listlessness, lassitude, poor appetite and poor memory.

Aetiology

Traditional Chinese medicine classifies neurosism as insomnia, *yu* syndrome, seminal emission, or sexual dysfunction, according to the primary manifestations of each case. It has several possible causes: febrile diseases or prolonged illness may consume the body *yin* with resulting insufficient nourishment of the heart; mental injury may damage the liver, heart, or spleen; or overexertion or excessive sexual activity may damage the kidney essence. Primarily affected are the heart, liver, spleen and kidneys.

Differentiation of syndromes

● Neurosism due to stagnation of the liver *qi*.
Characterized by depression, irritability, feeling of fullness in the chest and hypochondriac region, frequent sighing, insomnia, bad dreams, bluish complexion, thin whitish tongue coating and wiry pulse.

● Neurosism due to disturbance of the heart by the liver fire.
Characterized by restlessness, irritability, insomnia, nightmares, bitter taste in the mouth, dry throat, headache, scanty yellowish urine, red tongue with yellowish coating and rapid wiry pulse.

● Neurosism due to loss of coordination between the liver and stomach.
Characterized by restlessness, depression, insomnia and pain in the chest, hypochondriac region or abdomen; accompanied by anorexia, eructation, hiccups, listlessness, lassitude, loose stool or constipation, greasy whitish tongue coating and wiry pulse.

● Neurosism due to deficiency of the heart and spleen.
Characterized by palpitation, panic, poor memory, insomnia, bad dreams, listlessness, lassitude, poor appetite, abdominal distension, sal-

low complexion, emaciation, loose stool, pale tongue with whitish coating and weak thready pulse.

● Neurosism due to imbalance between the heart *yang* and kidney *yin*.
Characterized by refractory insomnia, bad dreams, palpitation, restlessness, dizziness, tinnitus and poor memory; accompanied by sensation of heat in the palms and soles, night sweating, seminal emission while dreaming, irregular menstruation, red tongue with little coating and rapid thready pulse.

● Neurosism due to deficiency of the kidney *yang*.
Characterized by listlessness, insomnia, premature ejaculation, sexual dysfunction, or seminal emission while awake; accompanied by dizziness, tinnitus, poor memory, sore and weak back and knees, sensation of cold in the extremities, thin whitish tongue coating and deep thready pulse.

● Neurosism due to disturbance of the heart by phlegm-heat.
Characterized by insomnia, restlessness, nightmares, heavy feeling in the head and vertigo; accompanied by feeling of fullness in the chest, nausea, vomiting, bitter taste in the mouth, red tongue with yellowish greasy coating and slippery wiry pulse.

Treatment

Body acupuncture

Main acupuncture points:

Baihui	(Du20)
Fengchi	(G20)
Neiguan	(P6)

The general therapeutic principle for treating neurosism is to tranquillize the mind. Baihui (Du20), the meeting point of the Du, Liver and six Yang Hand and Foot meridians located on the top of the head, is treated to tranquillize the mind. In clinical practice Baihui (Du20) is usually punctured alternately with Sishencong (Ex26) in order to increase stimulation. Fengchi (G20), an important point of the Gallbladder meridian located at the base of the skull, is effective for tranquillizing the mind. Neiguan (P6), the *luo* (collateral) point of the Pericardium meridian and one of the eight confluence points connecting with the Yinwei meridian, functions to open the chest and calm the mind.

Auxiliary points and appropriate methods of manipulation are chosen according to differentiation of syndromes.

● For neurosism due to stagnation of the liver *qi*, Taichong (Liv3) and Yanglingquan (G34) are added and punctured using the reducing method to promote the flow of the liver *qi*.

● For neurosism due to disturbance of the heart by the liver fire, Xingjian (Liv2) and Zulinqi (G41) are added and punctured using the reducing method to eliminate pathogenic fire.

● For neurosism due to loss of coordination between the liver and stomach, Taichong (Liv3), Zhongwan (Ren12) and Zusanli (S36) are added and punctured using the even method to harmonize the liver and stomach.

● For neurosism due to deficiency of the heart and spleen, Shenmen (H7), Sanyinjiao (Sp6), Zusanli (S36), Xinshu (B15) and Pishu (B20) are added and punctured using the reinforcing method to strengthen the heart and spleen.

● For neurosism due to imbalance between the heart *yang* and kidney *yin*, Shenmen (H7), Taixi (K3) and Sanyinjiao (Sp6) are added and punctured using the even method to nourish the kidney *yin* and subdue the heart *yang*.

● For neurosism due to deficiency of the kidney *yang*, the kidney *yang* is warmed by adding and puncturing Shenshu (B23), Mingmen (Du4), Guanyuan (Ren4) and Taixi (K3) using the reinforcing method, and adding moxibustion as needed.

● For neurosism due to disturbance of the heart by phlegm-heat, Fenglong (S40), Zhongwan (Ren12) and Sanyinjiao (Sp6) are added and punctured using the reducing method to eliminate phlegm and dispel heal.

Treat once a day or once every other day. Ten treatments constitute one course.

Electroacupuncture

Points used are the same as for body acupuncture. Select one or two pairs of points each time. Puncture the points until a needling sensation is achieved, then connect the needles to an electrical stimulator. Apply moderate intermittent wave stimulation for 15–20 minutes. Treat once a day or once every other day. Ten treatments constitute one course.

Auricular therapy

Main auricular points:

Subcortex: harmonizes excitation and inhibition of the cerebral cortex.

Anterior Ear Lobe (also called Neurosism Point): tranquillizes the mind.

Ear Shenmen, Occiput: tranquillize the mind.

Apex of Ear: blood-letting puncturing of this point with a three-edged needle tranquillizes the mind and clears the brain.

Auxiliary auricular points:

For stagnation of the liver *qi*, Liver and Chest are added to soothe the liver, regulate the flow of *qi* and open the chest.

For imbalance of the heart and kidneys, Heart and Kidney are added to cause the heart fire to descend and the kidney water to ascend, thus correcting the imbalance.

For loss of coordination between the liver and stomach; Spleen, Stomach, Abdomen and Liver are added to invigorate the spleen and stomach and promote the flow of *qi*.

Use auricular taping and blood-letting puncturing where indicated, twice a week. Five treatments constitute one course. Auricular pressure or self-massage may also be practiced twice a day.

Remarks

☙ Traditional therapies are very effective for treating all types of neurosism. Auricular therapy is particularly valuable due to its simplicity and acceptability to patients.

☙ Massage of the auriculae and acupuncture points located on the head, including Taiyang (Ex30), Baihui (Du20), Fengchi (G20) and Wangu (G12), before bed can help improve sleep.

87 Nocturnal enuresis

Nocturnal enuresis refers to unconscious urination during sleep. It occurs mainly in children. In the majority of cases it is a functional disorder which may occur due to developmental retardation of the micturition reflex, malnutrition or irregular sleeping habits. It may also occur as a symptom of diseases such as spina bifida or enterobiasis. Traditional therapies are suitable primarily for treating functional enuresis.

Aetiology and differentiation of syndromes

According to traditional Chinese medicine, urine is stored in the urinary bladder and urination is controlled by the kidney *qi*. If the kidney *qi* is deficient, control of urination will be affected. In mild cases, there are no symptoms other than urination during sleep once a night or every few nights. In severe cases, urination during sleep may occur several times a night, often accompanied by

lassitude, sore and weak back and knees, pale complexion, poor appetite, emaciation or even developmental disability. Nocturnal enuresis is characterized by pale tongue and deep, thready, weak pulse.

Treatment

Body acupuncture

Main acupuncture points:

Guanyuan	(Ren4)
Sanyinjiao	(Sp6)

Guanyuan (Ren4), the meeting point of the Ren and three Foot Yin meridians, is an important point for tonifying the kidney *qi* and *yang*. Sanyinjiao (Sp6), the meeting point of the three Foot Yin meridians, is punctured to reinforce the spleen and kidneys. Guanyuan (Ren4) is punctured obliquely downward until a needling sensation is felt in the external genitals.

- For mild cases, the two main points are punctured using the reinforcing method.
- For severe cases, the spleen and kidneys are warmed by adding and puncturing Shenshu (B23), Pangguangshu (B28), Zusanli (S36) and Baihui (Du20) using the reinforcing method; or puncturing and then applying moxibustion to Guanyuan (Ren4) and Shenque (Ren8) for 15 minutes.

Treat mild cases once a day; five treatments constitute one course. Treat severe cases once a day; ten treatments constitute one course.

Moxibustion

Points chosen are the same as for body acupuncture. Select two to four points each time. Apply moxa roll moxibustion to each point for 15–20 minutes. Treat once a day. Five treatments constitute one course.

Since this method is painless, it is usually well accepted by children. For children who are uncooperative, moxibustion may be given by the parents while the children are sleeping.

Point implantation therapy

Points chosen are the same as for body acupuncture. Using a triangular suture needle, implant surgical catgut on two to three points each time. Points may be treated repeatedly or alternately. Treat every three to four weeks. Three treatments constitute one course.

This method is usually not well accepted by children. Its use should be reserved for very severe cases or for adults.

Auricular therapy

Auricular points:

Kidney, Bladder, Lumbosacral Vertebrae: correspond to the affected area of the body; reinforce the kidneys to increase bladder capacity.

Subcortex, Forehead: regulate the function of the cerebral cortex to strengthen the micturition reflex.

Midpoint of Rim: corresponds to the pituitary gland; has antidiuretic properties.

Use auricular taping, twice a week. Five treatments constitute one course.

Remarks

- Acupuncture is an ideal therapy for treating nocturnal enuresis. There will generally be great improvement after three to five treatments. However, an additional course of treatment should be given after cessation of enuresis to consolidate the results and prevent relapse.
- The various methods discussed in this section may be used singly or in combination.
- Traditional therapies are ineffective in cases of enuresis with organic causes such as spina bifida or spinal cord injury. For cases caused by enterobiasis, acupuncture should be used auxiliary to aetiological treatment.
- Traditional therapies are suitable for treating elderly people with problems of frequent urination or urinary incontinence, or women experiencing post-partum urinary incontinence.

88 Obesity

Obesity is a commonly occurring condition. Its causes include nervous dysfunction, endocrine disorder, metabolic disturbance, improper diet, drugs, or heredity. It is marked by excessive fat deposits resulting in weight 20 per cent or more greater than standard.

Aetiology

Traditional Chinese medicine classifies obesity into excessive and deficient types. The excessive type may be either congenital, or caused by excessive consumption of fatty or sweet foods. The deficient type is due to deficiency of the spleen and stomach which results in accumulation of dampness and phlegm in the interior.

Differentiation of syndromes

● Excessive type.
Characterized by evenly distributed fat deposits, strong muscles, excessive appetite, flushed complexion, aversion to heat, profuse sweating, abdominal distension, constipation, normal or red tongue with thin yellowish coating and forceful pulse.
● Deficient type.
Characterized by unevenly distributed fat deposits, flaccid muscles, poor appetite, pale complexion, lassitude, drowsiness, aversion to cold, spontaneous sweating increasing with activity, hard or loose stool, scanty urine, pale tongue with thin whitish coating and deep thready pulse.

Treatment

Body acupuncture

Main acupuncture points:

Zhongwan	(Ren12)
Tianshu	(S25)
Zusanli	(S36)
Yinlingquan	(Sp9)
Sanyinjiao	(Sp6)

The spleen and stomach provide the material basis for the acquired constitution. Digestion and absorption of essential nutrients depend closely on the proper functioning of these organs. Therefore, points which function to regulate the spleen and stomach are selected to maintain normal weight.

Zhongwan (Ren12), the *hui* (influential) point of the *fu* organs and the front-*mu* point of the stomach; Tianshu (S25), the front-*mu* point of the large intestine; and Zusanli (S36), the *he* (sea) and lower *he* (confluent) point of the Stomach meridian, are treated in combination to regulate the stomach. Yinlingquan (Sp9), the *he* (sea) point of the Spleen meridian and Sanyinjiao (Sp6), the meeting point of the three Foot Yin meridians, are treated in combination to regulate the spleen.

Auxiliary points and appropriate manipulation are chosen according to differentiation of syndromes.

● For excessive type obesity, Quchi (LI11), Zhigou (SJ6), Neiting (S44) and Zhongji (Ren3) are added and punctured using the reducing method to decrease absorption and increase metabolism.
● For deficient type obesity, Qihai (Ren6), Guanyuan (Ren4) and Shenshu (B23) are added and punctured using the reinforcing method to strengthen the stomach, spleen and kidneys and remove dampness and phlegm.

Auricular therapy

Auricular points:

Endocrine, Midpoint of Rim: regulate endocrine function.

Spleen: strengthens the spleen to remove dampness and phlegm.

Kidney, San Jiao: promote drainage of water.

Lung, Large Intestine: increase excretion.

Subcortex, Forehead: regulate excitation and inhibition of the central nervous system.

Abdomen, Middle Superior Concha: remove dampness and phlegm.

Use auricular taping with strong manipulation, twice a week. Ten treatments constitute one course. Auricular self-massage and pressure may also be practised periodically during the day. Extended treatment should be pursued.

Remarks

◕ Traditional therapies are more effective for treating simple obesity than obesity due to nervous disorder, endocrine dysfunction, or metabolic disturbance. In cases of simple obesity, acquired obesity responds more readily to treatment than constitutional obesity.
◕ The effectiveness, simplicity and acceptability to patients of auricular therapy make it one of the most commonly used therapies for treating obesity.
◕ Body acupuncture is usually given in combination with auricular therapy in order to increase stimulation.
◕ It is necessary to regulate diet (more fruit and vegetables; less fatty, sweet and refined foods) and undertake an appropriate exercise programme during and after treatment in order to consolidate the results.

89 Otitis media suppurativa

Otitis media suppurativa is one of the most commonly seen infectious diseases of the ear. It is classified into acute and chronic types. Manifestations include intermittent or persistent secretion of pus from the ears, tinnitus and hearing loss.

Aetiology

Traditional Chinese medicine classifies otitis media suppurativa into excessive and deficient types. The excessive type is caused externally by invasion of damp-heat and internally by hyperactivity of the liver and gallbladder fire. The combination of external and internal factors results in the accumulation of damp-heat and toxic pathogens in the ears. The deficient type usually develops from the acute type following damage of the antipathogenic *qi* by long-standing presence of pathogens in the body.

Differentiation of syndromes

● Excessive type otitis media suppurativa.
  Characterized by ear pain with sticky yellowish pus and tinnitus; accompanied by headache, fever, bitter taste in the mouth, dry throat, restlessness, constipation, scanty urine, red tongue with yellowish coating and rapid wiry pulse.
● Deficient type otitis media suppurativa.
  Characterized by long-standing intermittent or persistent secretion of dilute or sticky pus from the ears and hearing loss; accompanied by dizziness, lassitude, sallow complexion, poor appetite, loose stool, pale tongue with whitish coating and weak pulse.

Treatment

Body acupuncture

Main acupuncture points:

Fengchi	(G20)
Yifeng	(SJ17)
Ermen	(SJ21)
Tinggong	(SI19)
Tinghui	(G2)

The San Jiao and Gallbladder meridians are closely connected with the ears, so main points for treating otitis media suppurativa are selected primarily from these meridians to activate antipathogenic *qi* and expel exogenous pathogens. Fengchi (G20), an important point of the Gallbladder meridian located at the base of the skull, functions to dispel heat and is a main point for treating various problems of the sensory organs. Yifeng (SJ17), the meeting point of the San Jiao and Gallbladder meridians, functions to dispel heat and benefit the ears. Ermen (SJ21), Tinggong (SI19) and Tinghui (G2) are three main local points effective for treating ear problems.

Auxiliary points and appropriate manipulation are chosen according to differentiation of syndromes.

● For excessive type otitis media suppurativa, Zulinqi (G41) and Zhongzhu (SJ3) are added and punctured using the reducing method to dispel excessive heat.
● For deficient type otitis media suppurativa, Zusanli (S36), Sanyinjiao (Sp6), Zhongwan (Ren12) and Baihui (Du20) are added and punctured using the reinforcing method to strengthen antipathogenic *qi*.

Treat the excessive type once a day; five treatments constitute one course. Treat the deficient type once a day or once every other day; ten treatments constitute one course.

Moxibustion

Acupuncture point:

Yifeng	(SJ17)

Apply moxa roll moxibustion for 15–20 minutes once a day. Ten treatments constitute one course. This method functions to strengthen the antipathogenic *qi* and is suitable for treating deficient type otitis media suppurativa.

Auricular therapy

Auricular points:

Internal Ear, External Ear, Temple: correspond to the affected area. Tape both frontal and dorsal surfaces of Internal Ear to increase stimulation.

San Jiao, Pancreas & Gallbladder: the San Jiao and Gallbladder meridians distribute to the ears, so these points are treated to clear and activate the meridians and collaterals.

Kidney: the kidneys open into the ears, so Kidney is treated to benefit the ears.

Endocrine, Adrenal Gland: relieve inflammation.

Subcortex: regulates the nervous and circulatory functions.

Apex of Ear: blood-letting puncturing of this point with a three-edged needle dispels heat and expels pathogens.

Use auricular taping with strong manipulation and blood-letting puncturing where indicated, twice a week. Five treatments constitute one course.

Remarks

☯ Traditional therapies are effective for treating otitis media suppurativa. Purulent secretions should be cleansed from the external auditory canal prior to treatment.

☯ These methods are also suitable for treating acute and chronic otitis media catarrhalis.

90 Pancreatitis

Pancreatitis refers to acute or chronic inflammation of the pancreas. Acute pancreatitis is caused by the overflow of pancreatic secretions from the pancreatic duct, resulting in inflammation of the pancreas and its surrounding tissues. It is marked by suddenly occurring, persistent stabbing pain in the left upper abdomen, with paroxysmal exacerbation and radiation to the lumbar region, back and left shoulder. It is usually accompanied by nausea, vomiting, fever, profuse perspiration and even tetany or toxic shock. Acute pancreatitis occurs primarily in adolescents and the elderly and is usually induced by biliary ascariasis, overindulgence in food or alcohol, or mental injury.

Chronic pancreatitis is marked by frequently recurring severe pain in the upper abdomen, radiating to the lumbar region, back and left shoulder and usually lasting for four to five hours. During the remission stage there may be no symptoms or minor dull pain in the upper abdomen. Some cases are marked by protracted, persistent, gradually worsening pain in the upper abdomen, while others may have no pain at all. Chronic pancreatitis occurs primarily in the middle-aged and more often in males than in females. Alcoholics and people with a history of cholecystitis, cholangitis, cholelithiasis or acute pancreatitis are at high risk for chronic pancreatitis.

Aetiology

Traditional Chinese medicine classifies pancreatitis as abdominal pain and considers it to be caused primarily by overindulgence in greasy food or alcohol, roundworm or mental injury, any of which can disturb the flow of *qi* in the interior. Mainly affected are the spleen, stomach, liver and gallbladder.

Differentiation of syndromes

● Pancreatitis due to stagnation of the liver *qi*.
  Characterized by persistent or paroxysmal pain in the upper abdomen with tenderness and mild or no muscular tension; accompanied by nausea, vomiting, poor appetite, loose stool, thin whitish or yellowish tongue coating and thready or tense pulse.
● Pancreatitis due to excessive heat in the spleen and stomach.
  Characterized by suddenly occurring, persistent stabbing pain in the upper abdomen with paroxysmal exacerbation and radiation to the lumbar region, back and left shoulder; horizontal tenderness and severe muscular tension in the upper abdomen; accompanied by high fever, chills, abdominal distension, nausea,

vomiting, thirst, constipation, scanty yellowish urine, red tongue with thick greasy or dry yellowish coating and full rapid pulse. There may be profuse perspiration and even tetany or toxic shock in severe cases.

● Pancreatitis due to accumulation of damp-heat in the liver and gallbladder.

Characterized by suddenly occurring distending pain in the upper abdomen slightly to the right, with paroxysmal exacerbation and radiation to the right lumbar region and shoulder and horizontal tenderness and mild muscular tension in the upper abdomen; accompanied by fever, dry throat and bitter taste in the mouth, thirst but no desire to drink, feeling of fullness in the chest, restlessness, dizziness, nausea, vomiting, constipation, scanty yellowish urine, jaundice, red tongue with greasy yellowish coating and rapid wiry or slippery pulse.

● Pancreatitis due to disturbance of the gallbladder by roundworm.

Characterized by suddenly occurring, paroxysmal colicky pain in the right upper abdomen, with horizontal tenderness but no muscular tension; dull pain during the remission stage; accompanied by nausea, vomiting, poor appetite, greasy whitish or yellowish tongue coating and wiry pulse.

Treatment

Body acupuncture

Main acupuncture points:

Zusanli	(S36)
Xiajuxu	(S39)
Pishu	(B20)
Weishu	(B21)
Zhongwan	(Ren12)
Neiguan	(P6)
Gongsun	(Sp4)
Liangqiu	(S34)

Main points are selected primarily from the Spleen and Stomach meridians to harmonize the spleen and stomach and relieve pain. Zusanli (S36) and Xiajuxu (S39), the lower *he* (confluent) points of the Stomach and Small Intestine meridians respectively, are punctured to regulate the stomach and intestines and relieve pain. Tender points usually found approximately 1 *cun* below Zusanli (S36) and Xiajuxu (S39) are punctured to increase the effectiveness of the treatment.

Pishu (B20) and Weishu (B21), the back-*shu* points of the spleen and stomach respectively and Zhongwan (Ren12), the front-*mu* point of the stomach, are treated in combination to regulate the stomach and spleen. Neiguan (P6) and Gongsun (Sp4), two of the eight confluence points connecting with the Yinwei and Chong meridians respectively, are treated in combination to regulate the flow of *qi* and relieve pain and vomiting. Liangqiu (S34), the *xi* (cleft) point of the Stomach meridian, is punctured to relieve pain.

Anywhere from four or five to all main points are selected each time, according to need.

Auxiliary points and appropriate methods of manipulation are chosen according to differentiation of syndromes.

● For pancreatitis due to stagnation of the liver *qi*, Taichong (Liv3) and Hegu (LI4) are added and punctured using the reducing method to harmonize the flow of the liver *qi*.

● For pancreatitis due to excessive heat in the spleen and stomach, Dazhui (Du14) is added and pricked with a three-edged needle and then cupped for 10–15 minutes to draw blood and clear away heat. Additional measures should be undertaken in emergency situations.

● For pancreatitis due to accumulation of damp-heat in the liver and gallbladder, Riyue (G24) and Yanglingquan (G34) are added and punctured using the reducing method to regulate the liver and gallbladder and eliminate damp-heat.

● For pancreatitis due to disturbance of the gallbladder by roundworm, Yanglingquan (G34) is added and punctured using the reducing method to tranquillize the roundworms and relieve pain.

Treat acute cases two to three times a day and chronic cases once a day or once every other day. Ten treatments constitute one course.

Electroacupuncture

Points used are the same as for body acupuncture. Select one or two pairs of points each time. Puncture using the reducing method until a needling sensation is achieved, then connect the needles to an electrical stimulator. Apply intermittent wave stimulation of the greatest bearable intensity for one hour. Treat once a day or once every other day. Ten treatments constitute one course.

Auricular therapy

Auricular points:

Pancreas & Gallbladder: corresponds to the affected organs. Locate positive points; tape both frontal and dorsal surfaces to increase stimulation. Concentrate on treating the left auricle.

Spleen, Stomach: regulate the spleen and stomach.

San Jiao: regulates the flow of *qi* to relieve pain.

Abdomen, Middle of Superior Concha: relieve abdominal pain.

Endocrine, Adrenal Gland: relieve inflammation.

Ear Shenmen, Sympathesis: relieve pain.

Use auricular taping with strong manipulation, twice a week. Five treatments constitute one course.

Remarks

- Acupuncture can immediately relieve symptoms of pancreatitis such as abdominal pain and vomiting; in most cases fasting and gastrointestinal decompression are unnecessary.
- Acupuncture can be used as the sole treatment for chronic pancreatitis and mild or moderate cases of acute pancreatitis. It can also be used as an effective auxiliary treatment for severe cases of acute pancreatitis.

91 Paralytic strabismus

Strabismus refers to a condition in which the visual line of one eye deviates from the visual target. The condition is called paralytic strabismus when it is caused by paralysis, either arising from damage to the nerves which control the extraocular muscles, or of the muscles themselves. In addition to double vision, symptoms caused by double vision such as dizziness, headache, vertigo, nausea or vomiting may occur. The causes of paralytic strabismus are various, including trauma, peripheral neuritis, cerebral diseases or tumours, diabetes mellitus or myasthenia gravis.

Aetiology and differentiation of syndromes

According to traditional Chinese medicine, paralytic strabismus is caused by trauma or invasion of the meridians by exogenous pathogens, either of which may obstruct the flow of *qi* and blood; or by insufficiency of the liver and kidneys which leads to insufficient nourishment of the extraocular muscles. Strabismus is usually differentiated according to meridian theory. For instance, the Urinary Bladder meridian stems from the inner canthus, so divergent strabismus is due to disorder

of the Urinary Bladder meridian; both the Hand and Foot Shaoyang meridians converge on the outer canthus, so convergent strabismus is due to disorder of the Gallbladder and San Jiao meridians.

Treatment

Body acupuncture

Main acupuncture points:

Fengchi	(G20)
Taichong	(Liv3)
Hegu	(LI4)
Taiyang	(Ex30)

Both the Liver and Gallbladder meridians connect with the eyes, so Fengchi (G20), an important point of the Gallbladder meridian located at the base of the skull, and Taichong (Liv3), the *yuan* (source) point of the Liver meridian, are treated in combination to activate the meridians. Hegu (LI4), the *yuan* (source) point of the Large Intestine meridian, functions to strengthen *qi* and blood. Taiyang (Ex30) has been proven through clinical experience to be effective for treating eye problems.

Auxiliary points and appropriate manipulation are chosen according to differentiation of syndromes.

- For divergent strabismus, Jingming (B1) and Zanzhu (B2) are added and punctured using the even method. Jingming (B1) is punctured perpendicularly to a depth of 0.5–1.0 *cun*; mild manipulation should be used in order to avoid bleeding. Zanzhu (B2) is punctured horizontally towards Yuyao (Ex28) to increase stimulation.
- For convergent strabismus, Qiuhou (Ex31) and Tongziliao (G1) are added and punctured using even manipulaton. Qiuhou (Ex31) is punctured perpendicularly to a depth of 1.0–1.5 *cun*; mild manipulation should be used in order to avoid bleeding. Tongziliao (G1) is punctured toward Sizhukong (SJ23) to increase stimulation.

Treat once a day or once every other day. Ten treatments constitute one course.

Electroacupuncture

Points used are the same as for body acupuncture, but electrical stimulation is not applied to Qiuhou (Ex31) and Jingming (B1). Select one or two pairs of points each time. Puncture until a needling sensation is achieved, then connect the needles to an electrical stimulator. Apply moderate continuous wave stimulation for 20–30 minutes, once a day or once every other day. Ten treatments constitute one course.

Remarks

- Traditional therapies are effective for treating some types of strabismus; the earlier treatment is instituted, the better the results will be.
- It is essential to establish the cause of the strabismus prior to instituting treatment.

92 Parkinson's disease

Parkinson's disease, also called shaking palsy, is an extrapyramidal disease marked by tremor, hypokinesis and muscle rigidity. It occurs primarily in the elderly and more often in males than in females. Although the cause of Parkinson's disease is not clear, the main pathogenic change is found in the black substance and striate body of the brain. Typically, tremor first occurs at the distal end of the unilateral upper limb, gradually spreading to the homolateral lower limb, contralateral limbs, jaw, lips, tongue and neck. Initially, the tremor occurs only in the static stage. It is aggravated by mental stress and disappears during voluntary movement and sleep. There may be no tremor in some cases, especially in people over 70 years old. Additional manifestations of functional autonomic nervous system disturbance include ptyalism, abnormal sweating, constipation, oculogyric crisis and orthostatic hypotension. Mental disorders such as depression or dementia may also occur.

Aetiology

Traditional Chinese medicine classifies Parkinson's disease as tremor. Mainly affected are the liver, kidneys and spleen. Primary pathogenesis is insufficient nourishment of the muscles and tendons. According to TCM, blood, which is stored in the liver and essence, which is stored in the kidneys, constitute the material basis of human life. Blood is produced by congenital essence and nourished by acquired essence. With ageing, the kidneys and liver become deficient and production of blood and essence becomes insufficient to nourish the muscles and tendons, resulting in tremor. The spleen provides the material basis for developing the constitution and dominates nourishing the muscles of the limbs. If the deficient spleen cannot produce sufficient *qi* and blood, or contributes to the accumulation of phlegm in the interior which then blocks the distribution of clear *qi*, insufficient nourishment of the muscles and resulting tremor may occur.

Differentiation of syndromes

- Parkinson's disease due to *yin* deficiency of the liver and kidneys.
  Characterized by tremor and stiffness, aggravated by mental stress and relieved by repetitive

movement such as walking and during sleep; accompanied by dizziness, tinnitus, dry eyes, restlessness, irritability, insomnia, constipation, red tongue with little or no coating and deep, thready, wiry pulse.

● Parkinson's disease due to deficiency of *qi* and blood.
  Characterized by frequent and severe tremor, not necessarily relieved by voluntary movement; accompanied by dizziness, blurred vision, pale complexion, lassitude, poor appetite, involuntary drooling, apathy, dementia, pale tongue and weak pulse.

● Parkinson's disease due to accumulation of phlegm in the interior.
  Characterized by mild or severe tremor and rigidity, accompanied by a feeling of stuffiness in the chest and upper abdomen, dizziness, ptyalism, poor appetite, depression, dementia, greasy whitish tongue coating and slippery pulse.

Treatment

Body acupuncture

Main acupuncture points:

Baihui	(Du20)
Fengchi	(G20)
Dazhui	(Du14)
Shousanli	(LI10)
Houxi	(SI3)
Hegu	(LI4)
Waiguan	(SJ5)
Zusanli	(S36)
Yanglingquan	(G34)
Sanyinjiao	(Sp6)
Taichong	(Liv3)

All Yang meridians are rich in *qi* and blood. Therefore main points are selected from these meridians to tonify the *qi* and blood and activate their flow, thus nourishing the muscles and tendons to relieve tremor. Hegu (LI4), the *yuan* (source) point of the Large Intestine meridian and Taichong (Liv3), the *yuan* (source) point of the Liver meridian, are treated in combination (called 'opening the four passes') to activate the flow of *qi* and blood and relieve tremor. Sanyinjiao (Sp6), the meeting point of the Spleen, Liver and Kidney meridians, is punctured to strengthen the functioning of these organs.

Select five to six main points each time.

Auxiliary points and appropriate manipulation are added according to symptoms and differentiation of syndromes.

● For Parkinson's disease due to *yin* deficiency of the liver and kidneys, Ganshu (B18), Shenshu (B23) and Taixi (K3) are added and punctured using the even method to tonify the liver and kidneys.

● For Parkinson's disease due to deficiency of *qi* and blood, *qi* and blood are nourished by adding and puncturing Qihai (Ren6) and Guanyuan (Ren4) using the reinforcing method, or applying moxibustion to Qihai (Ren6), Guanyuan (Ren4) and Zusanli (S36).

● For Parkinson's disease due to accumulation of phlegm in the interior, Zhongwan (Ren12), Danzhong (Ren17) and Fenglong (S40) are added and punctured using the even method to strengthen the spleen and remove phlegm.

● For cases involving refractory constipation, Tianshu (S25) and Shangjuxu (S37) are punctured to empty the bowels.

● For cases involving profuse sweating, Hegu (LI4) and Fuliu (K7) are punctured using the reinforcing method to arrest perspiration.

● For cases involving oculogyric crisis, Taiyang (Ex30) is punctured.

● For cases involving ptyalism, Dicang (S4) and Jiache (S6) are punctured.

● For cases involving mental disorders, Neiguan (P6) and Sishencong (Ex26) are punctured to regulate the mind.

Treat once a day or every other day. Twenty treatments constitute one course.

Scalp acupuncture

Scalp lines:

Dingzhongxian	(MS5)
Dingnie Qianxiexian	(MS6)
Dingpangxian 1	(MS8)
Dingpangxian 2	(MS9)

Select two or three lines each time. Twirl the needles using the even method for 5 minutes, or connect the needles to an electrical stimulator and apply moderate intermittent wave stimulation for 20–30 minutes. The needles should be retained for up to 24 hours to increase stimulation.

Treat once a day or once every other day. Ten treatments constitute one course.

Auricular therapy

Main auricular points:

Subcortex, Midpoint of Rim: correspond to the pathologically affected area. Locate and tape positive points.

Liver, Spleen, Kidney: locate positive points and tape both frontal and dorsal surfaces to strengthen these organs.

Ear Shenmen and Occiput: tranquillize the mind and relieve tremor.

Auxiliary auricular points:

● For cases involving profuse sweating, Sympathesis and Heart are added.

● For cases involving refractory constipation, Abdomen and Rectum are added.
● For cases involving mental disorders, Forehead and Heart are added.

Use auricular taping with strong manipulation, twice a week. Twenty treatments constitute one course. Auricular taping is seldom used alone, but is usually used as a supplement to body or scalp acupuncture in order to increase their effectiveness.

Remarks

☯ Acupuncture is a safe and effective method for treating Parkinson's disease. However, extended treatment must be given to achieve results.

---

93 Peptic ulcer

Peptic ulcer refers to circular or oval lesions on the wall of the stomach or duodenum, occurring primarily on the gastric pylorus or the duodenal bulb. Causes include physical, emotional and chemical factors, as well as some diseases. These conditions increase the corrosiveness of the gastric secretions while at the same time weakening the defensive functions of the gastric mucosa, leading to the formation of ulcers. Peptic ulcer is marked by regularly occurring pain in the epigastric region, accompanied by eructation, acid regurgitation, nausea, vomiting and poor appetite. Onset of pain is generally related to food intake. In cases of gastric ulcer, onset usually occurs 30 minutes to two hours after eating and disappears sometime before the next meal. In cases of duodenal ulcer, the pain usually starts two to three hours after eating and is relieved after eating the next meal.

Aetiology

Traditional Chinese medicine classifies peptic ulcer as epigastric pain. It is considered to be caused either by mental injury resulting in stagnation of the liver *qi* which then becomes hyperactive and attacks the stomach, or by improper eating habits such as irregular meals or overindulgence in

raw, cold or spicy foods. These conditions result in injury to the stomach and spleen. The main pathogenesis of peptic ulcer is stagnation of *qi* and blood which affects the stomach, spleen and liver.

Differentiation of syndromes

● Peptic ulcer due to attack on the stomach by hyperactive liver *qi*.
  Characterized by pain and distension in the epigastric region, radiating to the hypochondriac region; acid regurgitation, feeling of fullness in the chest, sighing, depression or irritability; all symptoms induced or aggravated by mental injury; whitish tongue coating and wiry pulse.
● Peptic ulcer due to blockage of the collaterals by stagnant blood.
  Characterized by severe fixed stabbing pain in the epigastric region, aggravated by pressure and worsening at night; haematemesis or melaena, purple or purple-spotted tongue and uneven thready pulse.
● Peptic ulcer due to burning of the stomach by hyperactive liver fire.
  Characterized by burning pain in the epigastric

region, possibly radiating to the hypochondriac region and induced or aggravated by mental injury; acid regurgitation, restlessness or irritability, bitter taste in the mouth and dry throat, haematemesis or melaena, red tongue with yellowish coating and rapid wiry pulse.

● Peptic ulcer due to *yang* deficiency of the spleen and stomach.
Characterized by intermittent dull pain in the epigastric region, aggravated by cold and alleviated by pressure or warmth or after eating; poor appetite, loose stool, aversion to cold, feeling of cold in the limbs, lassitude, pale complexion, pale tongue with whitish coating and deep thready pulse.

● Peptic ulcer due to deficiency of the stomach *yin*.
Characterized by dull or burning pain in the epigastric region, anorexia or bulimia, dry mouth, sensation of heat in the palms and soles, constipation or melaena, pale complexion, dry red tongue with little coating and rapid thready pulse.

Treatment

Body acupuncture

Main acupuncture points:

Zhongwan	(Ren12)
Weishu	(B21)
Zusanli	(S36)
Xiajuxu	(S39)
Liangmen	(S21) (left)
Shangwan	(Ren13)
Xiawan	(Ren10)
Juque	(Ren14)
Huatuojiaji	(Ex46) (T7-T12)

Zhongwan (Ren12) and Weishu (B21), the front-*mu* and back-*shu* points respectively of the stomach, are treated in combination to strengthen the stomach and spleen. Zusanli (S36), the *he* (sea) and lower *he* (confluent) point of the Stomach meridian and Xiajuxu (S39), the lower *he* (confluent) point of the Small Intestine meridian, are effective for treating problems of their corresponding *fu* organs. Liangmen (S21) (left), Shangwan (Ren13), Xiawan (Ren10) and Juque (Ren14) are local points for treating peptic ulcer.

Select four or five main points each time.

Auxiliary points and appropriate methods of manipulation are chosen according to symptoms and differentiation of syndromes.

● For peptic ulcer due to attack on the stomach by hyperactive liver *qi*, Neiguan (P6), Taichong (Liv3) and Yanglingquan (G34) are added and punctured using the reducing method to soothe the liver and regulate the flow of *qi*.

● For peptic ulcer due to blockage of the collaterals by stagnant blood, blood circulation is stimulated and pain relieved by adding and puncturing Liangqiu (S34), Hegu (LI4) and Taichong (Liv3) using the reducing method, pricking Geshu (B17) with a three-edged needle and then cupping for 10–15 minutes.

● For peptic ulcer due to burning of the stomach by hyperactive liver fire, Xingjian (Liv2) and Yanglingquan (G34) are added and punctured using the reducing method; Ganshu (B18) and Liangmen (S21) (left) are pricked with a three-edged needle and then cupped for 10–15 minutes.

● For peptic ulcer due to *yang* deficiency of the spleen and stomach, the spleen and stomach are warmed by adding and puncturing Pishu (B20) and Qihai (Ren6) using the reinforcing method and adding moxibustion to points of the back and abdomen.

● For peptic ulcer due to deficiency of the stomach *yin*, Sanyinjiao (Sp6), Pishu (B20) and Taixi (K3) are added and punctured using the even method to nourish the stomach *yin*.

● For cases with severe vomiting, Neiguan (P6) is added to subdue rebellious rising of the stomach *qi*.

● For cases with severe epigastric pain, Liangqiu (S34), the *xi* (cleft) point of the Stomach meridian, is added to relieve pain.

● For cases with constipation, Tianshu (S25), the front-*mu* point of the large intestine, is added to strengthen transportation by the large intestine.

● For cases with haematemesis or melaena, Geshu (B17), the *hui* (influential) point of the blood, is added to stimulate the blood circulation and arrest bleeding.

Treat once a day or once every other day. Ten treatments constitute one course.

Electroacupuncture

Points used are the same as for body acupuncture. Select one or two pairs of points each time. Puncture until a needling sensation is achieved, then connect the needles to an electrical stimulator. Apply moderate intermittent wave stimulation for 30 minutes. Treat once a day or once every other day. Ten treatments constitute one course.

Moxibustion

Points used are the same as for body acupuncture. Apply moxa roll moxibustion to four or five points for 10–15 minutes each time. Treat once a day or once every other day. Ten treatments constitute one course.

Moxibustion is suitable for treating all types of peptic ulcer except those due to burning of the stomach by hyperactive liver fire, or deficiency of the stomach *yin*. It is usually used in combination with body acupuncture.

Hot salt compress therapy

Points:

Zhongwan	(Ren12)
Weishu	(B21)
Shenque	(Ren8)

Heat 500–1000 g of salt in a hot dry pan. Put half of the hot salt in a small bag. Apply the bag to one point. Protect the skin by placing a towel under the bag while it is very hot; when it starts to cool down the towel can be removed. Change to a new hot bag when the first one is no longer hot. Apply for 30–60 minutes, once or twice a day. Ten treatments constitute one course.

This method functions to warm the spleen and stomach and promote the flow of blood and *qi*. It is therefore suitable for treating peptic ulcer due to *yang* deficiency of the spleen and stomach, attack on the stomach by hyperactive liver *qi* and blockage of the collaterals by stagnant blood.

Point implantation therapy

Points used are the same as for body acupuncture. Using a triangular surgical needle, implant surgical catgut on two or three points each time. (See Appendix 9.) Treat once every 20 or 30 days. Three treatments constitute one course.

Auricular therapy

Auricular points:

Stomach, Duodenum, Abdomen: correspond to the affected regions of the body; relieve pain and accelerate healing of ulcers.

Spleen: strengthens the spleen and stomach.

Liver: soothes the liver *qi* to relieve pain.

Sympathesis: relieves pain and inhibits gastric secretion.

Subcortex: regulates the function of the cerebral cortex.

Ear Shenmen and Occiput: tranquillize the mind and relieve pain.

Use auricular taping, twice a week. Ten treatments constitute one course.

Remarks

☯ Traditional therapies, especially point implantation therapy, can not only effectively relieve the symptoms of peptic ulcer, but also completely heal the lesion.

☯ In cases of peptic ulcer, there are usually positive signs such as streaky or nodular scleroma or tenderness on Weishu (B21), Pishu (B20) and Ganshu (B18).

☯ For cases of peptic ulcer involving perforation, traditional therapies, especially electroacupuncture, can be used as auxiliary treatments for healing the perforation, relieving infection and recovering gastrointestinal function as quickly as possible. Commonly used points are Zhongwan (Ren12), Liangmen (S21) (left), Zusanli (S36), Neiguan (P6), Hegu (LI4) and Taichong (Liv3).

94 Peripheral facial paralysis

Peripheral facial paralysis, or Bell's palsy, is caused primarily by acute non-suppurative inflammation of the facial nerves. It is marked by sudden onset of paralysis of the muscles controlling facial expression on the affected side, usually most apparent in the morning. Additional manifestations include incomplete closing of the eye, lacrimation, disappearance of the nasolabial groove, deviation of the mouth to the unaffected side, retention of food between the cheek and the gum and salivation; inability to frown, raise the eyebrow, puff out the cheek, pull back the lips to reveal the teeth, or whistle. There may be tenderness or pain in the mastoid region in the initial stage.

Aetiology and differentiation of syndromes

Traditional Chinese medicine catagorizes peripheral facial paralysis as deviation of the mouth. It is considered to be caused by deficiency of antipathogenic *qi* which allows invasion of the meridians by exogenous wind-cold, resulting in obstruction of the flow of *qi* and blood in the meridians and insufficient nourishment of the facial muscles. In addition to deviation of the mouth, there may be headache, tinnitus, aversion to cold, lassitude, poor appetite and tenderness or pain in the mastoid region during the initial stage. *Qi* and blood may be consumed in protracted cases. Primarily affected are the Stomach, Large Intestine, Gallbladder and San Jiao meridians.

Treatment

Body acupuncture

Acupuncture points:

Sibai	(S2)
Dicang	(S4)
Jiache	(S6)
Xiaguan	(S7)
Yangbai	(G14)
Chengjiang	(Ren24)
Taiyang	(Ex30)
Yifeng	(SJ17)
Fengchi	(G20)
Hegu	(LI4)
Fenglong	(S40)
Zhongzhu	(SJ3)

Both local and distal points are selected according to meridian theory. During the acute stage (the first week), the condition is still developing; therefore local points should not be punctured but only treated with moxa roll moxibustion and distal points should be punctured using the reducing method. Following the acute stage, both local points (primarily of the affected side) and distal points are punctured using the even method. Select five to eight points each time. Two adjacent local

points are usually punctured in one insertion in order to increase stimulation. For example, Dicang (S4) is punctured horizontally towards Jiache (S6); Sibai (S2) is punctured horizontally towards Jingming (B1); Zanzhu (B2) is punctured horizontally towards Yuyao (Ex28). For protracted cases, Zusanli (S36) and Baihui (Du20) are added and punctured using the reinforcing method to nourish the *qi* and blood.

Treat once a day for the first week and once every other day subsequently. Ten treatments constitute one course.

Electroacupuncture

Points used are the same as for body acupuncture. During the acute stage, only distal points are stimulated; subsequently both local points (primarily of the affected side) and distal points are treated. Select one or two pairs of points each time. Puncture the points until a needling sensation is achieved, then connect the needles to an electrical stimulator. Apply moderate intermittent wave stimulation for 20–30 minutes, once a day during the acute stage and once every other day thereafter. Ten treatments constitute one course.

Moxibustion

Primarily local points are used. Apply moxa roll moxibustion to each point for 10–15 minutes, once a day. Five treatments constitute one course. Moxibustion is usually used in combination with body acupuncture in order to increase stimulation and improve effectiveness.

Auricular therapy

Auricular points:

Cheek, Eye: correspond to the affected areas of the body. Locate positive points; tape both frontal and dorsal surfaces to increase stimulation.

San Jiao: the mixed branches of the glossopharyngeal, vagus and facial nerves pass through this auricular area, so San Jiao is an important point for treating facial paralysis.

Stomach, Large Intestine, Pancreas & Gallbladder: the Stomach, Large Intestine and Gallbladder meridians distribute to the face, so Stomach, Large Intestine and Pancreas & Gallbladder are taped to activate their corresponding meridians and promote the flow of of *qi* and blood.

Endocrine, Adrenal Gland: relieve inflammation.

Subcortex: regulates nervous function.

Use auricular taping with strong manipulation, twice a week. Five treatments constitute one course.

Remarks

☯ Acupuncture is effective for treating peripheral facial paralysis; the earlier treatment is instituted, the better the results will be.
☯ Long-standing cases (over six months) are very difficult to cure.
☯ The face should be kept warm during the course of treatment to shorten the course and improve effectiveness.

95 Phantom limb pain

Phantom limb pain occurs primarily in adult amputees, who continue to experience sensations of severe burning or stabbing pain at the site of the missing limb. Even the strongest analgesics, such as morphine or dilantin, are ineffective in many cases. Phantom limb pain is usually induced by secondary trauma or mental injury. Its cause is still not certain, but may be related to abnormality of peripheral nerve impulses at the site of the amputation, disorder of the sympathetic nervous system or altered body image in the central nervous system. Some researchers believe phantom limb pain may be related to mental disturbance following amputation.

Aetiology and differentiation of syndromes

According to traditional Chinese medicine, phantom limb pain is caused by severe trauma which disturbs the flow of *qi* and blood in the meridians.

Treatment

Auricular therapy

Auricular points:

Areas corresponding to the site of the pain: locate positive points; tape both frontal and dorsal surfaces to increase stimulation.

Ear Shenmen: main point for pain relief.

Occiput, Anterior Ear Lobe: tranquillize the mind and relieve pain.

Subcortex: regulates the central nervous function.

Apex of Ear: blood-letting puncturing of this point with a three-edged needle calms the mind.

Use auricular taping with strong manipulation and blood-letting puncturing where indicated, twice a week. Five treatments constitute one course.

Scalp acupuncture

Scalp lines:

Dingnie Houxiexian(MS7)

Puncture the contralateral side; manipulate using the reducing method for 5 minutes, or connect the needles to an electrical stimulator and apply intermittent wave stimulation for 20–30 minutes. The needles should be retained for up to 24 hours to increase stimulation. Treat once a day or once every other day. Five treatments constitute one course.

Electroacupuncture

Acupuncture points:

Huatuojiaji   (Ex46)

Select Huatuojiaji (Ex46) of the spinal segment corresponding to the site of the pain. Puncture until a needling sensation is achieved, then connect the needles to an electrical stimulator. Apply intermittent wave stimulation of the greatest bearable intensity for 30 minutes, once a day or once every other day. Five treatments constitute one course.

Remarks

๏ Traditional therapies are effective for treating phantom limb pain. They can be applied singly or in combination to increase stimulation and improve effectiveness.

๏ These methods are also effective for treating stump neuralgia.

96 Pharyngeal paraesthesia

Pharyngeal paraesthesia, also called globus hystericus, is a functional problem of the pharynx, caused by functional disturbance of the autonomic nervous system, irritative diseases of the oesophagus and gastrointestinal tract, cervical spondylopathy or disturbance of the metabolism or endocrine system. It occurs mainly in adult females. It is characterized by the subjective sensation of a foreign body or mass stuck in the throat, or of the throat being compressed. The sensation occurs or worsens when swallowing saliva, but there is no abnormal sensation or difficulty when swallowing food. Additional symptoms may include depression, a feeling of fullness in the chest, poor appetite, abdominal distension or acid regurgitation.

Aetiology and differentiation of syndromes

According to traditional Chinese medicine, pharyngeal paraesthesia is caused primarily by mental injury leading to stagnation of the liver *qi* which then attacks the spleen, resulting in accumulation of phlegm in the interior. The combination of stagnant *qi* and accumulated phlegm obstructs the throat. In addition to local manifestation, systemic manifestations include a feeling of fullness in the chest and hypochondriac region, frequent sighing, anxiety, doubt, or depression, greenish or sallow complexion, poor appetite, purple tongue with thick whitish coating and wiry pulse.

Treatment

Body acupuncture

Acupuncture points:

Taichong	(Liv3)
Neiguan	(P6)
Danzhong	(Ren17)
Pishu	(B20)
Zhangmen	(Liv13)
Zhongwan	(Ren12)
Zusanli	(S36)
Fenglong	(S40)
Tiantu	(Ren22)

The main pathogenesis of pharyngeal paraesthesia is stagnant *qi* and accumulated phlegm, so points are selected to promote the flow of the liver *qi* and strengthen the spleen to remove phlegm. Taichong (Liv3), the *yuan* (source) point of the Liver meridian, functions to promote the flow of the liver *qi*. Neiguan (P6), the *luo* (collateral) point of the Pericardium meridian and one of the eight confluence points connecting with the Yinwei meridian, functions to promote the flow of *qi* and open the chest. Danzhong (Ren17), the *hui* (influential) point of *qi*, regulates the flow of *qi*. Pishu (B20), the back-*shu* point of the spleen and Zhangmen (Liv13), the front-*mu* point of the spleen and *hui* (influential) point of the *zang* organs, are treated in combination to strengthen the spleen. Zusanli (S36), the *he* (sea) and lower *he* (confluent) point of the Stomach meridian and Zhongwan (Ren12), the front-*mu* point of the stomach and *hui* (influential) point of the *fu* organs, are treated in combination to strengthen the stomach and spleen. Fenglong (S40) is an important point for treating conditions involving phlegm. Tiantu (Ren22) is a local point of the Ren meridian used for treating throat problems; it is punctured first perpendicularly for 0.2 *cun* and then downward along the back of the sternum with mild manipulation for 0.5–1.0 *cun*.

Treat once a day or once every other day. Ten treatments constitute one course.

Auricular therapy

Auricular points:

Throat, Oesophagus: correspond to the affected area.

Liver, Chest: soothe the liver *qi* and open the chest.

Spleen, Abdomen: strengthen the spleen to remove phlegm.
San Jiao: regulates the flow of *qi* and drains water.

Subcortex, Ear Shenmen: tranquillize the mind.

Use auricular taping with strong manipulation, twice a week. Five treatments constitute one course.

Remarks

☯ Traditional therapies are effective for treating pharyngeal paraesthesia. Body acupuncture and auricular therapy are usually used in combination in order to increase stimulation.

☯ It is essential to encourage the patient to develop a positive attitude and confidence that traditional therapies can cure the disorder.

☯ Extreme care should be used when puncturing Tiantu (Ren22) to avoid damage to the lungs and trachea. There have been reports of improper manipulation of this point resulting in death.

97 Postconcussional syndrome

Postconcussional syndrome follows recovery from temporary loss of consciousness induced by cephalic trauma. Symptoms include poor memory, headache, dizziness, nausea, vomiting and drowsiness. In some cases, distending or pulsating headache or a girdling sensation around the head may persist for up to three months after trauma.

Aetiology

Traditional Chinese medicine categorizes postconcussional syndrome as headache, vertigo or insomnia and considers it to be caused by cephalic trauma leading to stagnation of the *qi* and blood and subsequent insufficient nourishment of the brain.

Differentiation of syndromes

● Postconcussional syndrome due to stagnation of the *qi* and blood.

Characterized by distending or pulsating headache, dizziness, nausea or vomiting, purple-spotted tongue with whitish coating and uneven pulse.

● Postconcussional syndrome due to deficiency of the *qi* and blood.

Characterized by dizziness, vertigo, tinnitus, poor memory, insomnia, sore and weak back and knees, thin tongue with whitish coating and weak thready pulse.

Treatment

Body acupuncture

Main acupuncture points:

Baihui	(Du20)
Fengchi	(G20)
Taiyang	(Ex30)

Baihui (Du20), the meeting point of the Du, Liver and six Yang Hand and Foot meridians, is punctured to tranquillize the mind. Fengchi (G20), an important point for treating problems of the brain, is punctured slightly downward towards the tip of the nose for 0.8–1.2 *cun*. Taiyang (Ex30) is an extraordinary point for treating headache. The three points are usually used in combination to treat problems of the brain.

Auxiliary points and appropriate methods of manipulation are chosen according to differentiation of syndromes.

- For postconcussional syndrome due to stagnation of the *qi* and blood, Taichong (Liv3) and Hegu (LI4) are added and punctured using the reducing method to activate the flow of *qi* and blood and relieve pain.
- For postconcussional syndrome due to deficiency of the *qi* and blood, the mind is refreshed and tranquillized by adding and puncturing Taixi (K3), Shenshu (B23) and Sanyinjiao (Sp6) using the reinforcing method, or replacing Baihui (Du20) with Sishencong (Ex26).

Treat once a day or once every other day. Five treatments constitute one course.

Electroacupuncture

Points used are the same as for body acupuncture. Select one or two pairs of points each time. Puncture the points until a needling sensation is achieved, then connect the needles to an electrical stimulator. Apply moderate intermittent wave stimulation for 30 minutes. Treat once a day or once every other day. Five treatments constitute one course.

Auricular therapy

Main auricular points:

Areas corresponding to the injured regions: tape both frontal and dorsal surfaces to increase stimulation.

Kidney: tonifies the kidneys to stimulate the production of marrow.

Liver: soothes the liver *qi* and promotes the blood circulation to relieve pain and dizziness.

Ear Shenmen, Subcortex: tranquillize the mind and relieve pain.

Apex of Ear: blood-letting puncturing of this point with a three-edged needle refreshes the mind.

Auxiliary auricular points:

For tinnitus, Internal Ear is added.

For nausea and vomiting, Cardia and Stomach are added.

For insomnia, Anterior Ear Lobe is added.

Use auricular taping with strong manipulation and blood-letting puncturing where indicated, twice a week. Five treatments constitute one course.

Remarks

- Traditional therapies are very effective for treating postconcussional syndrome. The sooner treatment is instituted, the better the results will be.
- The above three methods may be used singly or in combination.

98 Postpartum uterine contractions

Postpartum uterine contractions are a normal physiological transition between the highly distended state of the uterus during pregnancy and the normal state following parturition. They generally disappear spontaneously within three days to one week after delivery. However, treatment may be needed if the pains are very severe, last for longer than one week, or are accompanied by increased vaginal discharge.

Aetiology

According to traditional Chinese medicine, postpartum uterine contractions are caused either by major loss of blood during delivery leading to insufficient nutrition of the uterus, stagnation of lochia in the uterus which blocks the meridians, or invasion of the uterus by exogenous cold which contracts the meridians with resulting stagnation of the *qi* and blood.

Differentiation of syndromes

● Postpartum uterine contractions due to deficiency of blood.
  Characterized by dull pain in the lower abdomen and pale and scanty lochia; accompanied by dizziness, tinnitus, pale complexion, lassitude, pale tongue with thin whitish coating and weak thready pulse.
● Postpartum uterine contractions due to stagnation of lochia in the uterus.
  Characterized by severe stabbing pain in the lower abdomen, scanty dark red clotted lochia, spotted or dark red tongue and uneven pulse.
● Postpartum uterine contractions due to invasion of the uterus by exogenous cold.
  Characterized by severe pain and feeling of cold in the lower abdomen, aggravated by pressure and cold and alleviated by warmth; scanty dark red lochia, cold sensation in the extremities, dark red tongue with whitish coating and deep tense pulse.

Treatment

Body acupuncture

Main acupuncture points:

Guanyuan	(Ren4)
Sanyinjiao	(Sp6)

Guanyuan (Ren4), the meeting point of the Ren and three Foot Yin meridians and Sanyinjiao (Sp6), the meeting point of the three Foot Yin meridians, are treated in combination to regulate the Chong and Ren meridians and are the main points for treating gynaecological and obstetrical problems.

Auxiliary points and appropriate methods of manipulation are chosen according to differentiation of syndromes.

● For postpartum uterine contractions due to deficiency of blood, Qihai (Ren6) and Zusanli (S36) are added and punctured using the reinforcing method to tonify the blood.
● For postpartum uterine contractions due to stagnation of lochia in the uterus, Diji (Sp8) and Xuehai (Sp10) are added and punctured using the reducing method to promote the flow of blood.
● For postpartum uterine contractions due to invasion of the uterus by exogenous cold, moxibustion is added to Shenque (Ren8) to expel cold and relieve pain.

Treat once or twice a day. Three days constitute one course.

Moxibustion

Acupuncture points:

Guanyuan	(Ren4)
Qihai	(Ren6)
Shenque	(Ren8)
Guilai	(S29)

Select one point each time. Apply moxa roll moxibustion for 15–20 minutes, once or twice a day. Three days constitute one course. This method may be self-administered at home.

Hot salt compress therapy

Points used are the same as for moxibustion. Apply hot salt compress to one point for 30 minutes, once or twice a day. (See Appendix 9.) Three days constitute one course.

Remarks

☯ Traditional therapies are very effective for treating postpartum uterine contractions. In many cases one treatment is sufficient to relieve pain.
☯ The above methods are also suitable for treating lochiostasis.

99 Premenstrual syndrome

Premenstrual syndrome refers to a series of symptoms occurring in some women for several days before each menstrual period. It is caused by dysfunction of the cerebral subcortex and the automonic nervous system leading to disturbance of the sex hormones. Manifestations include nervousness, depression, anxiety, irritability, insomnia, headache; swelling of the hands, feet, or face;

nausea, vomiting, diarrhoea; cramps or sinking pain in the lower abdomen, lower back pain; and painful swelling, redness or inflammation of the breasts.

Aetiology

According to traditional Chinese medicine, premenstrual syndrome is caused primarily by mental injury. The liver functions to regulate the flow of *qi* and blood and acts on the spleen; when mental injury affects the liver, stagnation of *qi* and blood occur. With development of the condition, the stagnant *qi* may either transform into endogenous fire or adversely affect the spleen. Primarily affected are the liver and spleen.

Differentiation of syndromes

- Premenstrual syndrome due to stagnation of the liver *qi*.
  Characterized by distending pain in the breasts and lower abdomen; accompanied by feeling of fullness in the chest, restlessness, depression, insomnia, poor appetite, thin whitish tongue coating and wiry pulse.
- Premenstrual syndrome due to hyperactivity of the liver fire.
  Characterized by headache, painful swelling and redness of the breasts, epistaxis and fever; accompanied by restlessness, palpitation, shortness of breath, bitter taste in the mouth, dry throat, red tongue with yellowish coating and rapid wiry pulse.
- Premenstrual syndrome due to loss of coordination between the liver and spleen.
  Characterized by diarrhoea and abdominal pain, usually alleviated after defecation; accompanied by feeling of fullness in the chest and hypochondriac regions, restlessness, poor appetite, pale complexion, pale tongue with whitish coating and soft wiry pulse.
- Premenstrual syndrome due to accumulation of dampness arising from deficiency of the spleen.
  Characterized by swelling of the hands, face, or feet; accompanied by dizziness, lassitude, pale complexion, poor appetite, loose stool, swollen tongue with whitish coating and slippery pulse.

Treatment

Body acupuncture

Main acupuncture points:

Sanyinjiao	(Sp6)
Taichong	(Liv3)
Neiguan	(P6)
Hegu	(LI4)

Sanyinjiao (Sp6), the meeting point of the three Foot Yin meridians, functions to promote the flow of the liver *qi* and strengthen the spleen. Taichong (Liv3), the *yuan* (source) point of the Liver meridian, functions to promote the flow of the liver *qi*. Neiguan (P6), the *luo* (collateral) point of the Pericardium meridian and one of the eight confluence points connecting with the Yinwei meridian, functions to open the chest and promote the flow of *qi* and blood. Hegu (LI4), the *yuan* (source) point of the Large Intestine meridian, promotes the flow of *qi* and relieves pain.

Auxiliary points and proper manipulation are chosen according to differentiation of syndromes.

- For premenstrual syndrome due to stagnation of the liver *qi*, Danzhong (Ren17) and Yanglingquan (G34) are added and punctured using the reducing method to regulate the flow of *qi*.
- For premenstrual syndrome due to hyperactivity of the liver fire, Xingjian (Liv2) and Xiaxi (G43) are added and puctured using the reducing method to expel fire.
- For premenstrual syndrome due to loss of coordination between the liver and spleen, Zhongwan (Ren12) and Zusanli (S36) are added and punctured using the even method to strengthen the spleen and stomach.
- For premenstrual syndrome due to accumulation of dampness arising from deficiency of the spleen, Zusanli (S36), Pishu (B20) and Zhongwan (Ren12) are added and punctured using the reinforcing method to strengthen the spleen and remove dampness.

Treat once a day. Five treatments constitute one course.

Electroacupuncture

Points used are the same as for body acupuncture. Select one or two pairs of points each time. Puncture until a needling sensation is achieved, then connect the needles to an electrical stimulator. Apply moderate continuous wave stimulation for 20–30 minutes. Treat once a day. Five treatments constitute one course.

Auricular therapy

Main auricular points:

Internal Genitals, Endocrine, Midpoint of Rim: regulate the endocrine function.

Ear Shenmen, Subcortex: tranquillize the mind.

Liver: soothes the liver to promote the flow of *qi* and blood.

Auxiliary auricular points:

For mental symptoms, Heart is added.

For gastrointestinal problems, Stomach and Cardia are added.

For lower abdominal pain, Abdomen and Pelvis are added.

For painful swelling of the breasts, Chest is added.

Use auricular taping with strong manipulation, twice a week. Five treatments constitute one course. Auricular self-massage may also be practised twice a day.

Remarks

☯ Traditional therapies are effective for treating premenstrual syndrome; the above therapies may be used either singly, or in combination to increase stimulation and improve effectiveness.

☯ The onset, development and prognosis of premenstrual syndrome are closely related to psychological factors. It is essential to encourage a positive attitude and confidence that traditional therapies can relieve its symptoms and provide a cure.

100 Prolapse of the uterus

Prolapse of the uterus refers to descent of the uterus from its normal position, with the cervix dropping below the level of the ischial spine. In extreme cases, the entire uterus may protrude out of the vaginal opening. Prolapse of the uterus is usually accompanied by prolapse of both the anterior and posterior vaginal walls. In the initial stage, the prolapsed uterus may spontaneously return to normal when a horizontal position is assumed. But with development of the condition, it remains exposed outside the vaginal opening, with accompanying difficulty in defecation, urinary retention or incontinence, or urinary tract infection.

Aetiology

According to traditional Chinese medicine, primarily affected in cases of prolapse of the uterus are the spleen and kidneys. Prolapse of the uterus may occur if the spleen *qi* is damaged by improper diet or overstrain following delivery, or if the kidney *qi* is consumed by frequent pregnancies or excessive sexual activity. There may also be accompanying accumulation of damp-heat pathogens.

Differentiation of syndromes

● Prolapse of the uterus due to deficiency of the spleen *qi*.
Characterized by prolapse of the uterus and sinking sensation in the lower abdomen, aggravated by exertion; accompanied by lassitude, pale complexion, poor appetite, profuse thin vaginal discharge, pale tongue with whitish coating and weak pulse.

● Prolapse of the uterus due to deficiency of the kidney *qi*.
Characterized by prolapse of the uterus and sinking sensation in the lower abdomen; accompanied by dizziness, tinnitus, sore and weak back and knees, frequent urination, lack of vaginal lubrication, pale tongue with little coating and deep weak pulse.

● Prolapse of the uterus due to damp-heat.
Characterized by prolapse of the uterus and swelling, redness and pain of the cervix or body of the uterus; accompanied by feeling of fullness in the chest and epigastric region, poor appetite, bitter taste in the mouth, scanty or weak stream of yellowish urine, fever, greasy yellowish tongue coating and rapid slippery pulse.

Treatment

Body acupuncture

Main acupuncture points:

Guanyuan	(Ren4)
Sanyinjiao	(Sp6)
Baihui	(Du20)
Zigongxue	(Ex45)
Tituo	(Ex44)

Guanyuan (Ren4), the meeting point of the Ren and three Foot Yin meridians located on the lower abdomen, is an important point for tonifying the *yuan* (original) *qi* and treating gynaecological problems. Sanyinjiao (Sp6), the meeting point of the three Foot Yin meridians, functions to strengthen the spleen, liver and kidneys and is an important point for treating gynaecological and genital problems. Baihui (Du20), the meeting point of the Du, Liver and six Yang Hand and Foot meridians located on the top of the head, functions to lift sinking *qi*. Zigongxue (Ex45) and Tituo (Ex44) are clinically effective points for treating prolapse of the uterus. They are punctured obliquely downward towards the pubic symphysis for 2.0–2.5 *cun* until a needling sensation is experienced in the vulva.

Auxiliary points and proper manipulation are chosen according to differentiation of syndromes.

● For prolapse of the uterus due to deficiency of the spleen *qi*, Zusanli (S36) and Qihai (Ren6) are added and punctured using the reinforcing method to strengthen the spleen *qi*.
● For prolapse of the uterus due to deficiency of the kidney *qi*, Shenshu (B23), Ciliao (B32) and Qihai (Ren6) are added and punctured using the reinforcing method to tonify the kidney *qi*.
● For prolapse of the uterus due to damp-heat, Ligou (Liv5), Ququan (Liv8), Qugu (Ren2) and Yinlingquan (Sp9) are added and punctured using the reducing method to dispel heat and remove dampness. This is an emergency measure for treating the *biao* (branch or secondary aspect) of the condition. (See Glossary.)

The patient should empty the bladder before puncturing and the uterus manually returned to the proper position in severe cases. The patient should kneel in a knee to chest position with the head down for 20 minutes following treatment. Treat once a day or once every other day. Ten treatments constitute one course.

Moxibustion

Points used are the same as for body acupuncture. Select three to five points each time. Apply moxa roll moxibustion for 15–20 minutes, or three to five medium-sized moxa cones, to each point. Treat once or twice a day. Ten treatments constitute one course.

Moxibustion functions to tonify the *yuan* (original) *qi*; it is therefore suitable for treating prolapse of the uterus due to deficiency of the spleen or kidney *qi*.

Electroacupuncture

Points used are the same as for body acupuncture. Select one or two pairs of points each time. Puncture until a needling sensation is achieved, then connect the needles to an electrical stimulator. Apply intermittent wave stimulation of the strongest bearable intensity for 30 minutes. Treat once a day or once every other day. Ten treatments constitute one course.

Auricular therapy

Main auricular points:

Internal Genitals, Pelvis, Abdomen: correspond to the affected regions. Locate positive points; tape both frontal and dorsal surfaces to increase stimulation.

Kidney, Spleen: strengthen both congenital and acquired essence.

Liver: the Liver meridian passes through the external genitals and lower abdomen, so Liver is taped to activate the liver *qi*.

Auxiliary auricular points:

For difficulty in defecation, Lung and Large Intestine are added.

For urinary retention or incontinence, Urinary Bladder is added.

For urinary tract infection, Endocrine and Adrenal Gland are taped and Apex of Ear is punctured with a three-edged needle to cause bleeding.

Use auricular taping and blood-letting puncturing where indicated, twice a week. Ten treatments constitute one course.

Remarks

☯ Traditional therapies are very effective for treating mild (I) and moderate (II) prolapse of the uterus. However, in severe (III) cases they should only be used as auxiliary measures to other methods such as pessaries or surgery.

☯ Two or more methods are usually used in combination to increase stimulation and improve effect.
☯ It is helpful to excercise the levator ani muscle three times a day, 10–15 minutes each time.
☯ Heavy work and sexual activity are forbidden during the course of treatment.

101   Prostatitis

Prostatitis is an inflammation of the prostate gland. Acute prostatitis occurs primarily in adults and is marked by frequent, painful or dripping urination, sudden high fever, chills and distending or severe pain in the lumbosacral region and perineum. It is usually caused by overindulgence in alcohol; excessive sexual activity or suppression of ejaculation; injury of the perineum, acute urethritis or the common cold. Chronic prostatitis is marked by increased frequency of urination, burning sensation during urination, turbid terminal urine and sinking pain in the lumbosacral region, perineum and scrotum. It may be accompanied by sexual dysfunction including pain during ejaculation or impotence and neurosism. There is usually a history of acute prostatitis.

Aetiology

Traditional Chinese medicine classifies prostatitis as a *lin* syndrome and considers it to be caused primarily by accumulation of damp-heat in the Lower Jiao which affects the function of the urinary bladder. In protracted cases, the kidney *qi* may be damaged. Deficiency of the kidney *qi* and accumulation of damp-heat may occur concurrently, intensifying each other and resulting in refractory cases.

Differentiation of syndromes

● Prostatitis due to accumulation of damp-heat in the urinary bladder.
Characterized by sudden onset of frequent, painful, or dripping urination and distending pain in the perineum which may radiate to the

lumbosacral region, penis and thighs; usually accompanied by high fever, chills, soreness and pain of the entire body, headache, poor appetite, lassitude, greasy yellowish tongue coating and rapid slippery pulse.
● Prostatitis due to deficiency of the kidney *qi*.
Characterized by long-standing frequent burning urination; discomfort or pain in the perineum and anus which may radiate to the testes, groin and lumbosacral region; sometimes accompanied by lassitude, dizziness, sore and weak back and knees, hyposexuality, seminal emission, impotence or premature ejaculation, pale tongue with thin whitish coating and deep thready pulse.

Treatment

Body acupuncture

Main acupuncture points:

Zhongji	(Ren3)
Pangguangshu	(B28)
Sanyinjiao	(Sp6)

Zhongji (Ren3) and Pangguangshu (B28), the front-*mu* and back-*shu* points of the urinary bladder, are treated in combination to strengthen the urinary bladder and remove damp-heat. Sanyinjiao (Sp6), the meeting point of the three Foot Yin meridians, is punctured to strengthen the spleen and kidneys and eliminate dampness. When puncturing Zhongji (Ren3), it is essential that a needling sensation be felt in the external genitals.

Auxiliary points and appropriate methods of manipulation are chosen according to differentiation of syndromes.

- For prostatitis due to accumulation of damp-heat in the urinary bladder, Zhiyin (B67) is added and pricked with a three-edged needle to draw several drops of blood and dispel heat. The two sides should be pricked alternately.
- For prostatitis due to deficiency of the kidney *qi*, Guanyuan (Ren4), Taixi (K3), Shenshu (B23) and Zusanli (S36) are added and punctured using the even method to strengthen the kidneys and spleen.

Treat once a day or once every other day. Ten treatments constitute one course.

Electroacupuncture

Points used are the same as for body acupuncture. Select two or three pairs of points each time. Puncture until a needling sensation is achieved, then connect the needles to an electrical stimulator. Apply moderate intermittent wave stimulation for 30 minutes. Treat once a day or once every other day. Ten treatments constitute one course.

Auricular therapy

Main auricular points:

Angle of Superior Concha, Urethra: correspond to affected area of the body. Tape both frontal and dorsal surfaces to increase stimulation.

Kidney, San Jiao: drain water to dispel damp-heat.

Liver: the Liver meridian passes through the external genitals and lower abdomen, so Liver is taped to activate this meridian and relieve pain.

Endocrine, Adrenal Gland: relieve inflammation.

Ear Shenmen: relieves pain.

Apex of Ear: blood-letting puncturing of this point with a three-edged needle dispels damp-heat and relieves pain.

Auxiliary auricular points:

For pain in the lower abdomen, Abdomen and Pelvis are added.

For pain in the lumbosacral region, Lumbosacral Vertebrae is added.

For pain in the perineum and external genitals, External Genitals is added.

For sexual dysfunction, Internal Genitals is added.

For neurosism, Anterior Ear Lobe is added.

Use auricular taping with strong manipulation and blood-letting puncturing where indicated, twice a week. Ten treatments constitute one course.

Remarks

- The above therapies are effective for treating prostatitis.
- In acute cases, the patient should drink large amounts of water. In chronic cases, the patient should massage the prostate for 30 minutes once a week and sit in warm water for 20 minutes twice a day.
- Huiyin (Ren1) may be irradiated with a helium neon laser for 15 minutes once a day to increase effectiveness of treatment.
- These methods are also suitable for treating hyperplasia of the prostate.

102 Ptosis

Ptosis refers to drooping of one or both upper eyelids, which may cover the pupils and affect vision. It is classified into congenital and secondary types. Causes of the secondary types include oculomotor paralysis, trauma, trachoma or myasthenia gravis.

Aetiology and differentiation of syndromes

According to traditional Chinese medicine, ptosis may be caused by deficiency or congenital insufficiency of the spleen and stomach, or by trauma or invasion of the upper eyelids by exogenous pathogens, any of which result in flaccidity of the upper eyelids. Mainly affected are the Gallbladder and Urinary Bladder meridians.

Treatment

Body acupuncture

Acupuncture points:

Zanzhu	(B2)
Yangbai	(G14)
Sizhukong	(SJ23)
Fengchi	(G20)
Hegu	(LI4)
Zusanli	(S36)

Zanzhu(B2), Yangbai (G14) and Sizhukong (SJ23) are three local points for treating ptosis. They are punctured in combination from different directions toward Yuyao (Ex28) in order to increase stimulation. Fengchi (G20), an important point of the Gallbladder meridian located at the base of the skull, functions to expel exogenous pathogens and promote the flow of *qi* and blood. It is a main point for treating various eye problems. Hegu (LI4), the *yuan* (source) point of the Large Intestine meridian and Zusanli (S36), the *he* (sea) and lower *he* (confluent) point of the Stomach meridian, are punctured to activate the meridians and strengthen the *qi* and blood.

Puncture all points using the reinforcing method, once a day or once every other day. Ten treatments constitute one course.

Electroacupuncture

Points used are the same as for body acupuncture. Select one or two pairs of points each time. Puncture until a needling sensation is achieved, then connect the needles to an electrical stimulator. Apply moderate continuous wave stimulation for 20–30 minutes, once a day or once every other day. Ten treatments constitute one course.

Remarks

☯ Acupuncture is very effective for treating secondary ptosis.

103 Raynaud's disease

Raynaud's disease is a disorder of the peripheral circulation caused by spasm of the peripheral arterioles. It occurs primarily in adults, more often in women than men, and is usually induced by cold, mental injury or endocrine dysfunction. There may be a family history of the disease as well. Raynaud's disease is marked by symmetrical, intermittent change in the colour of the extremities, most often the hands. During onset, the skin of the affected area first becomes pale and then dark purple in colour, with accompanying localized coldness, numbness and stabbing pain. After a period ranging from several hours to several days, the skin becomes warm and its colour returns to normal.

Aetiology and differentiation of syndromes

Traditional Chinese medicine classifies Raynaud's disease as a *bi* syndrome and considers it to be caused primarily by exogenous cold or mental injury which result in obstruction in the meridians of the *qi* and blood and insufficient supply of warmth and nourishment to the extremities. Primarily affected are the Hand and Foot Yang meridians.

Treatment

Body acupuncture

Group 1:	
Quchi	(LI11)
Waiguan	(SJ5)
Hegu	(LI4)
Baxie	(Ex6)
Group 2:	
Zusanli	(S36)
Jiexi	(S41)
Bafeng	(Ex23)

Taichong   (Liv3)
Sanyinjiao   (Sp6)

Points of the Hand and Foot Yang meridians are selected as main points to promote the flow of *qi* and blood and warm and nourish the extremities. Group 1 is used for treating Raynaud's disease of the upper limbs and Group 2 for the lower limbs. Sanyinjiao (Sp6), the meeting point of the three Foot Yin meridians and Taichong (Liv3), the *yuan* (source) point of the Liver meridian, are treated in combination to promote the flow of blood and *qi* and relieve pain.

Treat once a day or once every other day. Use the reducing method for cases of short duration and the reinforcing method for long-standing cases. Ten treatments constitute one course.

Moxibustion

Points used are the same as for body acupuncture. Apply moxa roll moxibustion for 15–20 minutes to each point, once a day. Ten treatments constitute one course.

Moxibustion effectively warms the meridians, dispels cold and promotes the flow of *qi* and blood. It is therefore an ideal method for treating Raynaud's disease. It is usually used in combination with body acupuncture.

Electroacupuncture

Points used are the same as for body acupuncture. Select one or two pairs of points each time. Puncture until a needling sensation is achieved, then connect the needles to an electrical stimulator. Apply moderate intermittent wave stimulation for 30 minutes, once a day or once every other day. Ten treatments constitute one course.

Auricular therapy

Auricular points:

Auricular points corresponding to the affected areas of the body: locate positive points; tape both frontal and dorsal surfaces to increase stimulation.

Liver, Heart, Lung: regulate the flow of *qi* and blood.

Spleen: reinforces the spleen *qi* to improve blood circulation.

Sympathesis: alleviates spasm of the arterioles.

Subcortex: regulates nervous, circulatory and endocrine functions.

Ear Shenmen: relieves pain.

Apex of Ear: blood-letting puncturing of this point with a three-edged needle activates the meridians to relieve pain.

Use auricular taping with strong manipulation and blood-letting puncturing where indicated, twice a week. Ten treatments constitute one course.

Remarks

☯ Traditional therapies are very effective for treating Raynaud's disease; it can not only relieve symptoms but also treat the cause.
☯ Traditional therapies can also be used as auxiliary methods for treating Raynaud's symptoms appearing in other diseases including rheumatoid arthritis, thromboangiitis obliterans, peripheral neuritis and occupational diseases of typists, piano players, etc.
☯ Patients should abstain from tobacco and keep the extremities warm in order to prevent relapse.

104 Recurrent ulcer of the mouth

Recurrent ulcer of the mouth is the most commonly seen ulcerative condition of the mucous membrane of the mouth. It is marked by frequently recurring, painful, small circular or oval ulcers of the mucous membrane of the mouth. The pain is aggravated by exposure of the ulcers to heat, cold, acid or salt and may be severe enough to affect eating and sleep. The condition may become more severe or recur more frequently in the presence of insomnia, poor diet or overstrain.

Aetiology

According to traditional Chinese medicine, recurrent ulcer of the mouth is classified into excessive and deficient types. The excessive type is caused by overindulgence in spicy or greasy food or by mental injury, leading to accumulation of heat in the interior which flares up along the meridians to the mouth. The deficient type is caused by prolonged illness, overstrain, or excessive sexual activity which consume the kidney *yin*, leading to subsequent flaring up of deficient fire to the mouth.

Differentiation of syndromes

● Recurrent ulcer of the mouth due to excessive heat in the stomach.
  Characterized by small painful burning ulcers in the mouth; accompanied by thirst with preference for cold beverages, halitosis, constipation, scanty urine, red tongue with dry yellowish coating and rapid pulse.
● Recurrent ulcer of the mouth due to flaring up of deficient fire caused by deficiency of the kidney *yin*.
  Characterized by frequently recurring, mildly painful small ulcers in the mouth; accompanied by dry mouth and throat, a sensation of heat in the palms and soles, insomnia, restlessness, dry red tongue with little coating and thready rapid pulse.

Body acupuncture

Main acupuncture points:

Taichong	(Liv3)
Hegu	(LI4)
Fengchi	(G20)
Dicang	(S4)
Jiache	(S6)
Xiaguan	(S7)

The Liver meridian distributes to the inside of the cheeks and lips, so Taichong (Liv3), the *yuan* (source) point of the Liver meridian, is punctured to activate the meridians and relieve pain. Hegu (LI4), the *yuan* (source) point of the Large Intestine meridian, is a main point for treating oral diseases and disorders. Fengchi

(G20), an important point of the Gallbladder meridian located at the base of the skull, functions to dispel heat. Dicang (S4), Jiache (S6) and Xiaguan (S7), are local points of the Stomach meridian effective for treating oral problems.

Auxiliary points are chosen according to differentiation of syndromes.

● For recurrent ulcer of the mouth due to excessive heat in the stomach, Lidui (S45), Shangyang (LI1) and Shaoshang (L11) are added and pricked with a three-edged needle to let several drops of blood; main points are punctured using the reducing method to dispel excessive heat.
● For recurrent ulcer of the mouth due to flaring up of deficient fire caused by deficiency of the kidney *yin*, Taixi (K3), Zhaohai (K6), Sanyinjiao (Sp6) and Laogong (P8) are added and punctured using the even method to tonify the kidney *yin* and extinguish deficient fire.

Treat once a day or once every other day. Ten treatments constitute one course.

Auricular therapy

Main auricular points:

Tongue, Mouth: correspond to the affected area. Locate positive points; tape Tongue on both frontal and dorsal surfaces to increase stimulation.

Heart: the heart opens into the tongue, so Heart is taped to activate the Heart meridian and dispel heat.

Liver: the Liver meridian distributes to the internal cheek, so Liver is taped to clear and activate the Liver meridian.

San Jiao: clears passages to allow fire to descend.

Endocrine, Adrenal Gland, Wind Stream: relieve inflammation.

Ear Shenmen, Occiput: tranquillize the mind and relieve pain.

Auxiliary auricular points:

For excessive type recurrent ulcer of the mouth, Apex of Ear is added and punctured with a three-edged needle to cause bleeding.

For deficient type recurrent ulcer of the mouth, Kidney and Spleen are added to nourish the *yin*.

Use auricular taping with strong manipulation and blood-letting puncturing where indicated, twice a week. Five treatments constitute one course.

Remarks

☻ Both body acupuncture and auricular therapy are effective for treating recurrent ulcer of the mouth.
☻ These methods are also effective for treating acute and chronic cheilitis.

105 Retention of placenta

Retention of placenta refers to failure to expel the placenta from the uterus following parturition.

Aetiology

Traditional Chinese medicine classifies retention of placenta into two types. The *qi* deficiency type is caused by weak constitution or overstrain during delivery which consumes the *qi* and blood; the stagnant blood type is caused by stagnation of lochia in the uterus. Both types affect the ability of the uterus to contract and expel the placenta immediately following delivery.

Differentiation of syndromes

● Retention of placenta due to deficiency of *qi*.
  Characterized by failure to expel the placenta following delivery, mild distension and soft mass in the lower abdomen with no pain when palpated and profuse reddish lochia and blood; accompanied by pale complexion, lassitude, pale tongue with thin whitish coating and weak pulse.
● Retention of placenta due to stagnation of blood in the uterus.
  Characterized by failure to expel the placenta following delivery, hard mass and severe pain in the lower abdomen aggravated by pressure, scanty purple lochia, purple tongue and deep uneven pulse.

Treatment

Body acupuncture

Main acupuncture points:

Guanyuan	(Ren4)
Sanyinjiao	(Sp6)
Hegu	(LI4)
Duyin	(Ex24)

Guanyuan (Ren4), the meeting point of the Ren and three Foot Yin meridians located on the lower abdomen and Sanyinjiao (Sp6), the meeting point of the three Foot Yin meridians, are usually treated in combination. They are an important pair of points for treating gynaecological and obstetrical problems. Hegu (LI4) is punctured to accelerate delivery of the placenta and decrease haemorrhage. Duyin (Ex24) is a clinically effective point for treating placental retention.

Auxiliary points and appropriate methods of manipulation are chosen according to differentiation of syndromes.

● For retention of placenta due to deficiency of *qi*, *qi* is strengthened by puncturing the points using the reinforcing method and applying moxibustion to Shenque (Ren8), Yinbai (Sp1) and Duyin (Ex24).
● For retention of placenta due to stagnation of blood in the uterus, Qugu (Ren2) and Xuehai (Sp10) are added and punctured using the reducing method to promote the flow of blood.

Moxibustion

Point:

Shenque   (Ren8)

First apply a thin layer of salt to the umbilicus, then treat the point with 3–7 small moxa cones, or apply moxa roll moxibustion for 20–30 minutes. Moxibustion can effectively accelerate delivery of the placenta and decrease haemorrhage.

Electroacupuncture

Points used are the same as for body acupuncture. Select one or two pairs of points each time. Puncture until a needling sensation is achieved, then connect the needles to an electrical stimulator. Apply moderate continuous wave stimulation for 30 minutes.

Remarks

☯ Traditional therapies are very effective for treating retention of the placenta. In many cases, one treatment with one method is sufficient. In cases of partial retention of the placenta, acupuncture may be applied once a day. Five treatments constitute one course.

☯ It is suggested that Hegu (LI4) be punctured and moxibustion be applied to Shenque (Ren8) immediately following the expulsive stage in order to shorten the placental stage and decrease haemorrhage.

☯ For cases with profuse vaginal haemorrhage, additional measures should be undertaken concurrently.

☯ These methods are also suitable for cases of prolonged labour due to uterine atony; however, points on the lower abdomen may not be punctured.

106 Retention of urine

Retention of urine is a common symptom of various diseases and disorders. It is characterized by filling of the bladder with inability to voluntarily void urine. It is classified into three types, according to cause:

1. retention of urine due to sphincterismus of the urethra, caused by inflammation, injury, or pelvic, rectal or perineal surgery;
2. neurogenic retention of urine, caused by disturbance of the nerves which control urination, including encephalomyelopathy, mental injury or drug reactions;
3. retention of urine due to obstruction of the urinary tract caused by inflammation, stones or tumours of the urinary tract or its surrounding tissues.

Aetiology

According to traditional Chinese medicine, urine is stored in the urinary bladder and its excretion is controlled by the kidney *qi*. Difficulty in urination or retention of urine may be caused by accumulation of damp-heat in the bladder which obstructs the flow of *qi*, by trauma such as abdominal surgery which damages the *qi* in the meridians, or by deficiency of the kidney *yang* which affects the ability of the kidneys to excrete urine.

Differentiation of syndromes

● Retention of urine due to accumulation of damp-heat in the bladder.
Characterized by retention of urine or scanty urine with burning sensation while urinating; distension of the lower abdomen, bitter taste in the mouth, thirst but unwillingness to drink, poor appetite, constipation, red tongue with greasy yellowish coating and rapid slippery pulse.

● Retention of urine due to traumatic injury of the meridian *qi*.
Characterized by dribbling urination or complete retention of urine; history of trauma, parturition, or lower abdominal surgery; accompanied by distension and pain in the lower abdomen, whitish tongue coating and thready pulse.

● Retention of urine due to obstruction of the urinary tract.
Characterized by dribbling, weak, or suddenly stopping urinary stream; accompanied by distension and pain in the lower abdomen, purple-spotted tongue and uneven thready pulse.
● Retention of urine due to deficiency of the kidney *yang*.
Characterized by difficult urination or complete retention of urine; accompanied by listlessness, pale complexion, sensation of cold and weakness in the back and knees, pale tongue with whitish coating and deep, thready, weak pulse.

Treatment

Body acupuncture

Main acupuncture points:

| Zhongji | (Ren3) |
| Sanyinjiao | (Sp9) |

Retention of urine is a disorder of the urinary bladder, one of the six *fu* organs. Therefore Zhongji (Ren3), the front-*mu* point of the urinary bladder, is treated to stimulate the bladder and improve urination. The Liver, Spleen and Kidney meridians all pass through the lower abdomen, therefore Sanyinjiao (Sp6), the meeting point of these three meridians, is punctured to dredge the meridians and promote diuresis.

Auxiliary points and appropriate methods of manipulation are chosen according to differentiation of syndromes.

● For retention of urine due to accumulation of damp-heat in the bladder, Yinlingquan (Sp9) and Ligou (Liv5) are added and punctured using the reducing method to remove damp-heat.
● For retention of urine due to traumatic injury of the meridian *qi*, the meridians are activated to promote urination by adding and puncturing Xuehai (Sp10) and Taichong (Liv3) using the even method, or applying moxibustion as needed.
● For retention of urine due to obstruction of the urinary tract, acupuncture is used auxiliary to aetiological treatments.
● For retention of urine due to deficiency of the kidney *yang*, the kidney *yang* is tonified to promote diuresis by adding and puncturing Shenshu (B23) and Guanyuan (Ren4) using the reinforcing method and then applying moxibus-

tion to Shenshu (B23), Guanyuan (Ren4) and Shenque (Ren8) .

Treat once a day or once every other day. Ten treatments constitute one course.

Moxibustion

Points used are the same as for body acupuncture. Apply moxa roll moxibustion for 15–20 minutes to each point, once a day. Five treatments constitute one course.

Moxibustion is suitable only for treating retention of urine due to traumatic injury of the meridian *qi* or deficiency of the kidney *yang*.

Point injection therapy

Points used are the same as for body acupuncture. Inject 1.5 ml of proserine on each point, once a day. Five treatments constitute one course.

Electroacupuncture

Points used are the same as for body acupuncture. Select one or two pairs of points each time. Puncture the points until a needling sensation is achieved, then connect the needles to an electrical stimulator. Apply moderate intermittent wave stimulation for 20–30 minutes, once a day. Five treatments constitute one course.

Hot salt compress therapy

Points:

| Zhongji | (Ren3) |
| Guanyuan | (Ren4) |

Apply small bags filled with hot salt to both points. The bladder may be full or empty. Protect the skin by placing a towel under the bag while it is very hot; when it starts to cool down the towel can be removed. Change to a new hot bag when the first one is no longer hot. Apply for 30–60 minutes, once or twice a day. Ten treatments constitute one course.

This method functions to warm the kidney *yang* and strengthen the bladder. It is therefore suitable for treating retention of urine due to traumatic injury of the meridian *qi* or deficiency of the kidney *yang*.

Auricular therapy

Main auricular points:

Urinary Bladder, Urethra, Abdomen: correspond to the affected areas of the body. Locate positive points; tape both frontal and dorsal surfaces to increase stimulation.

Kidney: tonifies the kidneys and promotes urination.

San Jiao: dredges the water passages.

Subcortex, Sympathesis, Lumbosacral Vertebrae: regulate the nervous function.

Auxiliary auricular points:

For retention of urine due to accumulation of damp-heat in the bladder, Apex of Ear is added and punctured with a three-edged needle to dispel heat and remove dampness.

For retention of urine due to traumatic injury of the meridian *qi*, points corresponding to the site of the injury or surgery are added.

Use auricular taping and blood-letting puncturing where indicated, twice a week.

Remarks

☯ Acupuncture is an ideal method of treating reflex and some neurological types of retention of urine. For retention of urine due to obstruction of the urinary tract, the original problem should be treated.

☯ Many clinical reports indicate that acupuncture can cure retention of urine in one treatment. Body acupuncture and moxibustion, used either singly or in combination, are the usual methods chosen.

☯ When puncturing points located on the lower abdomen and in the lumbosacral region, a needling sensation should be felt in the perineal region for the greatest effectiveness to be achieved.

☯ Tapping Zhongji (Ren3) for 5–10 minutes while the bladder is full is useful for stimulating voiding.

107 Scapulohumeral periarthritis

Scapulohumeral periarthritis is a chronic retrograde inflammation of the soft tissues, including muscles, tendons and joint capsules, peripheral to the shoulder joint. It occurs primarily in people over 50 years old and more often in women than in men. It is marked by pain and limited abduction, outward rotation, backward extension and raising of the shoulder joint. The pain may radiate to the neck and upper arm, lessening during the day and worsening at night. In severe cases, the shoulder joint may become completely frozen, with resulting atrophy of the shoulder muscles.

Aetiology

According to traditional Chinese medicine, scapulohumeral periarthritis is caused by internal deficiency of *qi* and blood and external invasion by wind-cold, trauma or strain. The combination of internal and external factors results in obstruction of *qi* and blood in the meridians and insufficient

nourishment of the tendons and muscles. In clinical practice, scapulohumeral periarthritis is usually differentiated according to meridian theory. Primarily affected are the Lung, Large Intestine, San Jiao and Small Intestine meridians.

Differentiation of syndromes

● Scapulohumeral periarthritis of the Lung meridian type.
  Marked by limited backward extension of the affected arm and tenderness on Jianqian (Ex15).
● Scapulohumeral periarthritis of the Large Intestine meridian type.
  Marked by limited raising of the arm and tenderness on Jianyu (LI15).
● Scapulohumeral periarthritis of the San Jiao meridian type.
  Marked by limited abduction of the affected arm and tenderness on Jianliao (SJ14).

- Scapulohumeral periarthritis of the Small Intestine meridian type.

  Marked by limited abduction and raising of the affected arm and tenderness on Tianzong (SI11).

Clinically, these four types may occur singly or in combinations of two or more.

Treatment

Body acupuncture

Group 1:
Jianqian	(Ex15)
Chize	(L5)
Yuji	(L10)
Yinlingquan	(Sp9)

Group 2:
Jianyu	(LI15)
Shousanli	(LI10)
Hegu	(LI4)
Tiaokou	(S38)

Group 3:
Jianliao	(SJ14)
Waiguan	(SJ5)
Zhongzhu	(SJ3)
Jianjing	(G21)
Yanglingquan	(G34)

Group 4:
Jianzhen	(SI9)
Tianzong	(SI11)
Houxi	(SI3)
Shenmai	(B62)

Both local and distal points are chosen according to meridian theory to activate the meridians and relieve pain. The four groups are used for the four types of scapulohumeral periarthritis respectively. Distal points of the Foot meridians which correspond to the Hand meridians are treated to increase stimulation; they are punctured after the needles have been withdrawn from points of the Hand meridian. Patients should move the affected limbs during manipulation of the Foot meridian points in order to promote the circulation of *qi* and blood and relieve pain.

For acute cases with a strong constitution use strong manipulation; use moderate manipulation for chronic cases with a weak constitution. Treat once a day or once every other day. Ten treatments constitute one course.

Moxibustion

Select local and *ashi* points. Treat each point with moxa roll moxibustion for 15 minutes, or ginger and 10–15 medium-sized moxa cones, once a day or once every other day. Ten treatments constitute one course.

Electroacupuncture

Points used are the same as for body acupuncture. Select one or two pairs of points each time. Puncture the points until a needling sensation is achieved, then connect the needles to an electrical stimulator. Apply continuous wave stimulation of the highest bearable intensity for 30 minutes. Treat once a day or once every other day. Ten treatments constitute one course.

Point injection therapy

Local and tender points are injected with 2–4 ml of procaine, vitamin B_1, vitamin B_{12}, or dexamethasone, once every three days. Five treatments constitute one course.

Point implantation therapy

Select local or tender points. Using a triangular surgical needle, implant surgical catgut on two or three points each time. Treat once a week. Three treatments constitute one course. This method is used primarily for chronic or refractory cases.

Blood-letting puncturing and cupping

Prick one local or tender point each time with a three-edged needle, then cup for 15 minutes. Treat once every three to four days. Five treatments constitute one course. This method is usually used in combination with body acupuncture to increase stimulation.

Auricular therapy

Auricular points:

Shoulder, Clavicle: correspond to the affected areas of the body. Locate positive points; tape both frontal and dorsal surfaces to increase stimulation.

Lung, Small Intestine, Large Intestine, San Jiao: the meridians of these organs distribute to the shoulder, so these points are taped to activate the meridians and relieve pain.

Liver, Spleen, Kidney: these three organs nourish the tendons, so these points are taped to nourish the tendons and muscles and lubricate the shoulder joint.

Ear Shenmen: main point for pain relief.

Use auricular taping with strong manipulation, concentrating on the affected side for acute cases and bilateral sides for chronic cases, twice a week. Ten treatments constitute one course.

Remarks

☯ The above therapies can effectively relieve the pain of scapulohumeral periarthritis, but extended treatment should be given to improve the range of motion of the shoulder joint. The earlier treatment is instituted, the better the results will be.

☯ Two or more therapies are usually combined to increase stimulation and raise the effect of treatment.

☯ Doing shoulder range of motion exercises will increase the effectiveness of treatment and help prevent relapse.

108 Sciatica

Sciatica is a commonly occurring lumbocrural pain frequently seen in clinical practice. It is marked by stabbing or burning pain radiating along the pathway of the sciatic nerve, aggravated by walking, bending or coughing. Usually only one side is affected. Sciatica is classified into primary and secondary types. Primary sciatica is caused by infection affecting the sciatic nerve itself; secondary sciatica is caused by disease or disorder of the tissues adjacent to the sciatic nerve, such as prolapse of the lumbar intervertebral disc, sacroiliitis, coxitis or pelvic infection.

Aetiology

Traditional Chinese medicine classifies sciatica as a *bi* syndrome and considers it to be caused by stagnation of *qi* and blood in the meridians due to either exogenous wind-cold or damp-cold, or prolonged trauma or strain. The pain usually first manifests in the lumbosacral region or buttock, then radiates to the posterior side of the thigh, posterolateral side of the leg and lateral side of the dorsum. Primarily affected are the Urinary Bladder and Gallbladder meridians.

Differentiation of syndromes

● Sciatica due to invasion by damp-cold.
Characterized by lumbocrural pain and heaviness, possibly radiating to the lower limbs, aggravated in cold or damp weather and alleviated in warm or dry weather; greasy whitish tongue coating and deep pulse.

● Sciatica due to stagnation of the *qi* and blood.
Characterized by stabbing or lancinating pain in the lumbocrural region, possibly radiating to the lower limbs; purple or purple-spotted tongue and uneven pulse. There is usually a history of trauma or strain in the lumbosacral region.

● Sciatica due to deficiency of the kidney *qi*.
Characterized by frequently occurring or persistent pain in the lumbosacral region, possibly radiating to the lower limbs, aggravated by exertion and alleviated by rest; accompanied by sore and weak back and knees, lassitude, sensation of cold in the affected lower limb, pale tongue with whitish coating and deep thready pulse.

Treatment

Body acupuncture

Main acupuncture points:

Zhibian	(B54)
Chengfu	(B36)
Weizhong	(B40)

Chengshan	(B57)
Kunlun	(B60)
Shugu	(B65)
Huantiao	(G30)
Yanglingquan	(G34)
Huatuojiaji	(Ex46)(L1-L5)

Main points are chosen according to meridian theory. The distribution of sciatic pain is identical to the pathways of the Urinary Bladder and Gallbladder meridians, therefore main points are selected from these meridians. Three or four Urinary Bladder meridian points are selected each time. Huantiao (G30), the meeting point of the Gallbladder and Urinary Bladder meridians, is an important point for treating pain of the lower extremities. Yanglingquan (G34), the *he* (sea) point of the Gallbladder meridian and the *hui* (influential) point of the tendons, is closely related to the tendons and is an important point for treating pain of the lower extremities. There is usually tenderness on corresponding Huatuojiaji (Ex46) points, which are punctured to relieve pain.

Auxiliary points and appropriate methods of manipulation are chosen according to differentiation of syndromes.

● For sciatica due to invasion by damp-cold, Mingmen (Du4) and Yaoyangguan (Du3) are added and moxibustion is applied to warm the meridians and expel damp-cold.
● For sciatica due to stagnation of the *qi* and blood, tender points on the lumbosacral region are pricked with a three-edged needle and then cupped for 10–15 minutes to dredge the meridians and relieve pain.
● For sciatica due to deficiency of the kidney *qi*, Shenshu (B23), Taixi (K3) and Zusanli (S36) are added and punctured using the reinforcing method to strengthen the kidney *qi*.

Select five to seven points each time, concentrating on the affected side. Treat once a day or once every other day. Five treatments constitute one course.

Electroacupuncture

Points used are the same as for body acupuncture. Select one or two pairs of points each time. Puncture the points until a needling sensation is achieved, then connect the needles to an electrical stimulator. Apply intermittent wave stimulation of the strongest bearable intensity for 30 minutes. Treat once a day or once every other day. Ten treatments constitute one course.

Moxibustion

Points used are the same as for body acupuncture. Apply moxa roll moxibustion for 15–20 minutes to four to five points each time. Treat once a day or once every other day. Five treatments constitute one course.

Moxibustion is usually used in combination with other methods. Moxibustion is an ideal method of treatment in cases where acupuncture is contraindicated, such as during pregnancy or for people who tend to faint when given acupuncture.

Auricular therapy

Auricular points:

Sciatic Nerve, Lumbosacral Vertebrae, Buttock: correspond to the affected areas of the body. Locate positive points; tape both frontal and dorsal surfaces to increase stimulation.

Urinary Bladder, Pancreas & Gallbladder: clear and activate the meridians to relieve pain.

Kidney: the kidneys are connected both internally and externally with the urinary bladder and stored in the lumbus, so Kidney is taped to reinforce the kidney *qi* to strengthen the lumbus.

Ear Shenmen: main point for pain relief.

Use auricular taping with strong manipulation, twice a week. Five treatments constitute one course.

Remarks

☺ Traditional therapies can effectively relieve sciatic pain. In cases of secondary sciatica, concurrent treatment of the primary cause should be undertaken.
☺ The back and lower extremities should be kept warm to avoid relapse.

109 Seborrhoeic dermatitis

Seborrhoeic dermatitis is a chronic inflammatory condition of the sebaceous glands which occurs in conjunction with hypersteatosis, infection or metabolic dysfunction. It is classified into dry and moist types. The dry type is marked by yellowish-red patches covered with pityroid oleaginous scales. The moist type develops from the dry type, marked by eczematoid skin lesions with erosion, oozing and scabbing. Usually affected are the head, face, neck, axilla and chest.

Aetiology

According to traditional Chinese medicine, seborrhoeic dermatitis is caused either by exogenous wind-heat which invades the skin and consumes the blood, leading to insufficient nourishment of the skin, or by overindulgence in spicy or greasy foods, leading to accumulation of damp-heat in the interior and subsequent overflow to the skin.

Differentiation of syndromes

- Wind-heat seborrhoeic dermatitis.
  Characterized by yellowish-red patches covered with pityroid oleaginous scales; accompanied by itching, red tongue with dry whitish coating and rapid superficial pulse.
- Seborrhoeic dermatitis due to accumulation of damp-heat in the interior.
  Characterized by eczematoid skin lesions displaying erosion, oozing and scabbing; accompanied by constipation, dryness of the mouth, red tongue with greasy yellowish coating and rapid slippery pulse.

Treatment

Body acupuncture

Main acupuncture points:

Quchi	(LI11)
Hegu	(LI4)
Xuehai	(Sp10)
Sanyinjiao	(Sp6)

Fengchi	(G20)
Baihui	(Du20)

Quchi (LI11) and Hegu (LI4), the *he* (sea) and *yuan* (source) points of the Large Intestine meridian, are treated in combination to activate the meridians and expel pathogens. Xuehai (Sp10) (Sea of Blood in Chinese) functions to promote circulation and expel wind. It is one of the most important points for treating skin conditions. Sanyinjiao (Sp6), the meeting point of the three Foot Yin meridians, functions to strengthen the liver and spleen. Fengchi (G20) (Pool of Wind in Chinese) is an important point for expelling wind and relieving itching. Baihui (Du20), the meeting point on the top of the head of the Du, Liver and six Hand and Foot Yang meridians, functions to strengthen antipathogenic *qi* and expel pathogens.

Auxiliary points and appropriate manipulation are chosen according to differentiation of syndromes.

- For wind-heat seborrhoeic dermatitis, Dazhui (Du14) and Feishu (B13) are added and pricked with a three-edged needle, then cupped for 10–15 minutes to draw blood. The main points are punctured using the reducing method to expel wind and dispel heat.
- For seborrhoeic dermatitis due to accumulation of damp-heat in the interior, Dachangshu (B25), Tianshu (S25) and Zusanli (S36) are added and punctured using the reducing method to strengthen the stomach and intestines and remove damp-heat.

Treat once a day or once every other day. Ten treatments constitute one course.

Blood-letting puncturing

Acupuncture points:

Dazhui	(Du14)
Feishu	(B13)
Geshu	(B17)
Weizhong	(B40)
Quchi	(LI11)
Xuehai	(Sp10)

Select one or two points each time. Prick with a three-edged needle, then cup for 10–15 minutes to draw blood. Treat once every two to three days. This method is usually used in combination with other therapies.

Auricular therapy

Auricular points:

Areas corresponding to the affected regions: tap with a plum blossom needle to cause bleeding.

Lung: disperses the lung *qi* to expel exogenous pathogens.

Large Intestine, San Jiao: discharge damp-heat.

Liver, Spleen: strengthen the liver and spleen.

Endocrine, Subcortex: regulate endocrine and metabolic functions.

Sympathesis: inhibits secretion of the sebaceous glands.

Use auricular taping with strong manipulation and blood-letting puncturing where indicated, twice a week. Five treatments constitute one course.

Remarks

☯ Traditional therapies are very effective for treating seborrhoeic dermatitis.
☯ Avoid greasy and spicy foods; do not wash the skin with irritating soaps.

110 Seminal emission

Seminal emission refers to ejaculation in the male in the absence of sexual activity. Seminal emission that occurs while asleep is called oneirogmus; spontaneous seminal emission while awake is called spermatorrhoea. It is normal for healthy men to experience oneirogmus (popularly known as wet dreams) several times a month, but several times a week or every night is considered excessive. Excessive seminal emission is usually accompanied by weak and sore back and knees, dizziness, tinnitus, lassitude and poor memory.

Aetiology

According to traditional Chinese medicine, oneirogmus is caused by brooding which consumes the heart *yin*, resulting in imbalance between the heart and kidneys. Spermatorrhoea is caused by excessive masturbation or other sexual activity, or weakened constitution following prolonged illness, leading to deficiency of the kidney *qi*. Depression or anxiety which results in stagnation of the liver *qi* may also cause seminal emission. Primarily affected are the heart, liver and kidneys.

Differentiation of syndromes

● Seminal emission due to imbalance between the heart and kidneys.
Characterized by seminal emission while dreaming; accompanied by dizziness, palpitation, insomnia, dry mouth, night sweating, sensation of heat in the palms and soles, reddish tongue and rapid thready pulse.
● Seminal emission due to unconsolidated kidney *qi*.
Characterized by spontaneous seminal emission while awake; accompanied by dizziness, tinnitus, poor memory, listlessness, pale complexion, sore and weak back and knees, spontaneous sweating, coldness of the extremities, pale tongue with whitish coating and deep thready pulse.
● Seminal emission due to stagnation of the liver *qi*.
Characterized by seminal emission while either asleep or awake; accompanied by a feeling of fullness in the chest and hypochondriac region, depression or restlessness, frequent sighing, insomnia, poor appetite, loose stool, whitish tongue coating and wiry thready pulse.

Treatment

Body acupuncture

Main acupuncture points:

Guanyuan	(Ren4)
Sanyinjiao	(Sp6)
Yaoyangguan	(Du3)
Baihui	(Du20)

Guanyuan (Ren4), the meeting point of the Ren and three Foot Yin meridians located on the lower abdomen and Sanyinjiao (Sp6), the meeting point of the three Foot Yin meridians, are treated in combination to consolidate the *yuan* (original) *qi* and arrest the kidney essence. Yaoyangguan (Du3), a Du meridian point that corresponds to Guanyuan (Ren4), is treated in combination with Guanyuan (Ren4) to connect the *qi* of the Du and Ren meridians. Baihui (Du20), the meeting point of the Du and Hand and Foot Yang meridians, is punctured to tranquillize the mind and tonify the brain.

Auxiliary points and appropriate methods of manipulation are chosen according to differentiation of syndromes.

- For seminal emission due to imbalance of the heart and kidneys, Xinshu (B15), Shenmen (CH7) and Taixi (K3) are added and punctured using the even method to harmonize the heart and kidneys.
- For seminal emission due to unconsolidated kidney *qi*, the kidneys are tonified and essence arrested by adding and puncturing Shenshu (B23), Qihai (Ren4) and Zhishi (B52) using the reinforcing method, and adding moxibustion as needed.
- For seminal emission due to stagnation of the liver *qi*, Neiguan (P6) and Taichong (Liv3) are added and punctured using the reducing method to promote the flow of the liver *qi*.

Treat once a day or once every other day. Ten treatments constitute one course.

Electroacupuncture

Points used are the same as for body acupuncture. Select one or two pairs of points each time. Puncture until a needling sensation is achieved, then connect the needles to an electrical stimulator. Apply moderate intermittent wave stimulation for 30 minutes. Treat once a day or once every other day. Ten treatments constitute one course.

Moxibustion

Points:

Shenque	(Ren8)
Guanyuan	(Ren4)
Shenshu	(B23)
Zhishi	(B52)

Apply moxa roll moxibustion to all points for 15–20 minutes, or moxa cone moxibustion with salt to Shenque (Ren8) for 15–20 minutes, once a day or once every other day. Ten treatments constitute one course.

Moxibustion is suitable primarily for treating seminal emission due to unconsolidated kidney *qi*.

Auricular therapy

Main auricular points:

Kidney: tonifies the kidneys to arrest essence.

Liver: soothes the liver *qi* to regulate the emotions.

Spleen, Stomach: strengthen the spleen and stomach to increase acquired essence.

Subcortex: regulates the central nervous system.

Ear Shenmen, Occiput: calm the mind.

Auxiliary auricular points:

For seminal emission while dreaming, Heart and Anterior Lobe are added.

Use auricular taping twice a week. Five treatments constitute one course. Auricular self-massage and pressure may also be practised twice a day.

Remarks

- The above methods are effective for treating premature ejaculation as well as seminal emission. When puncturing Guanyuan (Ren4), it is essential that a needling sensation be experienced in the external genitals.
- Seminal emission is closely related to psychological factors. It is therefore essential to encourage a positive attitude and confidence that traditional therapies can provide a cure.

111 Sequelae of cerebrovascular accident

Cerebrovascular accident, including cerebral haemorrhage, thrombosis, embolism, subarachnoid haemorrhage, etc. is a leading cause of death among humans. Sequelae following the acute stage may include hemiplegia, deviation of the mouth, dysphasia or aphasia, dysphagia, urinary and fecal incontinence and mental disorders. These symptoms may exist singly or in conjunction. Experimental studies have shown that acupuncture can dilate the cerebral arteries, improve cerebral circulation and raise the partial pressure of oxygen in the brain, thus increasing the supply of oxygen to the cerebral cells surrounding the lesion and improving the repair of cerebral tissues. Treatment should be instituted immediately following the acute stage in order to alleviate symptoms and reduce sequelae.

Aetiology

Traditional Chinese medicine classifies cerebrovascular accident as windstroke and considers it to be caused primarily by mental injury or overindulgence in sexual activity, both of which may damage the liver and kidneys. The resulting overactivity and agitation of the liver *yang* in turn produce liver wind, which stirs up and disturbs the *qi*, blood, *yin* and *yang*. Another cause is overindulgence in alcohol and fatty foods leading to dysfunction of the spleen's functions of transportation and transformation, with subsequent accumulation of phlegm heat in the interior. Windstroke occurs when phlegm heat ascends to block the collaterals of the brain.

Post-acute stage sequelae, including hemiplegia, deviation of the mouth, stiff tongue, etc., occur due to obstruction of the meridians and collaterals by pathogenic phlegm and stagnant blood. Generally speaking, windstroke is deficient in origin and excessive in expression, that is, the liver, spleen and kidneys are deficient and pathogenic phlegm and stagnant blood are excessive. Acupuncture and related therapies improve the circulation of *qi* and blood, remove phlegm and strengthen the internal organs, thus treating both the cause and symptoms.

Differentiation of syndromes

- Sequelae of cerebrovascular accident due to hyperactivity of the liver *yang*.
  Characterized by headache, dizziness, flushed face, bitter taste in the mouth, restlessness, constipation, scanty yellowish urine, red tongue with yellowish coating and wiry thready pulse.
- Sequelae of cerebrovascular accident due to *yin* deficiency of the liver and kidneys.
  Characterized by dizziness, tinnitus, blurred vision, restlessness, insomnia, bad dreams, red tongue with little coating and rapid, wiry, thready pulse.
- Sequelae of cerebrovascular accident due to obstruction of the meridians and collaterals by turbid phlegm.
  Characterized by dizziness, drowsiness, involuntary drooling, wheezing sound in the throat, vomiting of fluid, poor appetite, greasy slimy tongue coating and wiry slippery pulse.
- Sequelae of cerebrovascular accident due to deficiency of *qi* and blood.
  Characterized by palpitation, shortness of breath, spontaneous sweating, lassitude, pale complexion, poor appetite, loose stool, pale or purple spotted tongue and deep, thready, weak pulse.
- Sequelae of cerebrovascular accident due to *yang* deficiency of the spleen and kidneys.
  Characterized by listlessness, drowsiness, swollen limbs, pale and dim complexion, anorexia, abdominal distension, swollen tongue with moist and glossy coating and deep, slippery, sometimes irregular pulse.

Treatment
Body acupuncture

Hemiplegia, points for the upper limbs

Jianyu	(LI15)
Quchi	(LI11)
Hegu	(LI4)
Waiguan	(SJ5)
Houxi	(SI3)
Baxie	(Ex6)
Huatuojiaji	(Ex46) (T1–T3)

Hemiplegia, points for the lower limbs

Zhibian	(B54)
Huantiao	(G30)
Zusanli	(S36)
Yanglingquan	(G34)
Xuanzhong	(G39)
Jiexi	(S41)
Bafeng	(Ex23)
Huatuojiaji	(Ex46) (L1–L5)

All Yang meridians, especially the Yangming meridians, are rich in *qi* and blood. Accordingly, points of these meridians are used to clear the meridians and activate the flow of *qi* and blood.

Puncture mainly the affected side, or the affected side in conjunction with the unaffected side, using the reducing method during the first three months and the reinforcing method thereafter.

Auxiliary points are added according to symptoms.

● For strephenopodia, Shenmai (B62) is punctured using the reinforcing method.
● For strephexopodia, Zhaohai (K6) is punctured using the reinforcing method.
● For spasm of the joints, local points are punctured using the even method. For instance, Yangchi (SJ4) and Daling (P7) are chosen for spasm of the wrist joint; Quze (P3) and Chize (L5) are chosen for spasm of the elbow joint, etc.

Deviation of the mouth

Dicang	(S4)
Jiache	(S6)
Xiaguan	(S7)
Yifeng	(SJ17)
Hegu	(LI4)

Both the Stomach and Large Intestine meridians distribute to the face, so points of these meridians are selected to activate the meridians. Dicang (S4) and Jiache (S6) are usually punctured simultaneously with one needle in order to increase stimulation. Yifeng (SJ17), located close to the facial canal, has been found through clinical experience to be effective for treating deviation of the mouth.

Dysphasia and aphasia

Jinjin and Yuye	(Ex33)
Lianquan	(Ren23)
Tongli	(H5)

The heart opens into the tongue, so Tongli (H5), the *luo* (collateral) point of the Heart meridian, is punctured to clear the meridians and eliminate phlegm. Jingjin and Yuye (Ex33) are pricked with a three-edged needle to draw several drops of blood; Lianquan (Ren23) is punctured toward the root of the tongue.

Dysphagia

Lianquan	(Ren23)
Tiantu	(Ren22)
Fengchi	(G20)
Fengfu	(Du16)

Puncture Tiantu (Ren22) perpendicularly for 0.2 *cun* and then vertically downward along the posterior wall of the sternum for 1.0–1.5 *cun* to regulate the flow of *qi*. With the patient's head lowered, puncture Fengfu (Du16) toward the base of the lower jaw to a depth of 0.5–0.8 *cun*. Manipulate the needle using the even method for 3–5 minutes, then withdraw.

Incontinence of urine and stool

Qihai	(Ren6)
Guanyuan	(Ren4)
Yaoshu	(Du2)

Puncture using the reinforcing method, then apply moxa roll moxibustion for 10–15 minutes to warm the *yuan* (primordial) *qi* and arrest urine and stool.

Mental disorders

Baihui	(Du20)
Sishencong	(Ex26)
Fengchi	(G20)
Neiguan	(P6)

Puncture using the reinforcing method to harmonize the flow of *qi* and tranquillize the mind.

All main acupuncture points are selected according to primary symptoms of the sequelae; auxiliary points are added according to differentiation of syndromes.

● For sequelae of cerebrovascular accident due to hyperactivity of the liver *yang*, Taichong (Liv3), Sanyinjiao (Sp6), Baihui (Du20) and Taiyang (Ex30) are added and punctured using the reducing method. Alternatively, Apex of Ear may be punctured with a three-edged needle to draw blood and soothe the liver *yang*.

● For sequelae of cerebrovascular accident due to *yin* deficiency of the liver and kidneys, Taichong (Liv3), Taixi (K3), Sanyinjiao (Sp6), Fengchi (G20) and Sishencong (Ex26) are added and punctured using the even method to tonify the liver and kidneys.

● For sequelae of cerebrovascular accident due to obstruction of the meridians and collaterals by turbid phlegm, Zhongwan (Ren12), Fenglong (S40), Sanyinjiao (Sp6) and Danzhong (Ren17) are added and punctured using the even method to strengthen the spleen and remove phlegm.

● For sequelae of cerebrovascular accident due to deficiency of *qi* and blood, Zusanli (S36), Sanyinjiao (Sp6), Qihai (Ren6) and Pishu (B20) are added and punctured using the reinforcing method, or moxibustion may be applied to the same points for 10–15 minutes, to tonify the *qi* and blood.

● For sequelae of cerebrovascular accident due to *yang* deficiency of the spleen and kidneys, Qihai (Ren6), Guanyuan (Ren4), Shenshu (B23), Mingmen (Du4), Taixi (K3) and Sanyinjiao (Sp6) are added and punctured using the reinforcing method and then treated with moxibustion for 10–15 minutes to warm the spleen and kidneys.

Choose main and auxiliary points as indicated; treat once a day or every other day. Ten treatments constitute one course.

Scalp acupuncture

Scalp lines:

Dingnie Qianxiexian (MS6)
Dingpangxian 1   (MS8)
Dingpangxian 2   (MS9)

Puncture the contralateral side; manipulate using the reducing method for five minutes, or connect the needles to an electrical stimulator and apply intermittent wave stimulation for 20–30 minutes. At the same time, have the patient move the affected limbs, providing assistance if necessary, in order to increase the effect. Several needles are applied along the appropriate line and usually retained for up to 24 hours to increase stimulation.

This method is suitable for treating hemiplegia resulting from cerebrovascular accident. For cases of cerebral haemorrhage, use scalp acupuncture only after the patient's blood pressure and general condition have stabilized. For cases of cerebral thrombosis, start treatment with scalp acupuncture as soon as possible after onset in order to increase effect and shorten the course of treatment. For cases accompanied by high fever, acute infection or heart failure, scalp acupuncture should be used with caution.

Treat once a day or once every other day. Ten treatments constitute one course.

Electroacupuncture

Points used are the same as for body acupuncture. Select two or three pairs of points each time. Puncture until a needling sensation in achieved, then connect the needles to an electrical stimulator. Apply moderate intermittent wave stimulation for hemiplegia and mild intermittent wave stimulation for other sequelae, for 15–30 minutes each time.

Treat once a day or every other day. Ten treatments constitute one course.

Remarks

😊 Acupuncture is an ideal method for treating sequelae of cerebrovascular accident.

😊 The earlier treatment is instituted, the better the results will be. Acupuncture may be started as soon as the intracranial hypertension and cerebral haemorrhage have been controlled, or immediately following onset of cerebral thrombosis.

😊 The various methods discussed above are usually used in conjunction in order to increase stimulation and raise effectiveness.

😊 When puncturing the unaffected side or giving scalp acupuncture, the patient should engage in passive or active exercise of the affected side both during and following treatment.

😊 It is recorded in the ancient literature that regular moxibustion on Zusanli (S36) and Xuanzhong (G39) may be used to prevent occurrence or recurrence of cerebrovascular accident in the elderly.

112 Simple glaucoma

Simple glaucoma is a disease of the eye marked by moderately or temporarily high intraocular pressure in the initial stage and by continuously high intraocular pressure in the advanced stage. Manifestations include distension of the eyeballs and easily tiring vision and headache. Hypopsia may occur in the advanced stage. There may be a family history of glaucoma.

Aetiology

According to traditional Chinese medicine, simple glaucoma is caused either by relative hyperactivity of the liver *yang* due to deficiency of the kidney *yin*, or by *yin* deficiency of the liver and kidneys.

Differentiation of syndromes

- Simple glaucoma due to hyperactivity of the liver *yang* caused by deficiency of the kidney *yin*.
  Characterized by distending pain in the eyeballs aggravated at night and alleviated during the day; blurred vision; accompanied by headache, restlessness, insomnia and wiry, thready, rapid pulse.
- Simple glaucoma due to *yin* deficiency of the liver and kidneys.
  Characterized by blurred vision and dryness and pain in the eyeballs; accompanied by dizziness, distending pain in the eyeballs, palpitation, insomnia, bad dreams, dry mouth and throat, sore and weak back and knees, red tongue with little coating and weak thready pulse.

Treatment

Body acupuncture

Main acupuncture points:

Fengchi	(G20)
Guangming	(G37)
Taichong	(Liv3)
Taiyang	(Ex30)
Qiuhou	(Ex31)

The liver opens into the eyes, the Liver and Gallbladder meridians connect with the eyes and the Liver and Gallbladder meridians are connected both internally and externally. Therefore main points for treating eye problems are selected from the Liver and Gallbladder meridians. Fengchi (G20), an important point of the Gallbladder meridian located at the base of the skull, functions to tranquillize the mind and brighten the eyes. Guangming (G37) (Brightness in Chinese) the *luo* (collateral) point of the Gallbladder meridian, functions to brighten the eyes. Taichong (Liv3), the *yuan* (source) point of the Liver meridian, functions to soothe the liver and subdue endogenous wind.

Taiyang (Ex30) and Qiuhou (Ex31) are two local extraordinary points for treating various eye problems. When puncturing Qiuhou (Ex31), support the eyeball with the thumb or index finger, then puncture the point below the eyeball to a depth of 0.5–1.0 *cun*.

Auxiliary points and appropriate manipulation are chosen according to differentiation of syndromes.

- For simple glaucoma due to hyperactivity of the liver *yang* caused by deficiency of the kidney *yin*, Baihui (Du20) is added and punctured using the even method to subdue the hyperactive liver *yang*.
- For simple glaucoma due to *yin* deficiency of the liver and kidneys, Sanyinjiao (Sp6) and Taixi (K3) are added and punctured using the even method to nourish the liver and kidneys.

Treat once a day or once every other day. Ten treatments constitute one course.

Auricular therapy

Auricular points:

Eye, Eye 2: correspond to the affected area.

Liver, Liver Yang: subdue hyperactive liver *yang*.

Kidney: nourishes the kidney *yin* to suppress the liver *yang*.

Occiput: corresponds to the visual centre.

Subcortex, Ear Shenmen: regulate the nervous function.

Apex of Ear: blood-letting puncturing of this point with a three-edged needle tranquillizes the mind and lowers the intraocular pressure.

Use auricular taping and blood-letting puncturing where indicated, twice a week. Five treatments constitute one course.

Remarks

☯ Traditional therapies can effectively alleviate the symptoms of simple glaucoma and lower intraocular pressure.
☯ Use mild manipulation when puncturing Qiuhou (Ex31) to avoid bleeding.
☯ These methods can also be used as auxiliary treatment for other types of glaucoma.

113 Stiff neck

Stiff neck refers to rigidity, pain and limited movement of the neck caused by improper sleeping position, strain, sprain, or attack by windcold. It usually occurs in the morning upon arising. It is marked by rigidity of the neck and pain which usually radiates to the homolateral shoulder and upper arm, accompanied by muscular tension of the neck, severe tenderness on the medial angle of the scapula and impaired neck movement.

Aetiology and differentiation of syndromes

According to traditional Chinese medicine, stiff neck is caused by obstruction of *qi* and blood in the meridians due to strain, sleeping with too many pillows or invasion of the neck by wind-cold. Usually affected are the Small Intestine, Urinary Bladder, Gallbladder, San Jiao and Du meridians. Cases due to disorder of the Gallbladder or San Jiao meridians are marked by difficulty in turning the head to the left and right; cases due to disorder of the Small Intestine, Urinary Bladder or Du meridians are marked by difficulty in bending the head forward and backward.

Treatment

Body acupuncture

Acupuncture points:

Group 1:
Yifeng	(SJ17)
Fengchi	(G20)
Zhongzhu	(SJ3)
Xuanzhong	(G39)

Group 2:
Tianzhu	(B10)
Dazhui	(Du14)
Houxi	(SI3)
Kunlun	(B60)

Both local and distal points are selected according to meridian theory. Points in Group 1 are used in cases due to disorder of the Gallbladder or San Jiao meridians. Yifeng (SJ17) and Fengchi (G20) are local points and Zhongzhu (SJ3) and Xuanzhong (G34) are distal points. There is usually tenderness present on the two local points.

Points in Group 2 are used in cases due to disorder of the Small Intestine, Urinary Bladder or Du meridians. Tianzhu (B10) and Dazhui (Du14) are local points; Houxi (SI3), one of the eight confluence points connecting with the Du meridian, is a distal point for treating neck problems. First puncture both local points and distal points and retain the needles for 20 minutes, then withdraw the needles from the local points and manipulate the distal points. Instruct the patient to move the neck while the distal points are being manipulated.

Manipulate using the reducing method for acute cases and the moderate method for chronic cases. Treat once a day for acute cases and once every other day for chronic cases. Five treatments constitute one course.

Electroacupuncture

Points used are the same as for body acupuncture. Select one or two pairs of points each time.

Puncture the points until a needling sensation is achieved, then connect the needles to an electrical stimulator. Apply continuous wave stimulation of the strongest bearable intensity for 30 minutes. Treat once a day or once every other day. Ten treatments constitute one course.

Auricular therapy

Auricular points:

Neck: corresponds to the affected area of the body. Locate positive points; tape both frontal and dorsal surfaces to increase stimulation.

Liver, Spleen: the liver nourishes the tendons and the spleen the muscles, so Liver and Spleen are taped to alleviate pain of the tendons and muscles.

Small Intestine, Pancreas & Gallbladder, Urinary Bladder: the meridians of these organs distribute to the neck, so Small Intestine, Pancreas & Gallbladder and Urinary Bladder

are taped to activate their corresponding meridians.

Subcortex, Ear Shenmen: relieve pain.

Use auricular taping with strong manipulation twice a week. Five treatments constitute one course.

Remarks

☯ The above treatments are very effective for treating stiff neck. Two to three treatments are often sufficient for acute cases.
☯ Many clinical reports indicate that it is sufficient to treat only the distal points. It is suggested that combining puncturing of the distal points and moxibustion or massage of the local points is an ideal method of treatment for stiff neck.
☯ Sleeping in a proper position, using a comfortable pillow and keeping the neck warm are essential for avoiding relapse.

114 Stye

Stye is classified into two types according to location. External stye refers to acute suppurative inflammation of the ciliary glands. It is marked by red and swollen eyelids with accompanying pain and scleroma, with an open sore appearing several days after onset. In severe cases, congestion and oedema of the bulbar conjunctiva may occur. Internal stye refers to acute suppurative inflammation of the tarsal glands, with manifestations similar to but more severe than those of external stye.

Aetiology

According to traditional Chinese medicine, stye is caused by exogenous wind-heat or overindulgence in spicy or greasy food, leading to stagnation of *qi* and blood in the eyelid.

Differentiation of syndromes

● Stye due to exogenous wind-heat.
  Characterized by red and swollen eyelids with pain and scleroma; accompanied by headache, fever, aversion to cold and rapid superficial pulse.
● Stye due to excessive heat in the stomach and spleen.
  Characterized by red and swollen eyelids with pain and scleroma; accompanied by thirst, restlessness, greasy yellowish tongue coating and rapid slippery pulse.

Treatment

Body acupuncture

Main acupuncture points:

Fengchi   (G20)

Hegu   (LI4)
Taiyang   (Ex30)

Fengchi (G20), a main point of the Gallbladder meridian located at the base of the skull, functions to expel wind, dispel heat and brighten the eyes. Hegu (LI4), the *yuan* (source) point of the Large Intestine meridian, functions to expel wind and dispel heat. Taiyang (Ex30) is an extraordinary point for treating eye problems; it is pricked with a three-edged needle to draw several drops of blood and dispel heat.

Auxiliary points and appropriate manipulation are chosen according to differentiation of syndromes.

● For stye due to exogenous wind-heat, wind is expelled and heat dispelled by adding and puncturing Dazhui (Du14) using the reducing method, or pricking Dazhui (Du14) with a three-edged needle and then cupping for 10–15 minutes to draw blood.

● For stye due to excessive heat in the spleen and stomach, Neiting (S44) is added and punctured using the reducing method to dispel heat.

Blood-letting puncturing

Auricular and acupuncture points:

Apex of Ear
Dazhui   (Du14)

Select one point each time. Prick Apex of Ear with a three-edged needle to draw several drops of blood. Prick Dazhui (Du14) with a three-edged needle and then cup for 10–15 minutes to draw blood.

This method functions to dispel heat, so it is very effective for treating stye.

Auricular therapy

Auricular points:

Eye, Eye 2: correspond to the affected tissues. Locate positive points; tape both frontal and dorsal surfaces to increase stimulation.

Spleen: according to Five Orbiculus theory, the spleen corresponds to the eyelid, so Spleen is taped to dispel heat in the eyelid.

Liver: the liver opens into the eyes, so Liver is taped to dispel wind-heat in the eyes.

Apex of Ear: blood-letting puncturing of this point with a three-edged needle dispels heat and relieves pain.

Use auricular taping with strong manipulation and blood-letting puncturing where indicated, twice a week.

Remarks

☯ Traditional methods are very effective for treating stye; in many cases one treatment will be sufficient to effect a cure.

☯ The above three methods may be used either singly, or in combination in severe or chronic cases to increase stimulation.

☯ For cases with no obvious general symptoms or signs, puncture only the main acupuncture points or use blood-letting puncturing therapy.

☯ These methods are also suitable for treating tarsal cyst, blepharitis or cyclitis.

115 Suppurative nasal sinusitis

Suppurative nasal sinusitis is an acute or chronic suppurative inflammation of the mucosa of the nasal sinuses. The acute type is caused by diseases of the nasal cavity, or may occur secondary to systemic disorders. It is marked by persistent nasal obstruction, pussy nasal discharge and pain in the nasal sinuses. General symptoms may include chills, fever, poor appetite and general malaise. The chronic type usually develops from the acute type and is marked by intermittent or persistent nasal obstruction, profuse nasal discharge, mild headache and hyposmia or anosmia.

Aetiology

According to traditional Chinese medicine, suppurative nasal sinusitis has three possible causes. The lungs may be invaded by wind-heat; mental injury may lead to stagnation of *qi*, which transforms into fire and flares up along the Gallbladder meridian; or overindulgence in spicy or greasy foods may lead to accumulation of heat in the interior, which then rises along the meridians.

Differentiation of syndromes

- Wind-heat type suppurative nasal sinusitis.
  Characterized by nasal obstruction and profuse yellowish nasal discharge; accompanied by aversion to heat, fever, headache, pain in the nasal sinuses, poor appetite, red tongue with yellowish coating and rapid superficial pulse.
- Suppurative nasal sinusitis due to hyperactive fire in the liver and gallbladder.
  Characterized by nasal obstruction and profuse foul-smelling sticky yellowish nasal discharge; accompanied by headache, vertigo, bitter taste in the mouth, dry throat, restlessness, red tongue with yellowish coating and rapid wiry pulse.

Treatment

Body acupuncture

Main acupuncture points:

Yingxiang	(LI20)
Hegu	(LI4)
Yintang	(Ex27)
Bitong	(Ex32)
Fengchi	(G20)

Yingxiang (LI20) (Welcoming Fragrance in Chinese), the meeting point of the Large Intestine and Stomach meridians located beside the nose, functions to open the nose. Hegu (LI4), the *yuan* (source) point of the Large Intestine meridian, functions to expel wind and dispel heat.

Yintang (Ex27) and Bitong (Ex32) are clinically effective points for treating various nasal problems. Yintang (Ex27) is punctured subcutaneously downward to a depth of 0.5–1.0 *cun*; Bitong (Ex32) is pricked with a three-edged needle.

Fengchi (G20), an important point of the Gallbladder meridian located at the base of the skull, is a main point for treating problems of the sensory organs.

Auxiliary points and appropriate manipulation are chosen according to differentiation of syndromes.

- For wind-heat type suppurative nasal sinusitis, Neiting (S44) is added and punctured using the reducing method to dispel heat.
- For suppurative nasal sinusitis due to hyperactive fire in the liver and gallbladder, Xiaxi (G43) and Xinjian (Liv2) are added and punctured using the reducing method to eliminate fire.

Treat once a day or once every other day. Ten treatments constitute one course.

Electroacupuncture

Points used are the same as for body acupuncture. Select one or two pairs of points each time. Puncture until a needling sensation is achieved, then connect the needles to an electrical stimulator. Apply moderate continuous wave stimulation for 20–30 minutes, once a day or once every other day. Ten treatments constitute one course.

Auricular therapy

Auricular points:

Internal Nose, Cheek: correspond to the affected area. Locate positive points; tape Cheek on both frontal and dorsal surfaces to increase stimulation.

Lung: regulates the flow of *qi* to clear the nose.

Pancreas & Gallbladder: dispels gallbladder fire.

Spleen, Stomach: regulate the spleen and stomach to remove dampness.

Endocrine, Adrenal Gland, Wind Stream: relieve inflammation.

Forehead: relieves pain in the forehead.

Ear Shenmen: relieves inflammation and pain.

Apex of Ear: blood-letting puncturing of this point with a three-edged needle dispels heat and relieves pain.

Use auricular taping with strong manipulation and blood-letting puncturing where indicated, twice a week. Five treatments constitute one course.

Remarks

❧ Traditional therapies are effective for treating suppurative nasal sinusitis; two or more therapies are usually combined to increase stimulation.

❧ For chronic or refractory cases, apply moxa roll moxibustion to Baihui (Du20), Shangxing (Du23), Yintang (Ex27) and Yingxiang (LI20) to activate the meridians and open the nose.

116 Thecal cyst

Thecal cyst is caused by strain or sprain which injures the joint capsule and tendon sheath, usually of the dorsum of the wrist, anterior aspect of the ankle or dorsum of the foot. It occurs primarily in adults and more often in males than in females. The cyst is hemispherical, soft and movable at first, later gradually becoming chondroid. The cyst may be unilocular or multilocular and contains clear, whitish or yellowish fluid. There may be soreness and weakness in the locally affected area, or no other subjective symptoms.

Aetiology

According to traditional Chinese medicine, thecal cyst is caused by strain or sprain which damages the meridians and tendons, with resulting stagnation of the *qi* and blood and subsequent accumulation of phlegm-damp. Primarily affected are the Hand and Foot Yang meridians.

Treatment

Body acupuncture

Main acupuncture points:

Ashi points

For small cysts, puncture using the surrounding method (called Five Tigers Catching One Sheep): insert one needle perpendicularly from the top of the cyst (if the cyst is multilocular, insert one needle on each surface) and another four needles obliquely from the edges of the cyst towards the centre. Manipulate using the reducing method; leave the needles in place for 20 minutes. Treatment is most effective when a discharge of yellowish fluid occurs upon withdrawal of the

needles. Treat once a day. Five treatments constitute one course.

For medium and large cysts, either withdraw the fluid with a syringe, or prick the top of the cyst (all surfaces if the cyst is multilocular) with a three-edged needle and then press to discharge fluid as thoroughly as possible. After discharging the fluid, insert four needles obliquely from the edges of the cyst towards the centre and leave in place for 20 minutes. Finally, apply a pressure binding for one week. If the cyst is not cured after one treatment, treat as for small cysts.

Auxiliary points are selected according to meridian theory.

● For cysts on the dorsum of the wrist, Waiguan (SJ5), Zhongzhu (SJ3) and Hegu (LI4) are added.

● For cysts on the anterior aspect of the ankle and dorsum of the foot, Zusanli (S36), Jiexi (S41), Neiting (S44) and Taichong (Liv3) are added.

Moxibustion

Apply moxa roll moxibustion to the cyst for 15–20 minutes, twice a day. Ten treatments constitute one course.

Moxibustion effectively warms the meridians and promotes the flow of *qi* and blood. It is therefore usually combined with body acupuncture in order to increase stimulation and improve effectiveness.

Remarks

❧ Traditional therapies are very effective for treating thecal cyst; in many cases there will be improvement after one to three treatments.

117 Thromboangiitis obliterans

Thromboangiitis obliterans refers to chronic, progressive and segmental inflammation of the arteries and veins of the entire body. It occurs mostly in adults, primarily in males. Usually affected are the lower extremities. There is frequently a history of trauma, mental injury, long-term smoking, or invasion of the body by cold or dampness. Thromboangiitis obliterans is marked in the initial stage by numbness and coldness of the extremities, fixed pain and intermittent claudication. The intermediate and advanced stages are marked by persistent severe pain worsening at night, myoatrophy and black pigmentation or dry or moist necrosis of the extremities.

Aetiology

According to traditional Chinese medicine, thromboangiitis obliterans is caused internally by deficiency of the kidneys due to excessive sexual activity and externally by stagnation of the *qi* and blood due to trauma, mental injury or invasion of the meridians by exogenous cold or dampness. The combination of internal and external factors results in insufficient supply of warmth to the extremities and nourishment to the muscles and bones.

Differentiation of syndromes

- Thromboangiitis obliterans due to damp-cold.
  Characterized by sensations of heaviness, numbness, soreness and cold in the affected limbs, aggravated by cold and alleviated by warmth; accompanied by intermittent claudication, greasy whitish tongue coating and deep thready pulse.
- Thromboangiitis obliterans due to stagnant *qi* and blood.
  Characterized by dark-red or purple colour or purple spots on the affected limbs, intensified when the limbs are lowered; persistent pain worsening at night, dry skin, muscle atrophy and thin or absent hair on the affected limbs; accompanied by sallow complexion, dark red, purple, or purple-spotted tongue with thin whitish coating and deep, thready, uneven pulse.

- Thromboangiitis obliterans due to toxic heat.
  Characterized by dark red colour and swelling of the affected limbs, dark purple colour or even diabrosis of the affected fingers or toes and persistent severe pain worsening at night and lessening during the day; accompanied by fever, restlessness, thirst, scanty yellowish urine, constipation, red tongue with dry or greasy yellowish coating and rapid full or thready pulse.
- Thromboangiitis obliterans due to deficiency of *qi* and blood.
  Characterized by myoatrophy, dry skin, desquamation and poorly healing lesions on the affected limbs; accompanied by sallow complexion, shortness of breath, palpitation, emaciation, lassitude, listlessness, pale tongue with thin whitish coating and deep, thready, weak pulse.

Treatment

Body acupuncture

Main acupuncture points:

Group 1:
Quchi	(LI11)
Hegu	(LI4)
Waiguan	(SJ5)
Baxie	(Ex6)
Taiyuan	(L9)

Group 2:
Zusanli	(S36)
Jiexi	(S41)
Chengshan	(B57)
Kunlun	(B60)
Xuanzhong	(G39)
Bafeng	(Ex23)
Sanyinjiao	(Sp6)
Taixi	(K3)
Taichong	(Liv3)

Main points are selected from the Hand and Foot Yang meridians to promote the flow of *qi* and blood, relieve pain and warm and nourish the extremities. Group 1 is used for treating thromboangiitis obliterans of the upper limbs. Taiyuan (L9), the *yuan* (source) point of the Lung meridian and the *hui* (influential) point of the blood vessels, is an important point for treating problems of the blood vessels. Group 2 is used for treating thromboangiitis obliterans of the lower limbs. Sanyinjiao (Sp6), the meeting point of the three Foot Yin meridians and Taixi (K3) and Taichong (Liv3), the *yuan* (source) points of the Kidney and Liver meridians respectively, are treated in combination to strengthen the liver, spleen and kidneys in order to promote the flow of *qi* and blood and nourish the muscles and bones.

Auxiliary points and appropriate methods of manipulation are chosen according to differentiation of syndromes.

- For thromboangiitis obliterans due to damp-cold, the meridians are warmed and dampness removed by using the heat-producing method of puncturing and adding moxibustion as needed.
- For thromboangiitis obliterans due to stagnant *qi* and blood, the meridians are dredged and pain relieved by adding and puncturing Xuehai (Sp10) using the reducing method, or using blood-letting puncturing on Baxie (Ex6) for the upper limbs and Bafeng (Ex23) for the lower limbs.
- For thromboangiitis obliterans due to toxic heat, Weizhong (B40) and Dazhui (Du14) are added and pricked with a three-edged needle, then cupped for 10–15 minutes to draw blood and eliminate toxic heat.
- For thromboangiitis obliterans due to deficiency of the *qi* and blood, *qi* and blood are tonified by adding and puncturing Qihai (Ren6) and Guanyuan (Ren4) using the reinforcing method, or adding moxibustion as needed.

Concentrate on treating points on the side of the affected limbs. Treat once a day or once every other day. Ten treatments constitute one course.

Moxibustion

Points used are the same as for body acupuncture. Apply moxa roll moxibustion for 15–20 minutes to three to five points each time, once a day. Ten treatments constitute one course.

Moxibustion effectively warms the meridians and promotes the flow of *qi* and blood. It is therefore especially suitable for treating thromboangiitis obliterans due to damp-cold or stagnant *qi* and blood. Moxibustion may by self-applied. It is usually combined with other methods in order to increase effectiveness of treatment.

Electroacupuncture

Points used are the same as for body acupuncture. Select two or three pairs of points each time. Puncture until a needling sensation is achieved, then connect the needles to an electrical stimulator. Apply moderate intermittent wave stimulation for 30 minutes, once a day. Ten treatments constitute one course.

Auricular therapy

Auricular points:

Auricular points corresponding to the affected areas of the body: locate positive points; tape both frontal and dorsal surfaces to increase stimulation.

Heart, Lung: improve circulation of the *qi* and blood.

Liver, Spleen: soothe the liver and strengthen the spleen to tonify the *qi* and blood.

Kidney: reinforces the kidney *yang* to warm the meridians.

Sympathesis, Subcortex: harmonize vasomotoricity to improve peripheral circulation.

Use auricular taping with strong manipulation, twice a week. Ten treatments constitute one course.

Remarks

- Thromboangiitis obliterans is a refractory problem; traditional therapies can relieve the pain it causes, but long-term treatment using a combination of two or three methods should be given in order to improve the peripheral circulation.
- The patient should adhere to the following guidelines which will help alleviate the condition and prevent relapse:
  - Wear loose shoes and socks.
  - Keep the feet warm and clean.
  - Avoid excessive sexual activity.
  - Abstain from smoking tobacco.
- The following exercises are helpful for improving the peripheral circulation.
  Lying in a supine position, raise the affected limbs to 45° for 2–3 minutes. Sitting on the side of the bed, lower the affected limbs for 5

minutes. Once again in the supine position, flex and extend the knee or elbow joints five to ten times. Keeping the limbs extended, move the hands or feet upward, downward, inward and outward, flexing and extending the fingers or toes, five to ten times. Rest with the limbs

extended for five minutes. Repeat the entire cycle five times, two or three times a day. This exercise is contraindicated for people with necrosis or infection of the affected limbs.

☯ The above methods are also suitable for treating thrombotic phlebitis.

118 Tinnitus and hearing loss

Tinnitus and hearing loss are two subjective symptoms of abnormal hearing. Tinnitus may be accompanied by hearing loss, or hearing loss may develop from tinnitus. Tinnitus and hearing loss are common symptoms of various diseases and disorders, including otitis externa, otitis media, perforation of the tympanic membrane, rupture of the tympanic membrane, auditory vertigo, acoustic neurinoma, meningitis, influenza, anaemia, hypertension and drug poisoning.

Aetiology

According to traditional Chinese medicine, the kidneys and San Jiao and Gallbladder meridians all open into the ears; normal hearing therefore depends closely on sufficient kidney essence and abundant flow of *qi* and blood in the meridians, especially the San Jiao and Gallbladder meridians. Tinnitus and hearing loss are classified clinically into excessive and deficient types. The excessive type is caused by exogenous pathogens, mental injury, or trauma; it is marked by sudden onset of rumbling tinnitus or hearing loss. The deficient type is due to ageing, weak constitution, excessive sexual activity, or prolonged illness, which consume the kidney essence or *qi* and blood. It is marked by gradual onset of chirping tinnitus or hearing loss.

Differentiation of syndromes

● Tinnitus and hearing loss due to invasion by exogenous wind-heat.
  Characterized sudden onset of ringing in the ears or hearing loss; accompanied by headache, fever, aversion to wind, itching or pain in the ears, otorrhoea, thin whitish or yellowish tongue coating and rapid superficial pulse.

● Tinnitus and hearing loss due to hyperactivity of fire in the liver and gallbladder.
  Characterized by rumbling ringing in the ears or hearing loss; accompanied by bitter taste in the mouth, dry throat, restlessness, bad dreams, scanty yellowish urine, constipation, red tongue with yellowish coating and rapid wiry pulse.

● Tinnitus and hearing loss due to accumulation of turbid phlegm in the Middle Jiao.
  Characterized by intermittent ringing in the ears or hearing loss; accompanied by vertigo, heavy muffled sensation in the head, drowsiness, poor appetite, nausea, vomiting, greasy whitish tongue coating and slippery pulse.

● Tinnitus and hearing loss due to deficiency of *qi* and blood.
  Characterized by intermittent or persistent chirping ringing in the ears or hearing loss; accompanied by pale complexion, lassitude, dizziness, poor memory, palpitation, pale tongue with thin coating and weak thready pulse.

● Tinnitus and hearing loss due to deficiency of the kidney essence.
  Characterized by intermittent or persistent chirping ringing in the ears or hearing loss; accompanied by dizziness, poor memory, seminal emission, sexual dysfunction, weak back and knees, pale tongue with thin whitish coating and deep, thready, weak pulse.

Treatment

Body acupuncture

Main acupuncture points:

Zhongzhu	(SJ3)
Fengchi	(G20)
Ermen	(SJ21)
Tinggong	(SI19)

Tinghui	(G2)
Yifeng	(SJ17)
Wangu	(G12)

Main points are selected according to meridian theory. The San Jiao meridian, called the Ear meridian in the *Silk Book Meridians* (circa 500 B.C.) and the Gallbladder meridian are closely connected with the ears. Both local and distal points of these two meridians are treated to activate the meridians and benefit the ears. Select two or three local main points each time.

Auxiliary points and appropriate methods of manipulation are chosen according to differentiation of syndromes.

● For tinnitus and hearing loss due to invasion by exogenous wind-heat, wind is expelled and heat dispelled by adding and puncturing Hegu (LI4), Waiguan (SJ5) and Dazhui (Du14) using the reducing method, or pricking Dazhui (Du14) with a three-edged needle and then cupping for 10–15 minutes.

● For tinnitus and hearing loss due to hyperactivity of fire in the liver and gallbladder, Taichong (Liv3), Xiaxi (G43) and Fengshi (G31) are added and punctured using the reducing method to extinguish fire in the liver and gallbladder.

● For tinnitus and hearing loss due to accumulation of turbid phlegm in the Middle Jiao, Fenglong (S40), Zhongwan (Ren12) and Baihui (Du20) are added and punctured using the even method to reduce phlegm.

● For tinnitus and hearing loss due to deficiency of *qi* and blood, *qi* and blood are tonified to benefit the ears by adding and puncturing Zusanli (S36), Guanyuan (Ren4) and Baihui (Du20) using the reinforcing method, or adding moxibustion to Baihui (Du20), Guanyuan (Ren4) and local points.

● For tinnitus and hearing loss due to deficiency of the kidney essence, Taixi (K3), Shenshu (B23) and Baihui (Du20) are added and punctured using the reinforcing method to strengthen the kidneys.

Treat once a day or once every other day. Ten treatments constitute one course.

Electroacupuncture

Points used are the same as for body acupuncture. Select one or two pairs of points each time. Puncture the points until a needling sensation is achieved, then connect the needles to an electrical stimulator. Apply moderate continuous wave stimulation for 15–20 minutes. Treat once a day or once every other day. Ten treatments constitute one course.

Scalp acupuncture

Scalp line:

| Niehouxian | MS11 |

Puncture from Shuaigu (G8) to Qubin (G7) for 1.5 *cun* using the reducing method for excessive syndromes and the reinforcing method for deficient syndromes. Retain the needles for 24 hours. Treat once every other day. Six treatments constitute one course.

Remarks

☙ Acupuncture is very effective for treating nervous tinnitus and hearing loss; there may be great improvement after one to three treatments.

☙ For cases of deafness accompanied by muteness, Yamen (Du15), Lianquan (Ren23), Tiantu (Ren22) and Tongli (H5) are added to activate the collaterals and improve speaking ability.

☙ The following ear exercise is very beneficial for improving hearing ability in chronic cases and the elderly.

– Step 1: Rub the palms together until they are warm.

– Step 2: With the hand in a loose fist, pinch the auriculae between the thumb and forefinger. Massage both the frontal and dorsal surfaces of the auriculae from top to bottom 24 times.

– Step 3: With a loose fist, massage the periauricular area from top to bottom, with the thumb on the posterior area following the San Jiao meridian (i.e. from Jiaosun (SJ20) to Yifeng (SJ17)) and the radial side of the index finger on the anterior area going downward from Ermen (SJ21) to Tinghui (G2). Repeat 24 times.

– Step 4: Use the fingers to fold the auricle forward to cover the auditory canal. Pressing heavily, tap with the index and middle fingers to vibrate the ear drum. Repeat 24 times. This is called 'Beating the Drum of the Sky', since the action resembles beating a drum.

– Step 5: Do the dry face washing exercise (see Myopia).

119 Tobacco withdrawal

Extensive research has shown that smoking tobacco is harmful to the health. Long-term exposure to the tar and nicotine contained in tobacco increases the incidence of bronchitis, coronary heart disease, emphysema, hypertension, fetal malformation and cancer of the lung, mouth, lips and pancreas. In addition, second-hand smoke pollutes the air breathed by non-smokers in the same room, resulting in harm to them as well as to the smokers themselves.

Tobacco is physically addictive as well as psychologically habit-forming. Long-term smokers often experience withdrawal symptoms including restlessness, anxiety, irritability, insomnia, feeling of emptiness and weight gain when they suddenly stop smoking. Acupuncture has been shown to be very effective in relieving these symptoms. A theoretical basis for this clinical finding has been provided by recent studies showing that electroacupuncture stimulates the release of endorphins and ACTH, which function to relieve pain and tranquillize the mind.

Treatment

Body acupuncture

Acupuncture points:

Baihui	(Du20)
Neiguan	(P6)
Danzhong	(Ren17)
Feishu	(B13)
Zhongwan	(Ren12)
Zusanli	(S36)
Sanyinjiao	(Sp6)
Sishencong	(Ex26)

The therapeutic principles for treating tobacco withdrawal are to tranquillize the mind, open the chest and strengthen the spleen and stomach. Baihui (Du20), the meeting point of the Du, Liver and six Yang meridians of the hand and feet located on the top of the head, is one of the most important points for tranquillizing the mind. Sishencong (Ex26) can be substituted for Baihui (Du20).

Neiguan (P6), the *luo* (collateral) point of the Pericardium meridian and one of the eight confluence points connecting with the Yinwei merid-

ian, functions to tranquillize the mind and open the chest. Danzhong (Ren17), the *hui* (influential) point for *qi*, functions to open the chest and promote the flow of *qi*. Feishu (B13), the back-*shu* point of the lungs, functions to open the chest and promote dispersal and descent by the lungs. Zhongwan (Ren12), the *hui* (influential) point of the *fu* organs and the front-*mu* point of the stomach; Zusanli (S36), the *he* (sea) and lower *he* (confluent) point of the Stomach meridian; and Sanyinjiao (Sp6), the meeting point of the three Foot Yin meridians, are treated in combination to strengthen the stomach and spleen.

Treat once a day or every other day. Ten treatments constitute one course.

Electroacupuncture

Points used are the same as for body acupuncture. Select one or two pairs of points each time. Puncture until a needling sensation is achieved, then connect the needles with an electrical stimulator. Apply moderate continuous wave stimulation for 20–30 minutes, once a day or once every other day. Ten treatments constitute one course.

Auricular therapy

Auricular points:

Mouth, Tongue, Trachea, Lung: correspond to areas of the body directly stimulated by the tar and nicotine contained in tobacco; inhibit the craving for tobacco.

Liver, Chest: soothe the liver and regulate the movement of *qi*.

Subcortex, Ear Shenmen, Occiput: tranquillize the mind.

Use auricular taping with strong manipulation twice a week. Five treatments constitute one course.

Remarks

☯ Traditional therapies are effective for treating tobacco withdrawal. Many people will experience subjective changes in the taste of tobacco smoke, which will seem to become bitter or astringent, with resulting aversion to smoking. There will generally be great improvement in withdrawal symptoms after three to five treatments.

- ☻ Auricular therapy is used especially often due to its special characteristics of effectiveness, simplicity and painlessness.
- ☻ Traditional therapies are only effective for those who are actively motivated to stop smoking.

120 Toothache

Toothache is a common symptom of various oral problems, including caries, pulpitis, apical periodontal inflammation, pericoronitis and periodontitis.

Aetiology

According to traditional Chinese medicine, the Large Intestine meridian enters the lower teeth and its collaterals distribute to all of the teeth. The Stomach meridian enters the upper teeth. Therefore, the Large Intestine and Stomach meridians are mainly affected in cases of toothache. Toothache may occur if heat accumulates in the stomach or large intestine and then flares up along the meridians, or if the Large Intestine and Stomach meridians are invaded by exogenous pathogens which obstruct the flow of *qi* and blood. Additionally, the teeth are terminals of the bones, which are nourished by the kidneys. Therefore, toothache may occur if deficient fire due to deficiency of kidney *yin* flares up.

Differentiation of syndromes

- Toothache due to excessive stomach fire.
  Characterized by severe toothache and red and swollen gums which may ooze pus and bloody fluid; accompanied by thirst with a preference for cold beverages, constipation, red tongue with dry yellowish coating and rapid pulse.
- Toothache due to pathogenic wind-heat.
  Characterized by severe paroxysmal toothache alleviated by cold and aggravated by heat and headache; accompanied by fever, aversion to heat, dry tongue with thin whitish coating and rapid superficial pulse.

- Toothache due to deficient kidney fire.
  Characterized by intermittent or persistent dull toothache, mild redness and swelling or atrophy of the gums and gomphiasis, or loss of teeth; accompanied by dry mouth and throat, sensation of heat in the palms and soles and rapid thready pulse.

Treatment

Body acupuncture

Main acupuncture points:

Hegu	(LI4)
Jiache	(S6)
Xiaguan	(S7)

Main points are selected according to meridian theory. Hegu (LI4), the *yuan* (source) point of the Large Intestine meridian, is the most important point for relieving toothache. Treatment of Hegu (LI4) alone is sufficient in many cases. Jiache (S6) and Xiaguan (S7) are two local points of the Stomach meridian effective for treating toothache.

Auxiliary points and appropriate manipulation are chosen according to differentiation of syndromes.

- For toothache due to excessive stomach fire, Lidui (S45), the *jing* (well) point of the Stomach meridian, is added and pricked with a three-edged needle. Main points are punctured using the reducing method to extinguish excessive fire.
- For toothache due to pathogenic wind-heat, Fengchi (G20) and Yifeng (SJ17) are added and punctured using the reducing method to dispel pathogenic wind-fire.

● For toothache due to deficient kidney fire, Taixi (K3) and Sanyinjiao (Sp6) are added and punctured using the even method to nourish the kidney *yin*.

Treat once a day. Five treatments constitute one course.

Electroacupuncture

Points used are the same as for body acupuncture. Select one or two pairs of points each time. Puncture until a needling sensation is achieved, then connect the needles to an electrical stimulator. Apply intermittent wave stimulation of the greatest bearable intensity for 20–30 minutes, once a day. Five treatments constitute one course.

Auricular therapy

Main auricular points:

Jaw, Teeth, Mouth: correspond to the affected area. Locate positive points; tape Jaw and Teeth on both frontal and dorsal surfaces to increase stimulation.

San Jiao: clinically effective point for treating toothache.

Adrenal Gland, Endocrine: relieve inflammation.

Ear Shenmen, Occiput: relieve inflammation and pain.

Auxiliary auricular points:

For lower toothache, Large Intestine is added.

For upper toothache, Stomach is added.

For toothache due to pathogenic wind-heat or hyperactive stomach fire, Apex of Ear is pricked with a three-edged needle to cause bleeding.

For toothache due to deficient kidney fire, Kidney is added.

Use auricular taping with strong manipulation and blood-letting puncturing where indicated, twice a week. Five treatments constitute one course. Auricular self-massage may also be practised twice a day.

Remarks

☯ Traditional therapies are very effective for treating toothache. In many cases there will be great improvement, or even complete cessation of pain, after only one or two treatments.

☯ The above treatments can be used either singly, or in combination to increase stimulation in refractory cases.

121 Trigeminal neuralgia

Trigeminal neuralgia refers to transient paroxysmal megalgia of the trigeminal nerve pathway. It occurs mainly in adults and more often in females than in males. Usually affected are the second and third branches of the trigeminal nerve; the first branch is rarely involved. Trigeminal neuralgia is marked by sudden onset of stabbing or burning pain along the pathway of the affected nerve, usually evoked by speaking, chewing, washing the face, brushing the teeth, catching cold or touching 'trigger points' on the face. Other manifestations include facial spasm, salivation and lacrimation. The pain usually disappears spontaneously after several seconds or minutes, with no discomfort between episodes.

Aetiology

Traditional Chinese medicine classifies trigeminal neuralgia as toothache and facial pain. It is considered to be caused by invasion of wind-cold or wind-heat, or by flaring up of endogenous fire, which obstruct the flow of *qi* and blood and result in pain in the teeth and face.

Differentiation of syndromes

● Trigeminal neuralgia caused by excessive stomach fire.

Characterized by pain in the cheek and toothache, accompanied by thirst with preference for

cold drinks, constipation, yellowish urine, red tongue with dry yellowish coating and rapid pulse.
- Trigeminal neuralgia caused by excessive heat in the gallbladder and liver.
  Characterized by pain in the supraorbital region and forehead; accompanied by feeling of fullness in the chest, restlessness, insomnia, bad dreams, bitter taste in the mouth, constipation, scanty yellowish urine, red tongue with yellowish coating and rapid wiry pulse.
- Trigeminal neuralgia caused by hyperactivity of deficient fire.
  Characterized by long-standing facial pain or toothache; accompanied by restlessness, insomnia, sensation of heat in the palms and soles, flushed cheeks, thin red tongue with little coating and rapid thready pulse.

Treatment

Body acupuncture

Main acupuncture points:

Group 1:
Zanzhu	(B2)
Yangbai	(G14)
Yuyao	(Ex28)
Taiyang	(Ex30)
Kunlun	(B60)

Group 2:
Sibai	(S2)
Kouheliao	(LI19)
Quanliao	(SI18)
Hegu	(LI4)

Group 3:
Jiachengjiang	(Ex34)
Jiache	(S6)
Xiaguan	(S7)
Zusanli	(S36)

Main points are selected according to both modern anatomical understanding of the trigeminal nerve and traditional meridian theory. The three groups of points are used for the three branches of the trigeminal nerve respectively.

Points of Group 1 are used to treat neuralgia of the first, or ocular, branch of the trigeminal nerve. This branch emerges from the supraorbital foramen (Zanzhu (B2)) and distributes to the upper eyelid and forehead. The Gallbladder and Urinary Bladder meridians also distribute to these areas,

therefore, Zanzhu (B2), Yangbai (G14) and Kunlun (B60), which are local and distal points of the Gallbladder and Urinary Bladder meridians, are punctured. Yuyao (Ex28) and Taiyang (Ex30) are clinically effective local points for treating trigeminal neuralgia.

Points of Group 2 are used to treat neuralgia of the second, or maxillary, branch of the trigeminal nerve. This branch emerges from the infraorbital foramen (Sibai (S2)) and distributes to the wings of the nose, upper lip and lower eyelid. The Large Intestine and Stomach meridians also distribute to these areas, therefore Sibai (S2), Kouheliao (LI19) and Hegu (LI4), which are local and distal points of the Large Intestine and Stomach meridians, are punctured. Quanliao (SI18) is a clinically effective local point for treating trigeminal neuralgia.

Points of Group 3 are used to treat neuralgia of the third, or mandibular, branch of the trigeminal nerve. This branch emerges from the mental foramen (Jiachengjiang (Ex34)) and distributes to the cheek, lower lip and mandible. The Stomach meridian also distributes to these points, therefore Jiache (S6), Xiaguan (S7) and Zusanli (S36), local and distal points of the Stomach meridian, are punctured. Jiachengjiang (Ex34) is effective for treating the neuralgia of the third branch of the trigeminal nerve due to its location.

Auxiliary points and appropriate methods are chosen according to differentiation of syndromes.

- For trigeminal neuralgia caused by excessive stomach fire, Neiting (S44) is added and punctured using the reducing method. Alternatively, Neiting (S44) may be pricked with a three-edged needle to let several drops of blood and remove excessive heat.
- For trigeminal neuralgia caused by excessive heat in the gallbladder and liver, Fengchi (G20), Xingjian (Liv2) and Xiaxi (G43) are added and punctured using the reducing method. Alternatively, Taiyang (Ex 30) may be pricked with a three-edged needle to let several drops of blood and eliminate excessive heat.
- For trigeminal neuralgia caused by hyperactivity of deficient fire, Sanyinjiao (Sp6) and Zhaohai (K6) are added and punctured using the even method to nourish the body's *yin* and subdue the hyperactive fire.

Treatment is concentrated on points of the affected side of the body. Treat once a day or once every other day. Ten treatments constitute one course.

Electroacupuncture

Points used are the same as for body acupuncture. Select one or two pairs of points each time. Puncture until a needling sensation is achieved, then connect the needles to an electrical stimulator. Apply intermittent wave stimulation, of the strongest bearable intensity, for 30 minutes. Treat once a day or once every other day. Ten treatments constitute one course.

Auricular therapy

Main auricular points:

Cheek, Jaw, Teeth: correspond to the affected area of the body. Tape both frontal and dorsal surfaces to increase stimulation.

San Jiao: dispels heat and relieves pain.

Subcortex: regulates the central nervous function.

External Ear, External Nose: correspond to the location of the trigeminal nerve pathway.

Ear Shenmen, Occiput: tranquillize the mind and relieve pain.

Apex of Ear: blood-letting puncturing of this point with a three-edged needle dispels heat and relieves pain.

Auxiliary auricular points:

For trigeminal neuralgia due to flaring up of the liver fire, Liver and Gallbladder are added.

For trigeminal neuralgia due to flaring up of the stomach fire, Stomach and Large Intestine are added.

Use auricular taping with strong manipulation and blood-letting puncturing where indicated, concentrating on the affected side, twice a week. Five treatments constitute one course.

Remarks

- Acupuncture is very effective for treating trigeminal neuralgia; in some cases the pain may be alleviated by the end of the treatment session.
- In cases of secondary trigeminal neuralgia, appropriate treatment of the primary disease should be undertaken and acupuncture used only as supplementary symptomatic treatment.

122 Urinary stones

Urinary stones occur in the urinary tract, including the kidneys, urinary bladder, ureters and urethra. Nephrolithiasis, or kidney stones, are marked by persistent dull pain or paroxysmal colicky pain in the lumbar region, radiating to the back and lower abdomen. Ureterolithiasis, or ureter stones, are marked by severe, paroxysmal, colicky pain radiating downward along the ureters to the perineum and medial side of the thighs, usually accompanied by restlessness, nausea, vomiting and profuse perspiration. Both kidney and ureter stones occur primarily in men 20–40 years old. Usually only one side is affected. The presence of stones in the urethra or bladder is marked by dripping or interrupted urination, accompanied by pain and blood in the urine. The pain may radiate to the perineum and glans of the penis in men or clitoris in women.

Acute retention of urine may occur if there are stones blocking the urethra. Bladder and urethral stones occur primarily in boys younger than 10 years old and older men with hyperplagia of the prostate.

Aetiology

Traditional Chinese medicine classifies urinary stones as *lin* syndrome. They are considered to be caused by accumulation of damp-heat in the Lower Jiao which consumes the *yin* fluid of the body and vaporizes the urine, resulting in the formation of stones. Colicky pain may occur if the stones obstruct the flow of *qi* and blood. In protracted cases, the kidney *qi* may be damaged.

Differentiation of syndromes

- Urinary stones which obstruct the flow of *qi*.
  Characterized by persistent dull or paroxysmal colicky pain in the lumbar region and lower abdomen, radiating to the perineum or medial side of the thighs; usually accompanied by nausea, vomiting, profuse perspiration, bloody urine, thin whitish tongue coating and wiry thready pulse.
- Urinary stones due to accumulation of damp-heat in the Lower Jiao.
  Characterized by frequent, painful or dripping urination; bloody urine, persistent pain in the lumbar region or lower abdomen; sometimes accompanied by fever, chills, headache, bitter taste in the mouth and poor appetite; greasy yellowish tongue coating and rapid slippery pulse.
- Urinary stones obstructing the urethra.
  Characterized by severe pain in the perineum, penis or vulva radiating to the glans or clitoris and difficulty in urination or sudden retention of urine. There are usually no accompanying symptoms.
- Urinary stones due to deficiency of the kidney *qi*.
  Characterized by long-standing dull pain in the lumbar region and frequent dripping urination aggravated by overstrain; accompanied by lassitude, dizziness, tinnitus, pale complexion, sore and weak back and knees, thin tongue with whitish coating and deep thready pulse.

Treatment

Body acupuncture

Main acupuncture points:

Shenshu	(B23)
Pangguangshu	(B28)
Zhongji	(Ren3)
Sanyinjiao	(Sp6)

Shenshu (B23) and Pangguangshu (B28), the back-*shu* and front-*shu* points of the kidney and urinary bladder respectively and Zhongji (Ren3), the front-*mu* point of the urinary bladder, are treated in combination to strengthen the function of the kidneys and urinary bladder to relieve pain and dispel stones. Sanyinjiao (Sp6) is an important point for treating urogenital problems.

Auxiliary points and appropriate methods of manipulation are chosen according to differentiation of syndromes.

- For urinary stones which obstruct the flow of *qi*, *ashi* points are added and punctured using the reducing method to activate the meridians and relieve pain.
- For urinary stones due to accumulation of damp-heat in the Lower Jiao, damp-heat is removed by pricking Zhiyin (B67) with a three-edged needle to draw several drops of blood and adding and puncturing Yinlingquan (Sp9) and Zusanli (S36) using the reducing method.
- For urinary stones obstructing the urethra, Ligou (Liv5) is added and punctured using the reducing method to relieve pain and discharge stones. If no improvement is seen, other methods may be alternated with acupuncture.
- For urinary stones due to deficiency of the kidney *qi*, the kidneys are strengthened by adding and puncturing Guanyuan (Ren4) and Zusanli (S36) using the reinforcing method, and applying moxibustion as needed.

Treat once a day or once every other day. Ten treatments constitute one course.

Electroacupuncture

Points used are the same as for body acupuncture. Select two or three pairs of points each time. Puncture until a needling sensation is achieved, then connect the needles to an electrical stimulator. Apply intermittent wave stimulation of the strongest bearable intensity for 30 minutes. Treat once a day or once every other day. Ten treatments constitute one course.

Auricular therapy

Main auricular points:

Kidney, Ureter, Urinary Bladder, Urethra: correspond to the affected organs. Select points according to the location of the stones; tape both frontal and dorsal surfaces to increase stimulation.

Abdomen, Lumbosacral Vertebrae: relieve pain in the lower abdomen and lumbosacral region.

San Jiao: promotes the passage of water to dispel damp-heat and discharge stones.

Sympathesis: relaxes spasm of the smooth muscles to relieve colicky pain in the internal organs.

Ear Shenmen: relieves pain.

Apex of Ear: blood-letting puncturing of this point with a three-edged needle dispels damp-heat and relieves pain.

Use auricular taping with strong manipulation and blood-letting puncturing where indicated, twice a week. Five treatments constitute one course.

Remarks

☯ The above methods are very effective for alleviating the pain of urinary stones; in many cases the pain is relieved by the end of the treatment session.

☯ Discharge of stones depends primarily on their size, shape and location. The following situations will respond most favourably to acupuncture and other traditional treatments:
   – Stones with a horizontal diameter less than 1 cm and vertical diameter less than 2 cm.
   – No deformity, stricture, or obstruction present in the urinary tract.
   – No stones embedded in the organ wall.

☯ Drinking large amounts of water and doing jumping exercises during the course of treatment will help discharge the stones.

☯ Comprehensive programme for discharging urinary stones:

Time	Method
6.30 a.m.	Drink 500 ml water or tea (tea is preferable)
7.00	50 mg dihydrochlorothiazide (oral administration)
8.00	500 ml water or tea
8.30	500 ml water or tea
9.30	0.5 mg atropine (intramuscular injection)
9.40	Electroacupuncture. Points are selected according to location of the stones: – For stones in the renal pelvis and middle and upper parts of the ureter, Shenshu (B23) and Pangguangshu (B28) are chosen. – For stones in the lower part of the ureter, Shenshu (B23) and Shuidao (S28) are chosen. – For stones in the bladder and urethra, Zhongji (Ren3) and Sanyinjiao (Sp6) are chosen. Puncture using the reducing method until a needling sensation is achieved, then connect the needles to an electrical stimulator. Apply intermittent wave stimulation of the strongest bearable intensity for 25 minutes.
10.05	Get up and do jumping exercises for 5 minutes.

The comprehensive programme is based on the theory that the increased volume of urine produced by diuretics in combination with drinking a large amount of water will flush the stones, while atropine and electroacupuncture both increase peristalsis and relax the smooth muscles of the ureter, thus promoting the discharge of stones.

This method is used primarily for treating cases in which ureter stones have a horizontal diameter of less than 1 cm, there are no obvious strictures or obstructions, only mild or no nephritis is present and renal function is normal.

Treat twice a week. Six to seven treatments constitute one course. If the stones descend or are not completely discharged after one course, another course should be given after a one- to two-week interval. Potassium chloride (1 g) should be given three times a day during the course of comprehensive treatment to prevent hypokalaemia.

123 Urticaria

Urticaria is an allergic skin reaction caused by sensitivity to environmental allergens. It is marked by itching reddish skin lesions of various sizes and shapes, quickly appearing and disappearing; accompanied by a feeling of fullness in the chest, shortness of breath, nausea, vomiting, abdominal pain or diarrhoea. Urticaria is classified into acute and chronic types. Acute urticaria may run its course in one to two weeks; chronic urticaria persists for six weeks or more.

Aetiology

According to traditional Chinese medicine, urticaria is caused either by internal deficiency of antipathogenic *qi* and subsequent invasion by wind-cold or wind-heat, or by improper diet leading to accumulation of heat in the interior.

Differentiation of syndromes

- Wind-cold urticaria.
  Characterized by reddish or whitish skin lesions of various sizes and shapes with severe itching; accompanied by aversion to cold, headache, soreness of the body, thin whitish tongue coating and tense superficial pulse.
- Wind-heat urticaria.
  Characterized by skin lesions of various sizes and shapes with severe itching; accompanied by fever, mild aversion to cold, sore throat, headache, thirst with preference for cold beverages, restlessness, dry whitish or yellowish tongue coating and superficial pulse.
- Urticaria due to accumulation of heat in the stomach and intestines.
  Characterized by red skin lesions of various sizes and shapes; accompanied by abdominal pain, nausea, vomiting, poor appetite, constipation or diarrhoea, greasy yellowish tongue coating and rapid slippery pulse.
- Urticaria due to endogenous wind resulting from deficiency of the blood.
  Characterized by long-standing frequent occurrence of urticaria, accompanied by lassitude, pale complexion, poor appetite, palpitation, shortness of breath, pale tongue with whitish coating and weak thready pulse.

Treatment

Body acupuncture

Main acupuncture points:

Hegu	(LI4)
Quchi	(LI11)
Xuehai	(Sp10)
Sanyinjiao	(Sp6)

According to traditional Chinese medicine, the main pathogenesis of urticaria is invasion of the blood by wind. Therefore, main points are selected from the Large Intestine and Spleen meridians to expel wind and promote the flow of blood in order to stop itching. Hegu (LI4) and Quchi (LI11), the *yuan* (source) and *he* (sea) points of the Large Intestine meridian respectively, are treated in combination to expel wind. Xuehai (Sp10) (Sea of Blood in Chinese) functions to dispel heat in the blood and is a main point for treating various skin conditions. Sanyinjiao (Sp6), the meeting point of the three Foot Yin meridians, regulates the flow of blood.

Auxiliary points and appropriate manipulation are chosen according to differentiation of syndromes.

- For wind-cold urticaria, Dazhui (Du14) and Fengchi (G20) are added and punctured using the reducing method to expel cold.
- For wind-heat urticaria, Shaoshang (L11) and Shangyang (LI1) are added and pricked using a three-edged needle to draw several drops of blood; main points are punctured using the reducing method to expel heat.
- For urticaria due to accumulation of heat in the stomach and intestines, Zhongwan (Ren12), Zusanli (S36) and Tianshu (S25) are added and punctured using the reducing method to regulate the stomach and intestines.
- For urticaria due to endogenous wind resulting from deficiency of the blood, Geshu (B17), Pishu (B20), Feishu (B13) and Qihai (Ren6) are added and punctured using the reinforcing method to tonify the blood and subdue endogenous wind.

Treat acute cases once a day; five treatments constitute one course. Treat chronic cases once every day or every other day; ten treatments constitute one course.

Blood-letting puncturing

Acupuncture points:

Geshu	(B17)
Weizhong	(B40)
Dazhui	(Du14)
Feishu	(B13)
Dachangshu	(B25)

Select two or three points each time. Prick with a three-edged needle, then cup for 10–15 minutes to draw a small amount of blood. This method functions to stimulate the circulation of blood and expel pathogens, so it is very suitable for treating urticaria. It is usually used in combination with other methods.

Cupping therapy

Shenque	(Ren8)

Cup the point for 10–15 minutes, once every other day. This method functions to strengthen anti-pathogenic *qi*, so it is especially suitable for treating urticaria due to endogenous wind resulting from deficiency of the blood.

Auricular therapy

Main auricular points:

Lung: the lungs nourish the skin, so Lung is treated to expel pathogens from the skin.

Spleen, Stomach: strengthen the spleen and stomach to remove dampness and heat from the exterior.

Heart: relieves itching.

Endocrine, Adrenal Gland, Wind Stream: relieve allergic reactions.

Ear Shenmen, Occiput: calm the mind and relieve itching.

Apex of Ear: blood-letting puncturing of this point with a three-edged needle expels wind and dispels heat to relieve itching.

Auxiliary auricular points:

For a feeling of fullness in the chest, Chest and Trachea are added.

For gastrointestinal symptoms, Stomach and Abdomen are added.

Use auricular taping with strong manipulation and blood-letting puncturing where indicated, twice a week. Five treatments constitute one course.

Remarks

- Traditional therapies are very effective for treating acute urticaria; in many cases there will be great improvement after only one or two treatments. For chronic urticaria, long-term treatment should be undertaken in order to achieve effective results.
- The various traditional therapies can be used either singly or in combination in order to increase stimulation.
- These methods are also effective for treating angioneurotic oedema.

124 Vomiting

Vomiting is a common symptom of many diseases and disorders including acute gastroenteritis, cardiospasm, pylorospasm, hepatitis, pancreatitis, cholecystitis and cerebral problems.

Aetiology

Traditional Chinese medicine classifies vomiting into excessive and deficient types. The excessive type may be caused by exogenous pathogens, mental injury, improper diet or consumption of contaminated food, any of which affect the stomach and result in rebellious rising of the stomach *qi*. The deficient type is caused by febrile diseases or protracted illness which consume the stomach *yin* so the stomach *qi* cannot descend. The excessive type is relatively mild, of short duration and easily cured; the deficient type is relatively severe, of longer duration and more difficult to treat.

Differentiation of syndromes

- Vomiting due to attack on the stomach by exogenous pathogens.
  Characterized by sudden onset of vomiting; accompanied by wind-cold, wind-heat, or summer-heat and dampness exterior syndrome:
  - Wind-cold type exterior syndrome includes chills, mild fever, headache, pantalgia (soreness of the entire body), stuffed or runny nose, thin whitish tongue coating and tense superficial pulse.
  - Wind-heat type exterior syndrome includes fever, headache, sweating, slight aversion to cold, sore throat, red tip and margin of the tongue with thin white or yellowish coating and rapid superficial pulse.
  - Summer-heat and dampness type exterior syndrome includes fever, sweating, restlessness, abdominal distension, thirst, red tongue with greasy yellowish coating and soft rapid pulse.
- Vomiting due to retention of phlegm and fluid in the Middle Jiao.
  Characterized by vomiting of phlegm and watery fluid, feeling of fullness in the chest, abdominal distension, borborygmi, poor appetite, dizziness, palpitation, greasy whitish tongue coating and slippery pulse.
- Vomiting due to attack on the stomach by hyperactive liver *qi*.
  Characterized by vomiting and acid regurgitation aggravated by mental injury, frequent belching, distension and pain in the chest and hypochondriac region, sighing, depression or restlessness, thin greasy tongue coating and wiry pulse.
- Vomiting due to *yang* deficiency of the spleen and stomach.
  Characterized by intermittent vomiting resulting from improper diet or attack by cold, poor appetite, lassitude, emaciation, preference for warmth and aversion to cold, feeling of coldness in the limbs, loose stool or stool containing undigested food, pale complexion, pale tongue with thin whitish coating and slow weak pulse.
- Vomiting due to deficiency of the stomach *yin*.
  Characterized by frequent scanty or dry vomiting, feeling of discomfort in the epigastric region, dry mouth and throat, anorexia, dry red tongue with little coating and rapid thready pulse.

Treatment

Body acupuncture

Main acupuncture point:

Neiguan   (P6)

The primary pathogenesis of vomiting is rebellious rising of the stomach *qi*. Neiguan (P6), the *luo* (collateral) point of the Pericardium meridian and one of the eight confluence points connecting with the Yinwei meridian, is selected as the sole main point to subdue rebellious rising of the stomach *qi* to halt vomiting. It is punctured obliquely upwards until the needling sensation ascends to the epigastric region. For patients who cannot accept acupuncture, or when vomiting prevents taking medicine, pressure can be applied to this point with the thumb instead of puncturing with a needle.

Auxiliary points and appropriate manipulation are chosen according to syndromes.

- For vomiting due to attack on the stomach by wind-cold, Fengchi (G20) and Hegu (LI4) are added and punctured using the reducing method to expel wind-cold.
- For vomiting due to attack on the stomach by wind-heat, Dazhui (Du14) is added, pricked with a three-edged needle and then cupped for 15 minutes to dispel wind-heat.
- For vomiting due to attack on the stomach by summer-heat and dampness, dampness is removed by adding and puncturing Zhongwan (Ren12) and Zusanli (S36) using the reducing method, or pricking Quze (P3) with a three-edged needle to draw blood and dispel heat.
- For vomiting due to retention of phlegm in the Middle Jiao, Zhongwan (Ren12) and Zusanli (S36) are added and punctured using the reducing method to strengthen transportation and transformation of the spleen and stomach and dispel phlegm and fluid.
- For vomiting due to attack on the stomach by hyperactive liver *qi*, Taichong (Liv3), Yanglingquan (G34) and Gongsun (Sp4) are added and punctured using the reducing method to regulate the flow of the liver *qi*.
- For vomiting due to *yang* deficiency of the spleen and stomach, the spleen and stomach are warmed by adding and puncturing Pishu (B20), Weishu (B21), Zusanli (S36) and Zhongwan (Ren12) using the reinforcing method and applying cupping or moxibustion to Zhongwan (Ren12) for 15 minutes.

● For vomiting due to deficiency of the stomach *yin*, Weishu (B21), Zusanli (S36) and Sanyin-jiao (Sp6) are added and punctured using the even method to nourish the stomach *yin*.

Treat once a day. Five treatments constitute one course for excessive cases; ten treatments constitute one course for deficient cases.

Auricular therapy

Auricular points:

Stomach, Cardia: correspond to affected areas of the body.

Spleen: the spleen is connected internally and externally with the stomach, so Spleen is treated to strengthen the spleen and regulate the stomach to stop vomiting.

Liver: soothes the liver *qi* and regulates the stomach to stop vomiting.

Sympathesis: alleviates spasm of the smooth muscles to stop vomiting.

Subcortex: regulates the digestive function.

Abdomen, Middle of Superior Concha: regulate the flow of *qi* to stop vomiting.

Use auricular taping, twice a week, or auricular self-massage or pressure, twice a day. Five treatments constitute one course for the excessive type; ten treatments constitute one course for the deficient type.

Remarks

☯ Traditional therapies are very effective for treating vomiting, especially the excessive type. Puncturing or pressing only Neiguan (P6) is sufficient in many cases.
☯ Vomiting is a general manifestation of various diseases and disorders, which should be treated after the vomiting has been halted.

125 *Wei* syndrome

Wei means flaccidity and atrophy in Chinese. *Wei* syndrome is characterized by flaccidity and atrophy of the muscles, especially those of the extremities, with accompanying motor impairment. It is a common symptom of various diseases and disorders such as neuritis, acute infective polyneuritis, acute myelitis, spinal arachnoiditis, myasthenia gravis, progressive myodystrophy, periodic paralysis and peripheral paralysis.

Aetiology

According to traditional Chinese medicine, *wei* syndrome is due primarily to dysfunction of the lungs, spleen, liver and kidneys. The main pathogenesis is insufficient nourishment of the muscles and tendons.

The lungs dominate respiration and distribute fluid and essence throughout the entire body. They are sensitive and easily damaged if warmth and heat pathogens consume the bodily fluid and essence. The remaining fluid and essence are insufficient for the lungs to distribute throughout the body, resulting in malnutrition of the muscles and tendons. This type of *wei* syndrome is found in cases of paralysis following infections of the central nervous system, such as acute infective polyneuritis, acute myelitis and spinal arachnoiditis.

The spleen determines the condition of the acquired constitution. It functions to transform and transport nutrients throughout the body, especially to the muscles and tendons of the limbs. It is especially susceptible to injury by damp pathogens. If the spleen becomes deficient, its function of transport and transformation of nutrients will be impaired. It may also be injured by exogenous damp pathogens which flow downward and obstruct the meridians and collaterals. In either case, flaccidity and atrophy of the muscles of the extremities will result. *Wei* syndrome involving deficiency of the spleen is found in cases of myasthenia gravis, progressive myodystrophy, or periodic paralysis. *Wei* syndrome involving injury by exogenous pathogens resembles multiple neuritis.

The liver nourishes the tendons and the kidneys the bones. In cases of congenital defect or if the liver and kidneys are damaged after birth, the tendons and bones receive insufficient nourishment. Flaccidity and atrophy are the result. This type of *wei* syndrome is found in cases of progressive myodystrophy or periodic paralysis.

Wei syndrome can also be caused by trauma which injures the meridians and obstructs the flow of *qi* and blood. This type of *wei* syndrome is found in cases of traumatic peripheral paralysis such as paralysis of the median, ulnar, radial, femoral, tibial and common peroneal nerves.

Differentiation of syndromes

● *Wei* syndrome due to injury of the lungs by exogenous warmth and heat pathogens.
Characterized by sudden onset of flaccidity and atrophy of the limbs or even the whole body; preceded by exterior warmth and heat syndrome marked by high fever, headache, cough, thirst with preference for cold drinks, restlessness, scanty yellowish urine, red tongue and rapid pulse. In the advanced stage, this syndrome may develop into deficiency of the liver and kidneys or deficiency of the spleen and stomach.
● *Wei* syndrome due to deficiency of the liver and kidneys.
Characterized by gradual onset of flaccidity and atrophy of the limbs or other parts of the body, gradually increasing in severity or frequently recurring; accompanied by dizziness, tinnitus, blurred vision, seminal emission, urinary incontinence, thin tongue with little coating and deep, thready, weak pulse.
● *Wei* syndrome due to deficiency of the spleen and stomach.
Characterized by gradual onset of flaccidity and atrophy of the limbs or even the whole body; accompanied by poor appetite, abdominal distension, sallow complexion, loose stool, pale tongue and weak pulse.
● *Wei* syndrome due to invasion of the spleen and lower limbs by exogenous damp-heat.
Characterized by gradual onset of flaccidity and atrophy of the limbs, especially the lower limbs; accompanied by mild swelling, itching, or stabbing pain of the affected hands or feet; feeling of stuffiness in the chest and upper abdomen, poor appetite, greasy yellowish tongue coating and rapid slippery pulse.
● *Wei* syndrome due to strain or trauma.
Characterized by flaccidity and atrophy of the limbs following strain or trauma. Position and degree of flaccidity and atrophy are related to location of strain or trauma. Accompanied by numbness, feeling of cold in the hands and feet, purple or purple-spotted tongue and uneven thready pulse. This type of *wei* syndrome may develop into deficiency of the liver and kidneys or spleen and stomach.

Treatment

Body acupuncture

Main acupuncture points:

For upper limbs

Jianyu	(LI15)
Quchi	(LI11)
Hegu	(LI4)
Waiguan	(SJ5)
Houxi	(SI3)
Baxie	(Ex6)
Huatuojiaji	(Ex46) (T1–T3)

For lower limbs

Baliao	(B31–B34)
Zhibian	(B54)
Huantiao	(G30)
Zusanli	(S36)
Yanglingquan	(G34)
Xuanzhong	(G39)
Jiexi	(S41)
Huatuojiaji	(Ex46) (L1–L5)

For ocular muscles

Taiyang	(Ex30)
Yuyao	(Ex28)
Zanzhu	(B2)

For muscles of the neck

Fengchi	(G20)
Tianzhu	(B10)
Dazhui	(Du14)

According to the therapeutic principles stated in *Neijing, the Classic of Medicine,* all main points for treating *wei* syndrome are selected from the Yang meridians, especially the Yangming meridians (including both the Stomach and Large

Intestine meridians), in order to promote the circulation of *qi* and blood and nourish the muscles and tendons. The stomach and spleen provide the material foundation of the acquired constitution. The stomach receives and transforms water and food into chyme and the spleen further transforms chyme into nutrients which are then transported to the lungs. The nutrients are then distributed from the lungs to all parts of the body.

Main points are selected according to the location of paralysis. Huatuojiaji (Ex46) can be punctured alternately with main points. Puncture points for paralysis using the even method in the acute stage and the reinforcing method in the post-acute stage in order to improve the flow of *qi* and nourish the muscles and tendons.

Auxiliary points and proper manipulation are chosen according to differentiation of signs and symptoms.

- For *wei* syndrome due to injury of the lungs by exogenous warmth and heat pathogens, Dazhui (Du14), Feishu (B13), Lieque (L7) and Zhaohai (K6) are added and punctured using the reducing method, or Shixuan (Ex1) is pricked with a three-edged needle to cause bleeding and dispel warmth and heat pathogens. Treat during the initial stage, once a day or in combination with other methods if necessary.
- For *wei* syndrome due to deficiency of the liver and kidneys, the liver and kidneys are tonified by adding and puncturing Ganshu (B18), Shenshu (B23), Taixi (K3) and Sanyinjiao (Sp6) using the reinforcing method, or adding moxibustion as needed.
- For *wei* syndrome due to deficiency of the spleen and stomach, the spleen and stomach are strengthened by adding and puncturing Zusanli (S36), Qihai (Ren6) and Guanyuan (Ren4) using the reinforcing method, or adding moxibustion as needed.
- For *wei* syndrome due to invasion of the spleen and lower limbs by exogenous damp-heat, Sanyinjiao (Sp6), Yinlingquan (Sp9) and Zhongwan (Ren12) are added in the initial stage. They are punctured using the reducing method to eliminate damp-heat. Points for local paralysis are punctured using the even method in the acute stage and the reinforcing method in the post-acute stage to improve the circulation of *qi* and blood and nourish the muscles and tendons.
- For *wei* syndrome due to strain or trauma, points are selected according to location of the paralysis. For instance, for injury of the radial nerve, points of the Large Intestine and San Jiao meridians are punctured, including Quchi (LI11), Shousanli (LI10), Hegu (LI4), Waiguan (SJ5), Yangchi (SJ4) and Kongzhui (L6). For injury of the median nerve, points of the Pericardium meridian are punctured, including Quze (P3), Jianshi (P5), Neiguan (P6), Daling (P7), Laogong (P8), Yuji (L10) and Baxie (Ex6). For injury of the ulnar nerve, points of the Heart and Small Intestine meridian are punctured, including Shaohai (H3), Xiaohai (SI8), Shenmen (H7), Shaofu (H8) and Houxi (SI3). For injury of the femoral nerve, points of the Stomach and Spleen meridians are punctured, including Biguan (S31), Futu (S32), Yinshi (S33), Liangqiu (S34), Zusanli (S36), Xuehai (Sp10) and Jimen (Sp11). For injury of the tibial nerve, points of the Urinary Bladder meridian are punctured, including Weizhong (B40), Chengshan (B57) and Kunlun (B60). For injury of the common peroneal nerve, points of the Gallbladder meridian are punctured, including Huantiao (G30), Fengshi (G31), Yanglingquan (G34), Xuanzhong (G39) and Qiuxu (G40).
- For cases involving retention of urine, Zhongji (Ren3) and Sanyinjiao (Sp6) are punctured using the reducing method to stimulate the function of the urinary bladder and void urine.
- For cases involving urinary incontinence, Guanyuan (Ren4) is punctured using the reinforcing method and moxibustion is applied to strengthen the urinary bladder and arrest urine.

Treat once a day or every other day. Fifteen treatments constitute one course. For cases of unilateral paralysis, concentrate on treating the affected side.

Electroacupuncture

Points chosen are the same as for body acupuncture. Select two to three pairs of points each time. Puncture until a needling sensation is achieved, then connect needles to an electrical stimulator. Apply moderate intermittent wave stimulation for 20–30 minutes. Treat once a day or every other day. Fifteen treatments constitute one course.

Point implantation therapy

Points chosen are the same as for body acupuncture. Select three to four points each time.

Use a triangular suture needle to implant surgical catgut on each point. (See Appendix 9.) Treat once a week, implanting points in turn or repeatedly. Three treatments constitute one course.

Because of the strong and long-term stimulation it provides, point implantation therapy is usually combined with body acupuncture in order to increase stimulation and improve effectiveness.

Remarks

- Acupuncture is an ideal method for treating *wei* syndrome. It is effective for treating both neuroparalysis and myogenic paralysis.

- *Wei* syndrome is a common manifestation of various diseases and disorders. In order to achieve effective results, it is necessary to both establish diagnosis according to modern medicine and to correctly differentiate symptoms and signs according to traditional Chinese medicine.

- Effectiveness of traditional therapies is closely related to type of disease and promptness of instituting treatment. The best results will be achieved in treating traumatic peripheral paralysis; followed by sequelae of infection of the central nervous system and hereditary paralysis.

- Several methods are usually used in combination in order to increase stimulation and effectiveness.

Appendices: Details of therapies and techniques

Appendix 1 The 14 meridians and their acupuncture points

1 Lung meridian of Hand Taiyin

Shoutaiyang Fei Jing

手太阴肺经

L1	中府	Zhōngfǔ	L7	列缺	Lièqūē
L2	云门	Yúnmén	L8	经渠	Jīngqú
L3	天府	Tiānfǔ	L9	太渊	Tàiyuān
L4	侠白	Xiábái	L10	鱼际	Yújì
L5	尺泽	Chǐzé	L11	少商	Shàoshāng
L6	孔最	Kǒngzuì			

2 Large Intestine meridian of Hand Yangming

Shouyangming Dachang Jing

手阳明大肠经

LI1	商阳	Shāngyáng	LI11	曲池	Qūchí
LI2	二间	èrjiān	LI12	肘髎	Zhǒuliáo
LI3	三间	Sānjiān	LI13	手五里	Shǒuwǔlǐ
LI4	合谷	Hégǔ	LI14	臂臑	Bìnào
LI5	阳溪	Yángxī	LI15	肩髃	Jiānyú
LI6	偏历	Piānlì	LI16	巨骨	Jùgǔ
LI7	温溜	Wēnliū	LI17	天鼎	Tiāndǐng
LI8	下廉	Xiàlián	LI18	扶突	Fútū
LI9	上廉	Shànglián	LI19	口禾髎	Kǒuhéliáo
LI10	手三里	Shǒusānlǐ	LI20	迎香	Yíngxiāng

3 Stomach meridian of Foot Yangming

Zuyangming Wei Jing

足阳明胃经

S1	承泣	Chéngqì		S24	滑肉门	Huáròumén
S2	四白	Sìbái		S25	天枢	Tiānshū
S3	巨髎	Jùliáo		S26	外陵	Wàilíng
S4	地仓	Dìcāng		S27	大巨	Dàjù
S5	大迎	Dàyíng		S28	水道	Shuǐdào
S6	颊车	Jiáchē		S29	归来	Guīlái
S7	下关	Xiàguān		S30	气冲	Qìchōng
S8	头维	Tóuwéi		S31	髀关	Bìguān
S9	人迎	Rényíng		S32	伏兔	Fútù
S10	水突	Shuǐtū		S33	阴市	Yīnshì
S11	气舍	Qìshě		S34	梁丘	Liángqiū
S12	缺盆	Qūēpén		S35	犊鼻	Dúbí
S13	气户	Qìhù		S36	足三里	Zúsānlǐ
S14	库房	Kùfáng		S37	上巨虚	Shàngjùxū
S15	屋翳	Wūyì		S38	条口	Tiáokǒu
S16	膺窗	Yīngchuāng		S39	下巨虚	Xiàjùxū
S17	乳中	Rǔzhōng		S40	丰隆	Fēnglóng
S18	乳根	Rǔgēn		S41	解溪	Jiěxī
S19	不容	Bùróng		S42	冲阳	Chōngyáng
S20	承满	Chéngmǎn		S43	陷谷	Xiàngǔ
S21	梁门	Liángmén		S44	内庭	Nèitíng
S22	关门	Guānmén		S45	厉兑	Lìduì
S23	太乙	Tàiyǐ				

4 Spleen meridian of Foot Taiyin

Zutaiyin Pi Jing

足太阴脾经

Sp1	隐白	Yǐnbái	Sp12	冲门	Chōngmén
Sp2	大都	Dàdū	Sp13	府舍	Fǔshè
Sp3	太白	Tàibái	Sp14	腹结	Fùjié
Sp4	公孙	Gōngsūn	Sp15	大横	Dàhéng
Sp5	商丘	Shāngqiū	Sp16	腹哀	Fùāi
Sp6	三阴交	Sānyīnjiāo	Sp17	食窦	Shídòu
Sp7	漏谷	Lòugǔ	Sp18	天溪	Tiānxī
Sp8	地机	Dìjī	Sp19	胸乡	Xiōngxiāng
Sp9	阴陵泉	Yīnlíngquán	Sp20	周荣	Zhōuróng
Sp10	血海	Xuèhǎi	Sp21	大包	Dàbāo
Sp11	箕门	Jīmén			

5 Heart meridian of Hand Shaoyin

Shoushaoyin Xin Jing

手少阴心经

H1	极泉	Jíquán	H6	阴郄	Yīnxì
H2	青灵	Qīnglíng	H7	神门	Shénmén
H3	少海	Shàohǎi	H8	少府	Shàofǔ
H4	灵道	Língdào	H9	少冲	Shàochōng
H5	通里	Tōnglǐ			

6 Small Intestine meridian of Hand Taiyang

Shoutaiyang Xiaochang Jing

手太阳小肠经

SI1	少泽	Shàozé		SI11	天宗	Tiānzōng
SI2	前谷	Qiángǔ		SI12	秉风	Bǐngfēng
SI3	后溪	Hòuxī		SI13	曲垣	Qūyuán
SI4	腕骨	Wàngǔ		SI14	肩外俞	Jiānwàishū
SI5	阳谷	Yánggǔ		SI15	肩中俞	Jiānzhōngshū
SI6	养老	Yǎnglǎo		SI16	天窗	Tiānchuāng
SI7	支正	Zhīzhèng		SI17	天容	Tiānróng
SI8	小海	Xiǎohǎi		SI18	颧髎	Quánliáo
SI9	肩贞	Jiānzhēn		LI19	听宫	Tīnggōng
SI10	臑俞	Nàoshū				

7 Bladder meridian of Foot Taiyang

Zutaiyang Pangguang Jing

足太阳膀胱经

B1	睛明	Jīngmíng	B35	会阳	Huìyáng
B2	攒竹	Zǎnzhú	B36	承扶	Chéngfú
B3	眉冲	Méichōng	B37	殷门	Yīnmén
B4	曲差	Qūchāi	B38	浮郄	Fúxì
B5	五处	Wǔchù	B39	委阳	Wěiyáng
B6	承光	Chéngguāng	B40	委中	Wěizhōng
B7	通天	Tōngtiān	B41	附分	Fùfēn
B8	络却	Luòquè	B42	魄户	Pòhù
B9	玉枕	Yùzhěn	B43	膏肓	Gāohuāng
B10	天柱	Tiānzhù	B44	神堂	Shéntáng
B11	大杼	Dàzhù	B45	譩譆	Yìxǐ
B12	风门	Fēngmén	B46	膈关	Géguān
B13	肺俞	Fèishū	B47	魂门	Húnmén
B14	厥阴俞	Juéyīnshū	B48	阳纲	Yánggāng
B15	心俞	Xīnshū	B49	意舍	Yìshè
B16	督俞	Dūshū	B50	胃仓	Wèicāng
B17	膈俞	Géshū	B51	肓门	Huāngmén
B18	肝俞	Gānshū	B52	志室	Zhìshì
B19	胆俞	Dǎnshū	B53	胞肓	Bāohuāng
B20	脾俞	Píshū	B54	秩边	Zhìbiān
B21	胃俞	Wèishū	B55	合阳	Héyáng
B22	三焦俞	Sānjiāoshū	B56	承筋	Chéngjīn
B23	肾俞	Shènshū	B57	承山	Chéngshān
B24	气海俞	Qìhǎishū	B58	飞扬	Fēiyáng
B25	大肠俞	Dàchángshū	B59	跗阳	Fūyáng
B26	关元俞	Guānyuánshū	B60	昆仑	Kūnlún
B27	小肠俞	Xiǎochángshū	B61	仆参	Púshēn
B28	膀胱俞	Pángguāngshū	B62	申脉	Shēnmài
B29	中膂俞	Zhōnglǚshū	B63	金门	Jīnmén
B30	白环俞	Báihuánshū	B64	京骨	Jīnggǔ
B31	上髎	Shàngliáo	B65	束骨	Shùgǔ
B32	次髎	Cìliáo	B66	足通谷	Zútōnggǔ
B33	中髎	Zhōngliáo	B67	至阴	Zhìyīn
B34	下髎	Xiàliáo			

8 Kidney meridian of Foot Shaoyin

Zushaoyin Shen Jing

足少阴肾经

K1	涌泉	Yǒngquán	K15	中注	Zhōngzhù
K2	然谷	Rángǔ	K16	肓俞	Huāngshū
K3	太溪	Tàixī	K17	商曲	Shāngqū
K4	大钟	Dàzhōng	K18	石关	Shíguān
K5	水泉	Shuǐquán	K19	阴都	Yīndū
K6	照海	Zhàohǎi	K20	腹通谷	Fùtōnggǔ
K7	复溜	Fùliū	K21	幽门	Yōumén
K8	交信	Jiāoxìn	K22	步廊	Bùláng
K9	筑宾	Zhùbīn	K23	神封	Shénfēng
K10	阴谷	Yīngǔ	K24	灵墟	Língxū
K11	横骨	Hénggǔ	K25	神藏	Shéncáng
K12	大赫	Dàhè	K26	彧中	Yùzhōng
K13	气穴	Qìxué	K27	俞府	Shūfǔ
K14	四满	Sìmǎn			

9 Pericardium meridian of Hand Jueyin

Shoujueyin Xinbao Jing

手厥阴心包经

P1	天池	Tiānchí	P6	内关	Nèiguān
P2	天泉	Tiānquán	P7	大陵	Dàlíng
P3	曲泽	Qūzé	P8	劳宫	Láogōng
P4	郄门	Xìmén	P9	中冲	Zhōngchōng
P5	间使	Jiānshǐ			

10 San Jiao (Triple Energizer) meridian of Hand Shaoyang

Shoushaoyang Sanjiao Jing

手少阳三焦经

SJ1	关冲	Guānchōng	SJ13	臑会	Nàohuì
SJ2	液门	Yèmén	SJ14	肩髎	Jiānliáo
SJ3	中渚	Zhōngzhǔ	SJ15	天髎	Tiānliáo
SJ4	阳池	Yángchí	SJ16	天牖	Tiānyǒu
SJ5	外关	Wàiguān	SJ17	翳风	Yìfēng
SJ6	支沟	Zhīgōu	SJ18	瘈脉	Chìmài
SJ7	会宗	Huìzōng	SJ19	颅息	Lúxī
SJ8	三阳络	Sānyángluò	SJ20	角孙	Jiǎosūn
SJ9	四渎	Sìdú	SJ21	耳门	ěrmén
SJ10	天井	Tiānjǐng	SJ22	耳和髎	ěrhéliáo
SJ11	清冷渊	Qīnglěngyuān	SJ23	丝竹空	Sizhúkōng
SJ12	消泺	Xiāoluò			

11 Gallbladder meridian of Foot Shaoyang

Zushaoyang Dan Jing

足少阳胆经

G1	瞳子髎	Tóngzǐliáo	G23	辄筋	Zhéjīn
G2	听会	Tīnghuì	G24	日月	Rìyuè
G3	上关	Shàngguān	G25	京门	Jīngmén
G4	颔厌	Hányàn	G26	带脉	Dàimài
G5	悬颅	Xuánlú	G27	五枢	Wǔshū
G6	悬厘	Xuánlí	G28	维道	Wéidào
G7	曲鬓	Qūbìn	G29	居髎	Jūliáo
G8	率谷	Shuàigǔ	G30	环跳	Huántiào
G9	天冲	Tiānchōng	G31	风市	Fēngshì
G10	浮白	Fúbái	G32	中渎	Zhōngdú
G11	头窍阴	Tóuqiàoyīn	G33	膝阳关	Xīyángguān
G12	完骨	Wángǔ	G34	阳陵泉	Yánglíngquán
G13	本神	Běnshén	G35	阳交	Yángjiāo
G14	阳白	Yángbái	G36	外丘	Wàiqiū
G15	头临泣	Tóulínqì	G37	光明	Guāngmíng
G16	目窗	Mùchuāng	G38	阳辅	Yángfǔ
G17	正营	Zhèngyíng	G39	悬钟	Xuánzhōng
G18	承灵	Chénglíng	G40	丘墟	Qiūxū
G19	脑空	Nǎokōng	G41	足临泣	Zúlínqì
G20	风池	Fēngchí	G42	地五会	Dìwǔhuì
G21	肩井	Jiānjǐng	G43	侠溪	Xiáxī
G22	渊腋	Yuānyè	G44	足窍阴	Zúqiàoyīn

12 Liver meridian of Foot Jueyin

Zujueyin Gan Jing

足厥阴肝经

Liv1	大敦	Dàdūn	Liv8	曲泉	Qūquán
Liv2	行间	Xíngjiān	Liv9	阴包	Yīnbāo
Liv3	太冲	Tàichōng	Liv10	足五里	Zúwǔlǐ
Liv4	中封	Zhōngfēng	Liv11	阴廉	Yīnlián
Liv5	蠡沟	Lígōu	Liv12	急脉	Jímài
Liv6	中都	Zhōngdū	Liv13	章门	Zhāngmén
Liv7	膝关	Xīguān	Liv14	期门	Qīmén

13 Du (Governor Vessel) meridian

Dumai

督　脉

Du1	长强	Chángqiáng	Du16	风府	Fēngfǔ
Du2	腰俞	Yāoshū	Du17	脑户	Nǎohù
Du3	腰阳关	Yāoyángguān	Du18	强间	Qiángjiān
Du4	命门	Mìngmén	Du19	后顶	Hòudǐng
Du5	悬枢	Xuánshū	Du20	百会	Bǎihuì
Du6	脊中	Jǐzhōng	Du21	前顶	Qiándǐng
Du7	中枢	Zhōngshū	Du22	囟会	Xìnhuì
Du8	筋缩	Jīnsuō	Du23	上星	Shàngxīng
Du9	至阳	Zhìyáng	Du24	神庭	Shéntíng
Du10	灵台	Língtái	Du25	素髎	Sùliáo
Du11	神道	Shéndào	Du26	水沟	Shuǐgōu
Du12	身柱	Shēnzhù	（人中）		Rénzhōng
Du13	陶道	Táodào	Du27	兑端	Duìduān
Du14	大椎	Dàzhuī	Du28	龈交	Yínjiāo
Du15	哑门	Yǎmén			

14 Ren (Conception Vessel) meridian

Renmai

任　　脉

Ren1	会阴	Huìyīn	Ren13	上脘	Shàngwǎn
Ren2	曲骨	Qūgǔ	Ren14	巨阙	Jùquè
Ren3	中极	Zhōngjí	Ren15	鸠尾	Jīuwěi
Ren4	关元	Guānyuán	Ren16	中庭	Zhōngtíng
Ren5	石门	Shímén	Ren17	膻中	Dànzhōng
Ren6	气海	Qìhǎi	Ren18	玉堂	Yùtáng
Ren7	阴交	Yīnjiāo	Ren19	紫宫	Zǐgōng
Ren8	神阙	Shénquè	Ren20	华盖	Huágài
Ren9	水分	Shuǐfēn	Ren21	璇玑	Xuánjī
Ren10	下脘	Xiàwǎn	Ren22	天突	Tiāntū
Ren11	建里	Jiànlǐ	Ren23	廉泉	Liánquán
Ren12	中脘	Zhōngwǎn	Ren24	承浆	Chéngjiāng

Appendix 2   Extraordinary acupuncture points

Locations and indications of commonly used extraordinary points

Shixuan (Ex1)

Location: On the tips of the fingers, approximately 0.1 *cun* from the top of the nails. There are a total of 10 points, one on each finger (Fig. 6).

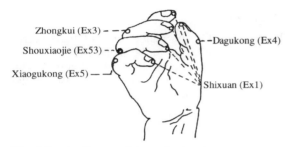

Fig. 6 Extraordinary points on the hand

Indications: High fever, sunstroke, loss of consciousness, numbness of the fingers, sore throat.
Procedure: Puncture superficially to a depth of 0.1–0.2 *cun*, or prick with a three-edged needle to draw several drops of blood. Puncture or prick each point.

Sifeng (Ex2)

Location: On the midpoint of the proximal interphalangeal creases on the palmar sides of the index to fifth fingers. There are a total of eight points, four on each hand (Fig. 7).
Indications: Malnutrition in children, childhood anorexia, indigestion, diarrhoea, whooping cough, asthma.
Procedure: Prick with a three-edged needle to draw several drops of blood or serum from each point.

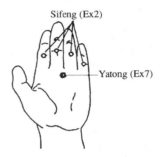

Fig. 7 Extraordinary points on the hand

Zhongkui (Ex3)

Location: On the midpoint of the proximal interphalangeal joint of the middle finger on the dorsal side (Fig. 6).
Indications: Nausea, vomiting, hiccups, poor appetite, epistaxis.
Procedure: Apply moxibustion, or puncture superficially to a depth of 0.2–0.3 *cun*.

Dagukong (Ex4)

Location: On the midpoint of the interphalangeal joint of the thumb on the dorsal side (Fig. 6).
Indications: Eye problems, vomiting, diarrhoea.
Procedure: Apply moxibustion, or puncture superficially to a depth of 0.2–0.3 *cun*.

Xiaogukong (Ex5)

Location: On the midpoint of the proximal interphalangeal joint of the little finger on the dorsal side (Fig. 6).
Indications: Eye problems, sore throat, pain and numbness of the little fingers.
Procedure: Apply moxibustion, or puncture superficially to a depth of 0.2–0.3 *cun*.

Baxie (Ex6)

Location: On the dorso-ventral boundary of the hand between the fingers. There are a

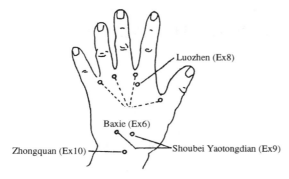

Fig. 8 Extraordinary points on the hand

total of eight points, four on each hand (Fig. 8).

Indications: Spasm, pain, numbness, or motor impairment of the fingers; inflammation or swelling of the hands.
Procedure: Puncture obliquely towards the palm for 0.5–0.8 *cun*.

Yatong (Ex7)

Location: On the palm between the third and fourth metacarpal bones, approximately 1 *cun* down from the dorsoventral boundary of the hand (Fig. 7).
Indications: Toothache, mandibular joint syndrome.
Procedure: Puncture perpendicularly for 0.5 *cun*.

Luozhen (Ex8)

Location: On the dorsal side of the hand between the second and third metacarpal bones, approximately 0.5 *cun* posterior to the metacarpophalangeal joints (Fig. 8).
Indications: Stiff neck, pain in the hands and forearms, stomachache.
Procedure: Puncture perpendicularly or obliquely for 0.5–0.8 *cun*.

Shoubei Yaotongdian (Ex9)

Location: On the back of the hand bilateral to the common extensor muscle of the

fingers, approximately 1 *cun* below the transverse crease of the wrist. There are two points on each hand (Fig. 8).
Indications: Acute lumbar sprain.
Procedure: Puncture obliquely towards the palm for 0.5–0.8 *cun*.

Zhongquan (Ex10)

Location: In the depression between Yangxi (CL25) and Yangchi (SJ4) (Fig. 8)
Indications: Feeling of fullness in the chest, stomachache, haematemesis.
Procedure: Puncture perpendicularly for 0.3–0.5 *cun*.

Erbai (Ex11)

Location: On the palmar side of the forearm bilateral to the radial flexor muscles of the wrist, approximately 4 *cun* above the transverse crease of the wrist. There are two points on each arm (Fig. 9).

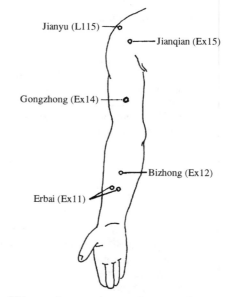

Fig. 9 Extraordinary points on the upper limb

Indications: Haemorrhoids, prolapse of anus.
Procedure: Puncture perpendicularly for 0.5–1.0 *cun*.

Bizhong (Ex12)

Location: On the palmar side of the forearm, midway between the transverse creases of the wrist and elbow (Fig. 9).
Indications: Paralysis or spasm of the upper limbs, neuralgia of the forearms, hysteria.
Procedure: Puncture perpendicularly for 1.0–1.5 *cun*.

Zhoujian (Ex13)

Location: On the tip of the olecranon of the flexed elbow (Fig. 10).

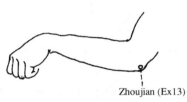

Zhoujian (Ex13)

Fig. 10 Extraordinary points on the upper limb

Indications: Scrofula.
Procedure: Apply moxibustion.

Gongzhong (Ex14)

Location: On the midline of the medial side of the upper arm, approximately 4.5 *cun* below the anterior axillary fold (Fig. 9).
Indications: Paralysis of the upper limbs, wristdrop.
Procedure: Puncture perpendicularly for 1–3 *cun*.

Jianqian (Ex15)

Location: Midway between the top of the anterior axillary fold and Jianyu (LI15) (Fig. 9).
Indications: Scapulohumeral periarthritis.
Procedure: Puncture perpendicularly for 1.0–1.5 *cun*.

Huanzhong (Ex16)

Location: On the midpoint between Huantiao (G30) and Yaoshu (Du2) (Fig. 11).
Indications: Sciatica, lumbago.

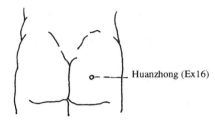

Huanzhong (Ex16)

Fig. 11 Extraordinary points on the buttocks

Procedure: Puncture perpendicularly for 2–3 *cun*.

Siqiang (Ex17)

Location: 4.5 *cun* directly above the midpoint of the base of the patella (Fig. 12).
Indications: Paralysis of the lower limbs.
Procedure: Puncture perpendicularly for 1.5–2.0 *cun*.

Baichongwo (Ex18)

Location: 1 *cun* above Xuehai (Sp10) (Fig. 12)
Indications: Urticaria, eczema, cutaneous pruritus.
Procedure: Puncture perpendicularly for 1.5–2.0 *cun*.

Heding (Ex19)

Location: In the depression above the midpoint of the base of the patella (Fig. 12).

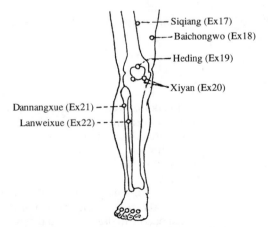

Siqiang (Ex17)
Baichongwo (Ex18)
Heding (Ex19)
Xiyan (Ex20)
Dannangxue (Ex21)
Lanweixue (Ex22)

Fig. 12 Extraordinary points on the lower limb

Indications: Knee pain, weakness or paralysis of the lower limbs.
Procedure: Puncture perpendicularly for 1.5–2.0 *cun*.

Xiyan (Ex20)

Location: In the depression between the apex of the patella and the patellar ligament. There are two points on each knee (Fig. 12).
Indications: Knee pain, weakness of the lower limbs, beriberi.
Procedure: Puncture obliquely towards the middle of the knee for 0.5–1.0 *cun*, or puncture towards contralateral Xiyan (Ex20) (Fig. 12).

Dannangxue (Ex21)

Location: Approximately 1–2 *cun* below Yanglingquan (G34) (Fig. 12).
Indications: Cholecystitis, gallstones, biliary ascariasis, *wei* or *bi* syndrome of the lower limbs.
Procedure: Puncture perpendicularly for 1–2 *cun*.

Lanweixue (Ex22)

Location: About 2 *cun* below Zusanli (S36) (Fig. 12).
Indications: Acute or chronic appendicitis, indigestion, *wei* or *bi* syndrome of the lower limbs.
Procedure: Puncture perpendicularly for 1.5–2.0 *cun*.

Bafeng (Ex23)

Location: On the dorsal-ventral boundary of the foot between the toes (see Fig. 21). There are a total of eight points, four on each foot.
Indications: Beriberi; redness, swelling, or pain of the feet.
Procedure: Puncture obliquely towards the sole for 0.5–0.8 *cun*, or prick with a three-edged needle to draw several drops of blood.

Duyin (Ex24)

Location: On the plantar side of the foot, on the midpoint of the transverse crease of the distal interphalangeal joint of the second toe (Fig. 13).

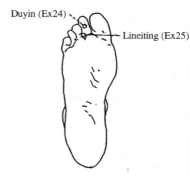

Fig. 13 Extraordinary points on the soles of the feet

Indications: Hernia, irregular menstruation.
Procedure: Apply moxibustion.

Lineiting (Ex25)

Location: On the plantar surface of the foot between the second and third toes, corresponding to Neiting (S44) (Fig. 13).
Indications: Acute stomachache, infantile convulsion, epilepsy, pain in the toes.
Procedure: Puncture perpendicularly for 0.3–0.5 *cun*.

Sishencong (Ex26)

Location: 1 *cun* anterior, posterior, left, and right to Baihui (Du20). There are four points altogether (Fig. 14).

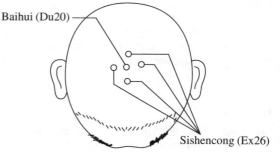

Fig. 14 Extraordinary points on the vertex

Indications: Headache, vertigo, insomnia, poor memory, epilepsy.
Procedure: Puncture horizontally for 0.5–0.8 *cun*.

Yintang (Ex27)

Location: On the middle of the glabella (also known as the ophryon) (Fig. 15).

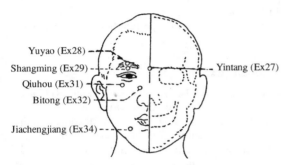

Fig. 15 Extraordinary points on the face

Indications: Headache, vertigo, epistaxis, rhinitis, infantile convulsion, insomnia.
Procedure: Puncture horizontally for 0.3–0.5 *cun*.

Yuyao (Ex28)

Location: On the midpoint of the eyebrow (Fig. 15).
Indications: Pain in the superciliary area, blepharoptosis, conjunctivitis.
Procedure: Puncture horizontally for 0.3–0.5 *cun*.

Shangming (Ex29)

Location: Below the midpoint of the supraorbital margin (Fig. 15).
Indications: Eye problems.
Procedure: Push the eyeball slightly downward, then slowly puncture perpendicularly for 0.5–1.5 *cun*. Lifting and thrusting manipulation may not be used on this point.

Taiyang (Ex30)

Location: In the depression approximately 1 *cun* posterior to the lateral end of the eyebrow and outer canthus (Fig. 16).

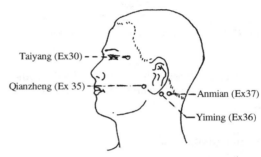

Fig. 16 Extraordinary points on the lateral side of the head

Indications: Headache, eye problems, toothache.
Procedure: Puncture perpendicularly or obliquely for 0.3–0.5 *cun*, or prick with a three-edged needle to draw several drops of blood.

Qiuhou (Ex31)

Location: On the junction between the lateral quarter and medial three-quarters of the infraorbital margin (Fig. 15).
Indications: Eye problems.
Procedure: Push the eyeball slightly upward, then slowly puncture perpendicularly for 0.5–1.5 *cun*. Lifting and thrusting manipulation may not be used on this point.

Bitong (Ex32)

Location: On the top of the nasolabial groove (Fig. 15).
Indications: Nose problems.
Procedure: Puncture horizontally to the medio-superior region for 0.3–0.5 *cun*.

Jinjin, Yuye (Ex33)

Location: On the sublingual veins, bilateral to the frenulum of the tongue. Left is Jinjin, right is Yuye (Fig. 17).
Indications: Aphtha, swelling of the tongue, vomiting, diabetes.

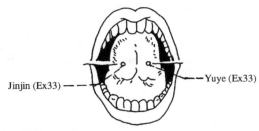

Fig. 17 Extraordinary points under the tongue

Procedure: Prick with a three-edged needle to draw several drops of blood.

Jiachengjiang (Ex34)

Location: Approximately 1 *cun* bilateral to Chengjiang (Ren24) (Fig. 15).
Indications: Deviation of the mouth, swelling of the gums and toothache.
Procedure: Puncture obliquely or horizontally for 0.5–1.0 *cun*.

Qianzheng (Ex35)

Location: Approximately 0.5–1.0 *cun* anterior to the earlobe (Fig. 16).
Indications: Deviation of the mouth, stomach-ache.
Procedure: Puncture obliquely or horizontally for 0.5–1.0 *cun*.

Yiming (Ex36)

Location: 1 *cun* posterior to Yifeng (SJ17) (Fig. 16).
Indications: Eye problems, tinnitus, insomnia.
Procedure: Puncture perpendicularly for 0.5–1.0 *cun*.

Anmian (Ex37)

Location: Midway between Yifeng (SJ17) and Fengchi (G20) (Fig. 16).
Indications: Insomnia, dizziness, headache, palpitation, *dian* or *kuang* syndrome.
Procedure: Puncture perpendicularly for 0.8–1.2 *cun*.

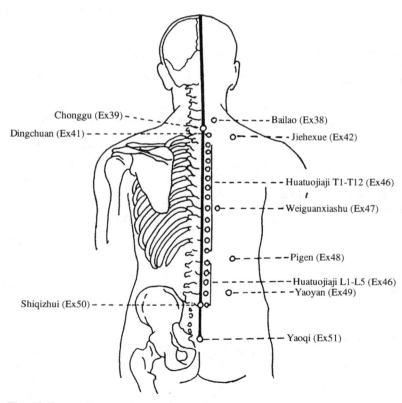

Fig. 18 Extraordinary points on the trunk

Bailao (Ex38)

Location: 2 *cun* above Dazhui (Du14) and 1 *cun* bilateral to the Du meridian (Fig. 18).
Indications: Scrofula, cough, asthma, stiff neck, night sweating.
Procedure: Puncture perpendicularly for 0.5–0.8 *cun*.

Chonggu (Ex39)

Location: Below the spinous process of the sixth cervical vertebra (Fig. 18).
Indications: Common cold, malaria, stiff neck, pulmonary tuberculosis, bronchitis, epilepsy.
Procedure: Puncture obliquely upward for 0.5–1.0 *cun*.

Jingbi (Ex40)

Location: 1 *cun* directly above the junction between the medial one-third and lateral two-thirds of the clavicle (Fig. 19).

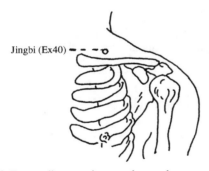

Fig. 19 Extraordinary points on the trunk

Indications: Pain, numbness or paralysis of the upper limbs.
Procedure: Puncture perpendicularly for 0.5–0.8 *cun*. To avoid damaging the lungs, do not puncture obliquely downward.

Dingchuan (Ex41)

Location: 0.5 *cun* bilateral to Dazhui (Du14) (Fig. 18).
Indications: Cough, asthma.
Procedure: Puncture perpendicularly for 0.5–0.8 *cun*.

Jiehexue (Ex42)

Location: 3.5 *cun* bilateral to Dazhui (Du14) (Fig. 18).
Indications: Tuberculosis.
Procedure: Puncture perpendicularly for 0.5–0.8 *cun*.

Sanjiaojiu (Ex43)

Location: Lay out an equilateral triangle with the top point on the umbilicus, and the length of the sides equal to the width of the patient's mouth. The two points of Sanjiaojiu (Ex43) are located on the bottom two points of the triangle (Fig. 20).

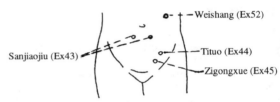

Fig. 20 Extraordinary points on the lower abdomen

Indications: Hernia, abdominal pain.
Procedure: Apply moxibustion.

Tituo (Ex44)

Location: 4 *cun* bilateral to Guanyuan (Ren4) (Fig. 20).
Indications: Prolapse of the uterus, hernia, abdominal pain.
Procedure: Puncture perpendicularly for 0.8–1.2 *cun*.

Zigongxue (Ex45)

Location: 3 *cun* bilateral to Zhongji (Ren3) (Fig. 20).
Indications: Prolapse of uterus, irregular menstruation, infertility.
Procedure: Puncture perpendicularly for 0.8–1.2 *cun*.

Huatuojiaji (Ex46)

Location: 0.5 *cun* bilateral to the spinous processes, from the first thoracic vertebra to the fifth lumbar vertebra (Fig. 18).

Indications: T1–T3 for problems of the upper limbs, T1–T8 for chest problems, T6–L5 for abdominal problems, L1–L5 for problems of the lower limbs.

Procedure: Puncture obliquely towards the spine for 0.5–1.0 *cun*.

Weiguanxiashu (Ex47)

Location: 1.5 *cun* bilateral to the spinous process of the eighth thoracic vertebra (Fig. 18).

Indications: Diabetes, dry throat.

Procedure: Puncture obliquely towards the spine for 0.5–0.8 *cun*.

Pigen (Ex48)

Location: 3.5 *cun* bilateral to the spinous process of the first lumbar vertebra (Fig. 18).

Indications: Lumps in the abdomen, lumbago.

Procedure: Puncture obliquely towards the spine for 0.8–1.2 *cun*.

Yaoyan (Ex49)

Location: In the depression approximately 3–4 *cun* bilateral to the spinous process of the fourth lumbar vertebra (Fig. 18).

Indications: Lumbago, irregular menstruation, leukorrhagia.

Procedure: Puncture perpendicularly for 1.0–1.5 *cun*.

Shiqizhui (Ex50)

Location: In the depression directly below the spinous process of the fifth lumbar vertebra (Fig. 18).

Indications: Lumbago, pain or paralysis of the lower limbs, dysfunctional uterine bleeding, irregular menstruation.

Procedure: Puncture obliquely upward for 1.0–1.5 *cun*.

Yaoqi (Ex51)

Location: In the depression of the sacral horn, approximately 2 *cun* directly above the end of the coccyx (Fig. 18).

Indications: Epilepsy, headache, insomnia, constipation.

Procedure: Puncture obliquely upward for 0.8–1.5 *cun*.

Weishang (Ex52)

Location: 2 *cun* above the umbilicus and 4 *cun* left of the Ren meridian (Fig. 20).

Indications: Gastroptosis.

Procedure: Puncture obliquely towards the umbilicus for 2.5–3.0 *cun*.

Shouxiaojie (Ex53)

Location: On the ulnar dorso-ventral boundary of the proximal interphalangeal joint of the ring finger (see Fig. 6).

Indications: Contusion, sprain.

Procedure: Puncture perpendicularly for 0.2–0.5 *cun*.

Zuxiaojie (Ex54)

Location: On the lateral dorso-ventral boundary of the proximal interphalangeal joint of the fourth toe (Fig. 21).

Indications: Contusion, sprain.

Procedure: Puncture perpendicularly for 0.2–0.3 *cun*.

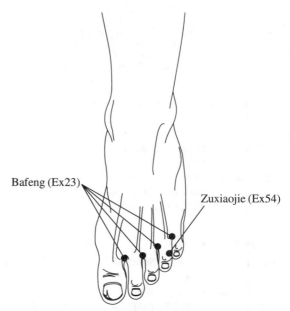

Bafeng (Ex23)

Zuxiaojie (Ex54)

Fig. 21 Extraordinary points on the dorsa of the feet

Appendix 3 Auricular therapy

Auricular therapy treats diseases and disorders by stimulating auricular points. It has several advantages over body acupuncture, including simplicity, practicality and easy acceptance by patients and is widely used as a primary or auxiliary method of treatment for over a hundred diseases and disorders.

Locations and indications of auricular points

The auricle is a miniature of the entire human body. Every part of the body has a corresponding point or area on the auricle. These points and areas are distributed in the shape of an upside-down fetus (the 'upside-down fetus' rule of distribution of auricular points and areas) (Fig. 22). Of the various auricular maps available, the *International Standard of Auricular Points* (ISAP) (Fig. 23), formulated by the China Acupuncture and Moxibustion Association with the assistance of the World Health Organization (WHO) in 1982, is recommended as the most practical. In order to simplify the location of points, this map presents points in relationship with areas. Each area consists of a group of points corresponding to a certain part of the body. The distribution of auricular points within each area, as well as the areas themselves, are upside down in relation to the body, in accordance with the 'upside-down fetus' rule of distribution. For example, within the Abdomen auricular area, the upper part corresponds to the lower abdomen, the middle part corresponds to the middle abdomen and the lower part corresponds to the upper abdomen.

Areas are not discrete units, but rather closely blend into one another. It is therefore possible to deduce the location of points and areas not depicted on the ISAP map by using the distribution rule of auricular points and areas. For instance, the auricular area corresponding to the lumbar muscles is found between Lumbosacral Vertebrae and the scaphoid fossa; the area corresponding to the forearm is located between Elbow and Wrist. Precise locations can be determined through auricular diagnosis.

A total of 90 points and areas are depicted on the ISAP map, as follows:

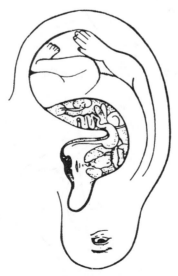

Fig. 22 Figurative drawing of the distribution of auricular points and areas viewed as an inverted fetus

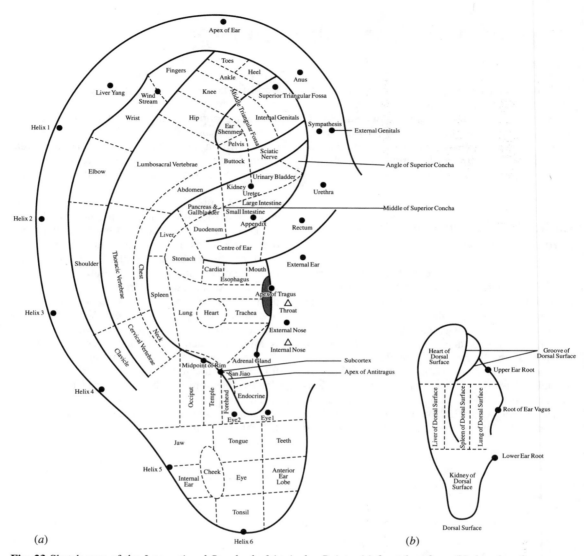

Fig. 23 Sketch map of the *International Standard of Auricular Points*: (a) frontal surface; (b) dorsal surface

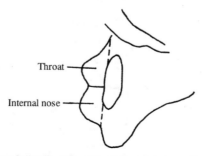

Fig. 24 Expanded view of distribution of auricular points on the tragus (internal side)

Names of auricular anatomy	Names of auricular points	Alternative names	Location	Indications
Crus of helix (1 point)	Centre of Ear	Zero Point, Diaphragm, Neurosis Point	On the crus of the helix	Hiccups, urticaria, cutaneous pruritus, childhood enuresis, haemoptysis
Helix (12 points)	Rectum	Lower Part of Rectum	On the helix close to the notch superior to the tragus and level with Large Intestine	Constipation, diarrhoea, prolapsed anus, haemorrhoids
	Urethra		On the helix superior to Rectum, level with Urinary Bladder	Frequent, painful, or dripping urination; retention of urine
	External Genitals		On the helix superior to Urethra, level with Sympathesis	Testitis, ovaritis, epididymitis, vulvar or scrotal pruritus
	Anus	Haemorrhoid Point	On the helix level with anterior border of the superior crus of the antihelix	Hemorrhoids, anal fissure
	Apex of Ear	Tonsil 1	On the top of the helix, level with the posterior border of the superior crus of the antihelix	Fever, hypertension, acute conjunctivitis, stye
	Liver Yang	Liver Yang 1, Liver Yang 2, Lesser Occipital Nerve	On the tubercle of the helix	Dizziness, headache, hypertension
	Helix 1–Helix 6		A line drawn on the helix from the lower border of tubercle of the helix to the midpoint of the lower rim of the lobe is separated into five equal sections. The six points thus delineated are from top to bottom Helix 1–Helix 6.	Tonsillitis, upper respiratory tract infection, fever
Scaphoid fossa (6 points)	Fingers	Appendix	The scaphoid fossa is separated into six equal horizontal sections. The uppermost section is Fingers.	Paronychia, pain and numbness of the fingers
	Wrist		On the second section from the top of the scaphoid fossa.	Wrist pain.
	Wind Stream	Allergy Area, Urticaria Point, Internal Tubercle	Between Fingers and Wrist	Urticaria, cutaneous pruritus, allergic rhinitis
	Elbow	Sleep Inducing Point	On the third section from the top of the scaphoid fossa.	Tennis elbow, elbow pain
	Shoulder	Appendix 2	On the fourth and fifth sections from the top of the scaphoid fossa	Scapulohumeral periarthritis
	Clavicle	Nephritis Point Appendix 3	On the lowermost section of the scaphoid fossa	Scapulohumeral periarthritis
Antihelix (14 points)	Toes		On the posterosuperior portion of the superior crus of the antihelix, close to Apex of Ear	Paronychia, pain in the toes
	Heel		On the anterosuperior portion of the superior crus of the antihelix, close to the upper portion of the triangular fossa	Heel pain
	Ankle		Between Heel and Knee	Strain of the ankle joint
	Knee		On the middle one-third of the superior crus of the antihelix	Swelling and pain of the knee joint
	Hip		On the lower one-third of the superior crus of the antihelix	Pain of the hip joint, sciatica

Names of auricular anatomy	Names of auricular points	Alternative names	Location	Indications
	Buttock		On the posterior one-third of the inferior crus of the antihelix	Sciatica, gluteal fasciitis
	Sciatic Nerve		On the anterior two-thirds of the inferior crus of the antihelix	Sciatica
	Sympathesis		On the juncture between the terminus of the inferior crus of the antihelix and the helix	Angina pectoris, gastrointestinal spasm, biliary colic, ureterolith, functional disturbance of the autonomic nervous system
	Cervical Vertebrae	Thyroid	The body of the antihelix (the area between the notch separating the antitragus and the antihelix, and the origin of the superior and inferior crus of the antihelix) is separated into five equal sections. Cervical Vertebrae is located on the lowermost section.	Stiff neck, cervical spondylopathy
	Thoracic Vertebrae	Mammary Gland	On the upper second and third sections as described above	Chest pain, premenstrual swelling of the breasts, mastitis
	Lumbosacral Vertebrae		On the top and upper second sections as described above	Pain in the lumbosacral region
	Neck		On the border of the concha anterior to Cervical Vertebrae	Stiff neck, neck pain or swelling
	Chest		On the border of the concha anterior to Thoracic Vertebrae	Pain in the chest or hypochondriac region, feeling of fullness in the chest, mastitis
	Abdomen		On the border of the concha anterior to Lumbosacral Vertebrae	Abdominal pain or distension, diarrhoea, acute lumbar strain
Triangular Fossa (5 points)	Ear Shenmen		On the triangular fossa superior to the origin of the superior and inferior crus of the antihelix	Insomnia, nightmares, withdrawal syndrome, pain
	Pelvis	Lumbago Point	On the triangular fossa inferior to the origin of the superior and inferior crus of the antihelix	Pelvic inflammation
	Middle Triangular Fossa	Asthma Point, Hepatitis Point	On the middle one-third of the triangular fossa	Asthma
	Internal Geneitals	Uterus, Essence Palace, Tiangui	On the anterior one-third of the triangular fossa	Dysmenorrhoea, irregular menstruation, leukorrhagia, dysfunctional uterine bleeding, seminal emission, premature ejaculation
	Superior Triangular Fossa	Blood Pressure Lowering Point	Anterosuperior to the triangular fossa	Hypertension

Names of auricular anatomy	Names of auricular points	Alternative names	Location	Indications
Tragus (6 points)	External Ear	Ear	Anterior to the notch superior to the tragus and close to the helix	Infection of the external auditory meatus, otitis media, tinnitus
	External Nose	Nose and Eye Cleaning Point, Hunger Point	Slightly anterior to the centre of the external side of the tragus	Nasal vestibulitis, rhinitis
	Apex of Tragus	Top of Tragus, Thirst Point	On the top of the upper eminence of the tragus	Fever, toothache
	Adrenal Gland		On the top of the lower eminence of the tragus	Hypotension, mumps, rheumatoid arthritis, intermittent malaria, vertigo caused by streptomycin poisoning
	Throat		On the upper half of the medial side of the tragus	Hoarseness, laryngopharyngitis, tonsillitis
	Internal Nose		On the lower half of the medial side of the tragus	Rhinitis, paranasal sinusitis, epistaxis
Antitragus (6 points)	Apex of Antitragus	Asthma Relief Point, Parotid Gland	On the upper portion of the antitragus	Asthma, parotitis, cutaneous pruritus, testitis, ovaritis, epididymitis
	Midpoint of Rim	Brain Point, Brainstem, Enuresis Point	On the midpoint between Apex of Antitragus and the notch between the antitragus and the antihelix	Nocturnal enuresis, Meniere's disease
	Occiput	Dizziness Point	On the posterosuperior portion of the external side of the antitragus	Dizziness, headache, asthma, epilepsy, neurosism
	Temple	Taiyang	On the middle portion of the external side of the antitragus	Migraine
	Forehead		On the anteroinferior portion of the external side of the antitragus	Dizziness, headache, insomnia, nightmares
	Subcortex	Ovary, Testicle, Excitation Point	On the medial side of the antitragus	Pain, intermittent malaria, neurosism, myopia
Inferior Concha (6 points)	Heart		On the centre of the inferior concha	Tachycardia, arrhythmia angina pectoris, pulseless disease, neurosism, hysteria, stomatoglossitis
	Lung	Pulmonary Point, Tuberculosis Point, Pulmonary Emphysema Point	On the inferior concha peripheral to Heart	Cough, asthma, feeling of fullness in the chest, hoarseness, acne, cutaneous pruritus, urticaria, flat wart, constipation, withdrawal syndrome
	Trachea		On the inferior concha between the foramen of the external auditory canal and Heart	Cough, asthma
	Spleen		On the posterosuperior portion of the inferior concha	Abdominal distension, diarrhoea, constipation, poor appetite, dysfunctional uterine bleeding, leukorrhagia, Meniere's disease

Names of auricular anatomy	Names of auricular points	Alternative names	Location	Indications
	Endocrine		On the base of the inferior concha close to the notch between the tragus and antitragus	Dysmenorrhoea, irregular menstruation, menopausal syndrome, acne, intermittent malaria
	San Jiao		On the base of the inferior concha superior to Endocrine	Constipation, abdominal distension, pain on the lateral side of the upper limbs
Superior Concha (7 points)	Liver		On the posteroinferior portion of the superior concha	Pain in the chest and hypochondriac region, vertigo, premenstrual syndrome, irregular menstruation, hypertension, pseudomyopia, simple glaucoma
	Pancreas & Gallbladder		Between Liver and Kidney	Gallstones, cholecystitis, biliary ascariasis, migraine, herpes zoster, otitis media, tinnitus, hearing loss, acute pancreatitis
	Kidney		On the superior concha inferior to the origin of the superior and inferior crus of the antihelix	Lumbago, tinnitus, neurosism, pyelitis, asthma, nocturnal enuresis, irregular menstruation, seminal emission, premature ejaculation
	Ureter		Between Kidney and Urinary Bladder	Urethral colic
	Urinary Bladder		Between Kidney and Angle of Superior Concha	Urocystitis, enuresis, retention of urine, lumbago, sciatica, occipital headache
	Angle of Superior Concha	Prostate	On the posterosuperior angle of the superior concha	Prostatitis, urethritis
	Middle of Superior Concha	Centre of Umbilicus, Ascites, Drunk Point, Anterior Peritoneum Posterior Peritoneum	On the centre of the superior concha	Abdominal pain or distension, biliary ascariasis parotitis
Peripheral Crus of Helix (8 points)	Mouth		The anterior one-third of the area inferior to the crus of the helix	Facial paralysis, stomatitis, cholecystitis, gallstones, withdrawal syndrome
	Oesophagus		The middle one-third of the area inferior to the crus of the helix	Oesophagitis, oesophagospasm, globus hystericus
	Cardia		The posterior one-third of the area inferior to the crus of the helix	Cardiospasm, neurogenic vomiting
	Stomach	Pylorus, Gastroptosis Point	On the area posterior to the terminus of the crus of the helix	Gastrospasm, gastritis, gastric ulcer, insomnia, toothache, indigestion

Names of auricular anatomy	Names of auricular points	Alternative names	Location	Indications
	Duodenum		The posterior one-third of the area superior to the crus of the helix	Duodenal ulcer, cholecystitis, gallstones, pylorospasm
	Small Intestine		The middle one-third of the area superior to the crus of the helix	Indigestion, abdominal distension, tachycardia, arrhythmia
	Large Intestine		The anterior one-third of the area superior to the crus of the helix	Abdominal distension, constipation, cough, acne
	Appendix		Between Small Intestine and Large Intestine	Simple appendicitis, diarrhoea
Frontal Surface of Earlobe (10 points)	Eye 1	Glaucoma Point	On the frontal surface of the earlobe, anteroinferior to the notch between the tragus and the antitragus	Pseudomyopia
	Eye 2	Astigmia Point	On the frontal surface of the earlobe, posteroinferior to the notch between the tragus and the antitragus	Pseudomyopia
	Teeth	Anaesthesia Point for Dental Extraction, Toothache Point, Blood Pressure Raising Point	A grid of nine equal portions is laid out on the frontal surface of the earlobe by drawing two equidistant horizontal lines and two equidistant vertical lines below the lower border of the cartilage of the notch between the tragus and the antitragus. The sections are numbered from anterior to posterior and top to bottom. Teeth is located on the first section of the earlobe grid	Toothache, periodontitis, hypotension
	Tongue	Palate, Lower Palate	On the second section of the earlobe grid	Glossitis, stomatitis
	Jaw	Upper Jaw Mandible	On the third section of the earlobe grid	Toothache, dysfunction of the tempomandibular joint
	Anterior Ear Lobe	Anaesthesia Point for Dental Extraction, Neurosism Point	On the fourth section of the earlobe grid	Neurosism, toothache
	Eye		On the fifth section of the earlobe grid	Acute conjunctivitis, electric ophthalmitis, stye, pseudomyopia
	Internal Ear		On the sixth section of the earlobe grid	Meniere's disease, tinnitus, hearing loss
	Cheek		On the border between the fifth and sixth sections of the earlobe grid	Peripheral facial paralysis, trigeminal neuralgia, acne, flat wart
	Tonsil	Tonsil 4	On the eighth section of the earlobe grid	Tonsillitis, pharyngitis
Dorsal surface of auricle (9 points)	Upper Ear Root	Spinal Cord 1, Stagnation in the Interior	On the upper portion of the ear root	Epistaxis
	Root of Ear Vagus		On the juncture of the dorsal surface of the auricle and the mastoid process, corresponding to the crus of the helix	Cholecystitis, gallstones, biliary ascariasis, nasal obstruction, tachycardia, abdominal pain, diarrhoea

Names of auricular anatomy	Names of auricular points	Alternative names	Location	Indications
	Lower Ear Root		On the lower portion of the ear root	Hypotension
	Groove of Dorsal Surface	Blood Pressure Lowering Groove	The groove formed by the antihelix and its two branches on the dorsal surface of the auricle	Hypertension, cutaneous pruritus
	Heart of Dorsal Surface		On the upper portion of the dorsal surface of the auricle	Palpitation, insomnia, nightmares
	Spleen of Dorsal Surface		On the dorsal surface of the auricle close to the terminus of the crus of the helix	Gastric pain, indigestion, poor appetite
	Liver of Dorsal Surface		On the dorsal surface of the auricle lateral to Spleen of Dorsal Surface	Cholecystitis, gallstones, pain in the hypochondriac region
	Lung of the Dorsal Surface		On the dorsal surface of the auricle medial to Spleen of Dorsal Surface	Cough, asthma, cutaneous pruritus
	Kidney of Dorsal Surface		On the lower portion of the dorsal surface of the auricle	Dizziness, headache, neurosism

Supplemental: The distribution of points and areas on both frontal and dorsal surfaces of the auricle is identical, so main points and areas are often taped on both surfaces simultaneously in order to increase stimulation. For example, Knee is taped on both frontal and dorsal surfaces to treat pain in the knee joint; Anterior Lobe is taped on both frontal and dorsal surfaces to treat neurosism. Increasing stimulation in this way is especially effective for treating pain in various parts of the body.

Selection of auricular points

Achieving good results in auricular therapy depends on the correct selection of points to be treated. The following rules should be followed when selecting points in clinical practice.

● Choose points according to location of the diseased or affected area of the body.
This is a fundamental principle of auricular therapy. Every currently used auricular treatment adheres to this method. For example, Forehead is the major auricular point used for treating frontal headache, Eye is used for all eye diseases and Large Intestine for all diseases of the large intestine.

● Choose points according to principles of traditional Chinese medicine.
The eleven auricular areas corresponding to the five *zang* and six *fu* organs are especially significant in Chinese auricular therapy. They are used extensively in clinical practice, not only to treat disorders of their corresponding *zangfu* organs, but also to treat problems of the tissues with which the *zangfu* organs are considered by the principles of TCM to be connected. For example, the liver opens into the eyes, so Liver can be used to treat eye problems such as glaucoma, pseudomyopia and conjunctivitis. The Urinary Bladder meridian distributes to the occiput, back of the neck, lumbus, anus and back of the lower limbs, so Urinary Bladder can be used to treat pain in the occipital region, stiff neck, backache, lumbago, haemorrhoids and sciatica.

● Choose points according to principles of modern medicine.
For example, the sympathetic nervous system functions to relax spasm of the visceral smooth muscles, regulate vasomotion and inhibit glandular secretion; therefore Sympathesis is an important point for treating visceralgia, bronchial asthma, Raynaud's disease and hyperhydrosis. The major pathogenesis of Meniere's

disease is labyrinthine hydrops, so Internal Ear and External Ear are used to treat this condition.

● Choose points according to specific effect.

For instance, blood-letting puncturing of Apex of Ear functions to dispel heat, lower blood pressure, tranquillize the mind, relieve allergic reactions, restore consciousness and brighten the eyes; therefore Apex of Ear is widely used to treat fever, hypertension, insomnia, allergies, headache, poor memory and blurred vision. Centre of Ear functions to expel wind and improve the blood circulation, so it is used to treat urticaria and cutaneous pruritus. Ear Shenmen is useful for calming the mind and relieving pain, so it is used for treating mental problems and all kinds of pain.

Auricular diagnosis

Auricular diagnosis is an important aspect of auricular therapy. When disease or disorder is present in the *zangfu* organs or tissues of the body, positive signs may occur on the corresponding areas of the auricle. For example, discoloration, deformities, desquamation, pimples, angioparesis, tenderness, or lowered auricular electrical resistance may be present. These positive signs are not only used to diagnose the position, nature and clinical development of the problem, but also provide reliable evidence for determining the selection of auricular points to be used in its treatment.

In clinical practice, the following three methods of auricular diagnosis – inspection, palpation and measurement of electrical resistance – are used in combination with modern diagnostic methods and the differentiation of signs and symptoms to establish an accurate diagnosis and provide reliable evidence for determining the selection of auricular points to be treated.

Auricular inspection

Auricular inspection consists of carefully checking for discoloration, deformities, desquamation or pimples on the auricle in order to diagnose disease or disorder. It can be used to diagnose both acute and chronic diseases, as well as the acute onset of chronic diseases.

Procedure

1. In adequate light, carefully examine the auricle from top to bottom and inside to outside.
2. When a positive sign is found, use the fingers to first stretch and then slowly loosen the dorsal surface of the auricle. Repeat the manipulation several times in order to distinguish the size, shape and colour of the positive sign.
3. When an eminence is found, determine its size, shape, hardness, mobility and whether there is tenderness when it is palpated with the fingers or a probe.
4. Compare the positive signs on the bilateral auriculae in order to determine the exact position of the disease or disorder and to confirm whether or not the signs are genuine.
5. When examining the triangular fossa and the superior and inferior concha, a detection probe should be used to open and completely expose these areas.

Positive signs and their clinical significance

1. Discoloration

Red: including bright, light or dark red. The discoloured area may be spotty, patchy or irregular. Bright red indicates acute disease or pain; light or dark red indicates chronic disease or recovery from severe disease. For example, cases of chronic lumbago may show patchy dark red or light red signs on Kidney or Lumbosacral Vertebrae.

White: may be spotty, patchy, or spotty white in the centre with reddish border. White usually indicates chronic or deficient disease or disorder. For example, cases of chronic bronchitis or asthma may show spotty white eminences on Lung and Trachea; cases of rheumatic cardiac disease may show white patches with reddish border on Heart.

Dark brown: resembling freckles. This usually indicates chronic disease, especially refractory or proliferative problems. For instance, cases of prolapse of the intervertebral disc may show brown streaky pigmentation on Lumbosacral Vertebrae.

2. Deformities

Eminence: including nodular eminences the size of a grain of wheat or small bean and streaky or patchy eminences. Nodular eminences usually indicate headache, or proliferative or chronic problems. Streaky eminences usually indicate proliferative or organic diseases, for instance, cases of gastric ulcer may show streaky eminence on Stomach. Patchy eminence indicates acute problems, for instance, cases of neurosism may show patchy eminence on Anterior Lobe or Occiput and cases of tonsillitis may show patchy eminence on Tonsil.

Pitting or depression: may be spotty, patchy or thread-like. Spotty pitting usually indicates tinnitus or astigmia; patchy pitting indicates chronic or organic problems such as gastro-duodenal ulcer; thread-like pitting indicates tinnitus or coronary heart disease.

Pimples: whitish spotty pimples indicate chronic inflammatory conditions such as chronic bronchitis, chronic diarrhoea, pelvitis, annexitis or cholecystitis. Patchy dark brown pimples usually indicate skin disease such as neurodermatitis or contact dermatitis.

3. Desquamation
Patchy desquamation usually indicates chronic inflammatory conditions or skin diseases. For example, desquamation on Wind Stream, Lung, or the entire auricle indicates skin diseses such as seborrhoeic dermatitis or psoriasis; desquamation on Lung indicates chronic bronchitis; desquamation on the triangular fossa indicates chronic genital or gynaecological problems.

Points to remember

1. Take into account differences in age, sex, constitution and season; distinguish pre-existing non-pathological deformities of the auricle from genuine positive signs.
2. Use adequate light; natural light is best.
3. Distinguish false from genuine positive signs. When a detection probe (any instrument with a blunt point approximately the size of a match-head) is used to press an eminence, discoloured area or pimple, genuine positive signs will show soreness, distension, or even stabbing pain, while false positive signs will show no reaction.

Auricular palpation

Auricular palpation consists of palpating auricular positive signs such as discoloured areas, eminences, pimples or tender spots with a detection probe (any instrument with a blunt point approximately the size of a match-head) in order to diagnose disease or disorder of corresponding body parts.

Procedure

Holding the auricle with one hand, palpate auricular points with a detection probe to detect positive signs such as tenderness, discoloration, or deformities (eminence, pitting, or pimples).

● Positive signs and their clinical significance

Tenderness: Tenderness is a positive sign commonly seen in auricular diagnosis. It is classified into three grades: mild tenderness, with no other pain reaction when palpated; moderate tenderness, accompanied by frowning and blinking when palpated; and severe tenderness, accompanied by stabbing pain and flinching when palpated. Obvious auricular tenderness is usually present in cases of acute disease, pain or tumours, so auricular palpation is suitable for the diagnosis of these conditions.

Eminence: Eminence includes spotty, patchy or streaky scleroma, or proliferation of the auricular cartilage. Scleroma usually indicates chronic, organic or proliferative conditions. For example, cases of chronic cholecystitis may show patchy scleroma on Pancreas & Gallbladder; cases of cervical spondylopathy may show proliferation of cartilage on Cervical Vertebrae.

Indentation when palpated: Carefully observe depth, colour and recovery time of the indentation after palpation. Generally speaking, deep whitish indentations with long recovery time indicate deficient syndromes such as oedema and asthma; superficial reddish indentations with a short recovery time indicate excessive syndromes such as acute tonsillitis and gastritis.

Points to remember

1. Palpate all points with even pressure and for the same length of time in order to avoid false positive or negative signs.
2. Compare tender points with adjacent points several times.
3. Carefully observe patients' reactions during palpation; inquire whether there are other sensations present such as soreness, distension, radiating pain, etc.
4. There may be several tender points on one auricle, but the most severe tenderness usually occurs on the area which corresponds to the major problem area of the body.

5. Positive signs usually indicate homolateral disease or disorder, so it is important to compare bilateral auriculae in order correctly to diagnose the location of the problem.
6. Take into account differences in age, sex and constitution. According to clinical experience, the pain threshold of women and children is usually relatively lower than that of men and the elderly; pressure used when palpating should be adjusted accordingly. Some people have a very high pain threshold, so it is almost impossible to locate tender points even when they have very severe problems; on the other hand, others have such a low pain threshold that many tender points may exist on their auriculae even though they have no problems at all.

Measurement of auricular electrical resistance

This diagnostic method uses an electrical detector to measure auricular electrical resistance. When disease or disorder is present in the body, there may be an obvious decrease in electrical resistance on corresponding auricular points. This phenomenon allows measurement of auricular electrical resistance to be an effective tool in establishing a diagnosis.

Procedure

Each individual's basic electrical resistance is different, so a basic standard should be established in each case before proceeding with auricular diagnosis. It has been found that the electrical resistance of the upper root of the auricle can be taken as the basic electrical resistance. It is found by placing one electrode of the detector on the upper root of the auricle and regulating the potentiometer until a faint sound is heard. The resulting measurement is used as the standard when measuring other auricular points. Areas where the electrical resistance is lower than standard are referred to as positive, or highly conducive, electrical resistance points.

Positive electrical resistance points and their clinical significance

Positive electrical resistance points are classified into two grades according to their degree of electrical resistance. *Intensely positive points* have the lowest electrical resistance and stabbing pain is usually experienced on the points during measurement. *Positive points* have electrical resistance

somewhat lower than standard; stabbing pain is sometimes experienced on the points during measurement.

Intensely positive points generally correspond to the primary affected area of the body. Cases of acute disease usually show an obvious decrease of auricular electrical resistance; cases of chronic disease often do not. Measurement of auricular electrical resistance can therefore be helpful in distinguishing the course and stage of the problem.

Points to remember

Auricular electrical resistance is affected by many factors, including constitution, season, dampness of the skin and manipulation. Measures should be taken to avoid influencing the results of measurement with extraneous factors.

1. Do not wash or rub the auriculae prior to measurement in order to avoid false positive points caused by increased conduction due to congestion of blood. If the auriculae must be washed because they are seborrhoeic, a 10-minute interval should be allowed before beginning measurement.
2. During the winter, a short interval should be allowed before beginning measurement after coming in from outdoors. Auricular blood vessels contract and electrical resistance increases in the presence of cold, so measuring electrical resistance on a cold auricle may give false negative results.
3. Electrical resistance may vary among different areas of the auricle. For instance, the triangular fossa, the superior and inferior concha and the scapha often show relatively lower electrical resistance. Therefore, light pressure should be used when measuring these areas and points of lower electrical resistance should be compared with other areas. The results of inspection and palpation should also be considered in order to assist in distinguishing genuine from false positive signs.
4. Electrical resistance on the auricle corresponding to the affected side will be much lower than that on the healthy side, so a comparison of bilateral electrical resistance should be made to establish location of the problem.
5. Individual differences should be taken into account. Some people's electrical resistance is relatively high, making it difficult to detect positive points with this method; on the other

hand, that of other people may be very low, resulting in easily occurring false positive points.

Therapeutic methods

Auricular therapy stimulates auricular points to regulate the meridians, *qi*, blood and *zangfu* organs and balance *yin* and *yang* ☯. Proper and sufficient stimulation must be provided if good effects are to be achieved. Generally speaking, sufficient stimulation refers to the greatest intensity the patient can bear. There should be sensations of heat, distension, or radiating pain in the auricle being treated.

With the development of modern technology, new methods such as the use of electricity and lasers have been developed to stimulate the auricle. However, only four traditional methods noted for their effectiveness, simplicity and convenience are introduced here.

Auricular taping

Auricular taping consists of taping small, round, hard, smooth objects such as mustard seeds, pills or ball bearings to particular auricular points that have been selected through the process of auricular diagnosis. The taped objects are then pressed in order to stimulate the points to treat disease or disorder in corresponding areas of the body. This method has gained wide acceptance due to its safety, simplicity, effectiveness, wide range of indications and lack of contraindications.

Procedure

1. Choose small, round, hard, smooth objects of the appropriate size for stimulating auricular points. The objects chosen should have no toxic properties or side effects. Seeds of *Vaccaria segetalis* (mustard) or other plants, small beans, pills or small ball bearings are all suitable for use in auricular taping.
2. Prepare sufficient adhesive tape, cut into squares 0.5 cm square.
3. Sterilize the auricle with tincture of iodine or alcohol.
4. Holding the auricle with one hand, use a detection probe (any instrument with a blunt point the size of a match-head) to press the auricular point hard enough to leave a depression. Tape the seed, etc. to the positive point and press for several minutes until a needling sensation of heat, distension or radiating pain is achieved.
5. Tape the points in the order of upper to lower and frontal to dorsal; tape primarily the auricle of the affected side of the body. Bilateral auriculae may be taped simultaneously or during alternate treatment sessions.
6. The distribution of auricular points on the frontal and dorsal surfaces is identical. Therefore, main auricular points may be taped on both sides simultaneously in order to increase stimulation and improve effectiveness. This method is especially effective for treating pain such as headache, backache and sore joints.
7. Allow the tape and seeds, etc. to remain on the auricle for 3–7 days. Each point should be pressed for 3–5 minutes two or three times each day, until a needling sensation of heat, distension or radiating pain is achieved.
8. Remove the tape and seeds, etc. the evening before the next treatment and clean the auricle with soap and warm water.

Indications

Auricular therapy is safe, effective and easily accepted by a wide range of patients. It is widely used in clinical practice for the treatment of pain, inflammation, endocrine disturbance, functional disorders, motion sickness and allergic reactions. It is especially suitable for children, the elderly and people with weak constitutions or drug allergies.

Normal reactions to auricular taping therapy

Reactions to auricular taping therapy are varied owing to differences in constitution, age and sex. The most common reactions include localized sensations of heat, distension, radiating pain, or numbness. Some people may experience reflex muscle reactions or a sensation of flowing heat and comfort in the corresponding body area. Many people feel vigorous, have a good appetite and sleep well after taping. All of these reactions indicate that the therapeutic method and points chosen were correct and that the prognosis is favourable.

Abnormal reactions in auricular taping, their prevention and management

As in acupuncture, abnormal reactions may occur during or after auricular taping. They include the following:

1. Fainting. Various degrees of fainting may occur due to nervousness, hunger, weak constitution due to prolonged illness, overstrain or use of inappropriate points of stimulation:

    Mild fainting: manifesting as dizziness, sensation of fullness or discomfort in the chest, or nausea.

    Moderate fainting: manifesting as palpitation, vertigo, nausea and vomiting, pale complexion, perspiration, coldness of the limbs and rapid thready pulse.

    Severe fainting: manifesting as coldness of the entire body, profuse sweating, low blood pressure, very weak and thready pulse and even loss of consciousness.

    Mild and moderate fainting is common but severe fainting is quite rare in auricular therapy. Fainting may occur either during or after taping. In mild cases, the patient should lie down, drink some hot water or hot sugar water and relax. Treatment may be continued when the patient recovers. In moderate or severe cases, the tape and seeds etc. should first be removed. Place the patient in Trendelenburg's position and loosen the collar and belt. Be careful to keep the patient warm, especially in winter. Puncture Subcortex and Adrenal Gland auricular points. Additional emergency treatment should be undertaken if necessary.

    Auricular therapy differs from acupuncture in that fainting due to overstrain, hunger or weak constitution due to prolonged illness is much more common than fainting due to nervousness. Therefore, care should be taken when treating patients with these predisposing conditions. In these cases, a period of rest in the clinic before and after taping should be allowed, fewer points are selected, a horizontal position is adopted during taping and moderate manipulation is utilized. These patients should be informed of the possibility of fainting and how to manage it if it occurs.

    Moderate and severe fainting generally occur during treatment, while mild fainting may occur well after. Mild fainting is usually induced by obvious factors or predisposing conditions such as hunger, overstrain or severe motion. Therefore, adequate rest after taping is essential.

2. Infection of the auricle. The main causes of infection following auricular taping are allergic reactions to the adhesive tape or incomplete sterilization. In mild cases, there may be itching and pain in the taped areas, sometimes accompanied by a reddish rash or pimples. In severe cases, there may be swelling or redness of the auricle, ulcerative infection of the taped areas, or even necrosis and atrophy of the auricular cartilage resulting in deformity of the auricle.

    Because of the relatively poor blood circulation in the auriculae, auricular infections are difficult to cure. Hypoallergenic tape should be used when treating people with adhesive allergies. Since infection may still occur in these cases relatively easily, alternative auricular therapies such as auricular blood-letting, auricular pressure or auricular massage should be considered.

Precautions

1. Avoid exposing the adhesive tape to moisture. In order to achieve a strong bond, apply the tape only after the alcohol used to sterilize the auricle has evaporated completely from the skin of the ear.
2. Use hypoallergenic tape for people with adhesive allergies. At the time of treatment, also tape Adrenal Gland and Wind Stream and prick Apex of Ear with a three-edged needle to let several drops of blood. Or use alternative methods such as auricular blood-letting, auricular pressure or auricular massage.
3. Auricular therapy is contraindicated in cases of inflamed or frostbitten auriculae.
4. If sleep is affected because bilateral auriculae have been taped simultaneously, tape each side alternately.
5. Auricular taping is contraindicated in cases of severe cardiac disease.
6. Mild manipulation should be used with pregnant women. Do not tape points which may cause the uterus to contract. Auricular taping is contraindicated for pregnant women who have a history of repeated miscarriage.
7. During the summer, points should be taped for a shorter period (three days) because of increased perspiration. During the winter, pay attention to keeping the auriculae warm.
8. To prevent injury to the auricle, do not rub in a sideways or circular motion while pressing the taped auricular points.

Auricular blood-letting puncturing

Auricular blood-letting puncturing uses a three-edged needle, plum blossom needle, or ensiform needle to draw blood from selected auricular points, areas or collaterals to treat disease and disorder of corresponding parts of the body. Blood-letting puncturing of the auriculae, especially Apex of Ear and Helix 1 to Helix 6, stimulates blood circulation to the auriculae, thus improving the metabolism of the entire body. Blood-letting puncturing is indicated primarily for excessive or heat syndromes, although it is also useful in some deficient syndromes such as insomnia or dizziness.

Procedure

1. Massage the auricle to cause congestion of blood.
2. Strictly sterilize the needles and area to be treated.
3. Holding the auricle with one hand, either puncture the selected points to a depth of 2 mm with a three-edged needle, heavily tap the points with a plum blossom needle, or incise the selected collaterals of the dorsal surface with an ensiform needle.
4. Pinch the auricle to express five to eight drops of blood. Absorb the blood with dry sterile cotton.
5. Puncture bilateral auriculae alternately for general cases and simultaneously for acute cases.
6. Treat twice a week for general cases and once every other day for acute cases.

Indications

1. Apex of Ear. Blood-letting puncturing of Apex of Ear with a three-edged needle relieves heat, eliminates wind and benefits the ears. This method is widely used in clinical practice for treating fever, inflammatory reactions, neuroses, hypertension, skin diseases, allergic reactions, pain, eye problems, tinnitus and deafness. Plentiful blood vessels and ease of manipulation on this point make it the most ideal point for auricular blood-letting.
2. Liver Yang. Blood-letting puncturing of Liver Yang with a three-edged needle calms the liver to arrest endogenous wind. This method is used to treat headache, vertigo and tinnitus due to hyperactivity of the liver *yang*.
3. Apex of Tragus. Blood-letting puncturing of

Apex of Tragus with a three-edged needle relieves heat and pain and has a tranquillizing effect. This method is used to treat fever, inflammatory infections and neuroses.
4. Groove of Dorsal Surface. Tapping Groove of Dorsal Surface with a plum blossom needle lowers the blood pressure. This method is used to treat dizziness, vertigo, headache, blurred vision and tinnitus due to hypertension.
5. Collaterals on the Dorsal Surface. Incising the collaterals with an ensiform needle to draw blood eliminates wind and relieves heat. This method is used to treat skin diseases and inflammatory infections.
6. Helix 1 to Helix 6. Blood-letting puncturing of Helix 1 to Helix 6 with a three-edged needle relieves heat. This method is used to treat inflammatory infections such as tonsillitis, conjunctivitis, laryngopharyngitis and mumps.
7. Other points. Blood-letting puncturing can be used on all auricular points to treat excessive or heat syndromes. Needles are chosen according to the position of the point to be treated. For instance, Cheek is tapped with a plum blossom needle to treat acne, flat wart, chloasma, or for cosmetic purposes. Lung is punctured with a three-edged needle to treat lung diseases.

Precautions

1. Massage the auricle before treatment to dilate the blood vessels and make blood-letting easier.
2. Strictly sterilize the needles and the areas to be punctured in order to avoid infection of the auricle.
3. To prevent damage to the auricular cartilage, do not puncture too deeply with a three-edged needle (2 mm is sufficient).
4. Sufficient blood should be expressed, usually five to eight drops. For severe excessive or heat syndromes, slightly more blood should be let. It is very easy to cause bleeding in patients with heat syndrome because the circulation is quite rapid. If the blood spurts like a fountain, the prognosis is very good.
5. If it is necessary to draw blood repeatedly on the collaterals of the auricular dorsal surface, the distal end should be incised first.
6. Auricular blood-letting puncturing is contra-indicated in cases of immunological insufficiency, or haemorrhagic diseases such as haemophilia, primary thrombocytopenic purpura or aplastic anaemia.

Auricular pressure

Auricular pressure employs pressure on selected auricular points with a detection probe (any instrument with a blunt point the size of a match-head) to treat disease or disorder in corresponding parts of the body. It has been found in clinical practice that there is often immediate improvement in symptoms such as pain, nausea and vomiting when tender points are located and pressed with the detection probe during the diagnostic process. Auricular pressure activates the meridians and collaterals, regulates the *qi* and blood and calms the mind, so it is suitable for treating pain, chronic illnesses, injury of the soft tissues and neurosism.

Procedure

Press each point with a detection probe for 2–3 minutes until a sensation of heat, distension or radiating pain is achieved. Pressure may vary from light to heavy. This method may be self-applied at home two or three times a day.

Precautions

Sharply pointed instruments should not be used to apply auricular pressure in order to prevent injury to the auricle.

Auricular massage

Long-term massage of the auriculae with the hands can activate the meridians and collaterals, regulate the *qi* and blood, restore the functions of the *zangfu* organs, nourish the brain, brighten the eyes and benefit the ears. It is used to treat problems such as neurosism, headache, dizziness, blurred vision or tinnitus, as well as to raise the intelligence and improve general fitness. It was recorded in *The Effective Prescriptions of Sushen* (Song dynasty circa 907–1279 A.D.) that massage of the ears can strengthen antipathogenic *qi*. There are also records of early Taoists using this method for health preservation and longevity.

Procedure

1. Rub the palms together until they are warm. Massage both the frontal and dorsal auricular surface between them.
2. With the thumb on the dorsal surface and the index finger on the frontal surface, massage both the frontal and dorsal auricular surfaces from top to bottom. The index finger should massage the auricular areas in the following order: helix, scapha, triangular fossa, antihelix, superior concha, inferior concha, peripheral crus of the helix, medial side of the antitragus, medial side of the tragus, lobe. The index finger should remain longer on areas specific to the patient's condition.
3. The procedure should be repeated several times until the auriculae are hot. The results will be greatly improved if the patient's mind is focused and attention concentrated during the massage.

Concluding note

For a detailed explanation of the theory and clinical application of auricular therapy, see *Chinese Auricular Therapy* and its accompanying *Practical Auricular Point and Area Map* by Dr Bai Xinghua, published by the Scientific and Technical Documents Publishing House, Beijing, 1994.

Appendix 4　Blood-letting puncturing

Blood-letting puncturing treats diseases and disorders by puncturing and drawing blood from acupuncture points, superficial collaterals, or affected areas with a three-edged needle. Use of this method was first recorded in *Neijing, The Classic of Medicine*, which recommended it for treating refractory problems and heat syndromes. The three-edged needle is one of the nine types of needles discussed in this work. The needle is marked by a thick round handle, three-edged body and sharp tip (Fig. 25).

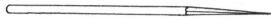

Fig. 25 A three-edged needle

Procedure

Hold the handle of the three-edged needle with the thumb and index finger, leaving 0.1–0.2 cm of the tip exposed. Stabilize the tip with the middle finger to control depth of insertion (Fig. 26).

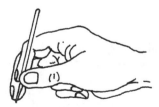

Fig. 26 How to hold a three-edged needle

There are three methods of puncturing, each used for different areas.

1. *Pricking points*. This method is suitable for use on all body acupuncture points, especially those on the extremities such as Shixuan (Ex1) and *jing* (well) points. First rub the area to be pricked to cause localized congestion of blood. Holding the area steady with one hand, quickly prick the point to a depth of 0.3 cm with the other. Withdraw the needle immediately and squeeze the surrounding area to express several drops of blood.

2. *Piercing collaterals*. This method is suitable for use on stagnant superficial collaterals and collaterals of the cubital and popliteal fossae, such as Chize (L5) and Weizhong (B40). To treat stagnant superficial collaterals, first pierce, then squeeze the surrounding area to express the stagnant blood. Finally cover the hole with sterilized cotton. For collaterals of the cubital and popliteal fossae, apply a ligature above the fossae. Sterilize the local area; press below the area to be pierced with the thumb of one hand and pierce with the other. Withdraw the needle immediately and allow 0.5–2.0 ml of blood to flow spontaneously. Then remove the ligature and press with sterilized cotton to arrest bleeding.

3. *Leopard-spot pricking*. This method is used to treat superficial localized problems. Sterilize the lesion and surrounding area, then lightly prick the surrounding area to cause some bleeding.

Indications

Blood-letting puncturing functions to activate the meridians, dredge the collaterals, dispel heat, restore consciousness and relieve swelling and pain. It is suitable for treating excessive and heat syndromes and cases due to stagnation of blood. For instance, pricking Shixuan (Ex1) or *jing* (well) points is effective for treating sunstroke, infantile convulsion; numbness, swelling or pain of the hands and feet; and high fever. Piercing collaterals of the cubital fossa is effective for treating acute gastroenteritis; piercing collaterals of the popliteal fossae is effective for treating lumbago. Leopard-spot pricking is commonly used for treating skin diseases, soft tissue injury and thecal cyst.

Precautions

● Strictly sterilize needles and the areas to be punctured in order to avoid infection.
● Prick the points, lesions, or surrounding area lightly, superficially and quickly to draw several drops of blood and avoid injury to major arteries. When piercing the collaterals of the

cubital and popliteal fossae, avoid causing excessive bleeding.

- Blood-letting puncturing is contraindicated in cases of compromised immune system, or for haemorrhagic diseases such as haemophilia, primary thrombocytopenic purpura or aplastic anaemia.

- Treat once a day or once every other day for general cases and twice a day for acute conditions. Five treatments constitute one course.

- Cupping is usually applied following blood-letting puncturing in order to draw more stagnant blood, increase stimulation and improve effectiveness.

Appendix 5 Chiropractic

Chiropractic uses the massage of the areas on either side of the spinal column to treat diseases and disorders. The back-*shu* points of the *zangfu* organs fall along the first and second lines of the Urinary Bladder meridian, located on the back bilateral to the spinal column. Massage of these areas can both invigorate the body's antipathogenic *qi* and strengthen the functions of the *zangfu* organs. This method is commonly used for treating indigestion and malnutrition in children.

Procedure

Have the patient lie prone with the hands resting on either side of the head, so the back is flat and the back muscles relaxed. Using the thumb and index fingers, knead the muscles on either side of the spinal column from Changqiang (Du1) to Dazhui (Du14) four or five times (Fig. 27). Starting with the second time, lift the back-*shu* points of the *zangfu* organs obliquely upwards while kneading to increase stimulation. After kneading and lifting, strike the kneaded area repeatedly with the side of the hand. Finally, roll the loose fist back and forth from top to bottom three or four times. Treat once a day. Ten treatments constitute one course.

Indications

Chiropractic functions to strengthen the functions of the *zangfu* organs, especially the stomach and spleen. It is very effective for treating indigestion, malnutrition and weak constitution in children, as well as chronic digestive problems in adults such as chronic gastritis and peptic ulcer.

Remarks and precautions

- Chiropractic is an ideal 'do-it-yourself' method for treating diseases and disorders and keeping

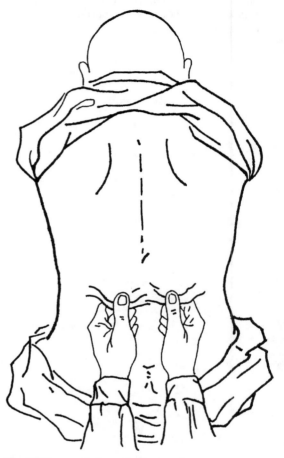

Fig. 27 Demonstration of chiropractic

fit. Long-term practice of chiropractic can improve the constitution and promote growth and development in children.
- Chiropractic is contraindicated in cases of severe heart disease, skin lesions on the back and haemorrhagic diseases such as haemophilia, primary thrombocytopenic purpura and aplastic anaemia.

Appendix 6 Cupping

Cupping treats diseases and disorders by applying jars with negative pressure to affected areas or acupuncture points in order to induce local congestion and stasis of blood and activate the meridians. Cupping has a very long history. It is easily accepted by a wide range of people due to its simplicity of application.

Instruments

It is recorded that horn was the material first used for cupping. Jars made of various materials including clay, bamboo, metal and glass later became available (Fig. 28). Glass jars are now used most often, since their transparency allows the degree of congestion and bleeding occurring inside to be observed and duration of application more easily regulated. Either specially made jars, or any jar of the appropriate size with a smooth and even mouth, may be used for cupping.

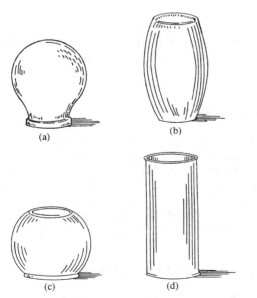

Fig. 28 Cups made of glass (a), bamboo (b), china (c) and bronze (d)

Procedure

There are three stages to cupping.

Step 1

Use fire to expel the air from the jar and form a vacuum in one of the following three ways.

1. Holding a piece of alcohol-soaked cotton with a pair of forceps, ignite it and circle it around the inside of the jar one to three times. Withdraw the cotton and immediately apply the jar to the chosen area. This method is very safe since there is no fire inside the jar during the cupping. In order to avoid burning the skin, do not using excessive alcohol which might drip on the skin and keep the ignited cotton away from the mouth of the jar (Fig. 29).

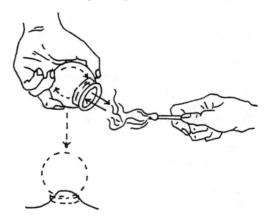

Fig. 29 Flash-fire cupping

2. Put a piece of burning paper into the jar and immediately apply the jar to the chosen area before the paper burns out. When using this method, the jar is usually applied horizontally to prevent the burning paper from falling onto the skin (Fig. 30).
3. Put a thin layer of dry cotton in the bottom of the jar, ignite and immediately apply the jar to the chosen area. This method is simple and safe, but the cotton should not be too thick in order to avoid burning the skin or losing suction.

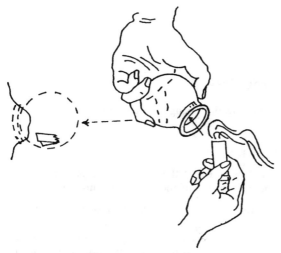

Fig. 30 Fire-insertion cupping

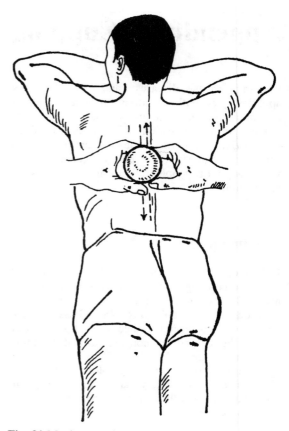

Fig. 31 Moving cupping

Step 2

Apply the jar to the chosen area using one of the following three methods.

1. Leave the jars in place for 8–15 minutes, until the skin becomes dark red (observable when using glass jars). When using larger jars with stronger suction, leave in place for a shorter time in order to avoid causing blisters. When using smaller jars with less suction, leave in place longer in order to increase stimulation. This method is commonly used and is suitable for all indications of cupping therapy.
2. Moving cupping. Coat the chosen areas with a thin layer of lubricant, apply the jar and move up and down or back and forth several times until the local skin becomes dark red (Fig. 31). This method is suitable for cupping large areas which are rich in muscle, such as the back, lumbar region, buttocks and thighs.
3. Blood-letting puncturing and cupping. Prick the chosen area with a three-edged needle or tap with a plum blossom needle, then cup for 8–15 minutes to draw blood. The combination of blood-letting puncturing and cupping increases stimulation and is especially suitable for treating excessive and heat syndromes such as *bi* syndrome, high fever and skin diseases.

Step 3

Withdraw the jars. Holding the jar with one hand, press the skin next to the mouth of the jar to release some air and break the suction. The jar will then spontaneously drop off. Do not pull or rotate the jar when breaking the seal in order to avoid injury to the skin.

Indications

Cupping functions to expel wind, dispel cold and eliminate dampness; activate the meridians and dredge the collaterals; subdue swelling and relieve pain; and dispel pathogenic heat and fire. It is commonly used to treat *bi* syndrome, the common cold, abdominal pain or distension, diarrhoea, headache, furuncles, urticaria and herpes zoster.

Remarks and precautions

● The patient should be in a comfortable position. Cup areas which are even and rich in muscle; do

- not cup areas with hair, joints or large blood vessels.
- Select jars of appropriate size according to the size of the area to be cupped. Apply the cups steadily, accurately and quickly.
- Apply a thin layer of lubricant to the areas to be cupped in order to avoid burns and increase suction.
- The lower abdomen and lumbosacral region may not be cupped and moving cupping may not be used in pregnant women.

- Cupping is contraindicated in cases of severe heart disease and haemorrhagic problems such as haemophilia, primary thrombocytopenic purpura and aplastic anaemia.
- If blisters or scalding occur, prick the blister with a sterilized needle if large, then coat with gentian violet and cover with sterilized gauze.
- Treat once every other day. Cup the same points until congestion and stasis of blood no longer result from the treatment.

Appendix 7 Electroacupuncture

Electroacupuncture, developed from traditional acupuncture, treats diseases and disorders using a combination of acupuncture and stimulation with electrical current. It is more effective than traditional acupuncture for treating some diseases. Electroacupuncture is also commonly used in acupuncture anaesthesia and scientific research, since parameters such as wave form, frequency and intensity can be controlled and standardized.

Instruments

Various electrical stimulators are available, but their basic principle is the same. An impulse generator is used to produce low-frequency impulse current similar to the bio-electricity of the human body. Three types of wave form may be selected: continuous wave, including dispersed wave (2–5 per second) and dense wave (50–100 per second); combined dense and dispersed wave; and intermittent wave. Appropriate wave forms and intensity are chosen according to the clinical requirements of each case.

Procedure

- The selection of points for electroacupuncture is similar to that for body acupuncture, however, at least two points must be used in order to form a closed circuit. Usually two to three pairs of points are used each time. It is better to attach the two poles of each pair of electrodes to two points on the same side of the body in order to prevent the impulse current from passing through the heart. This is especially important when puncturing points on the chest and back and for cases with severe heart diseases.
- Needles of the highest quality should be used in order to avoid bending or breakage. Set all knobs of the stimulator on '0'.
- Puncture the points until a needling sensation is achieved, then connect the needles with the electrical stimulator. For each pair of electrodes, the negative pole should be attached to a main point and the positive pole to an auxiliary point. Select the appropriate wave form, turn on the stimulator and gradually turn up the intensity

until it reaches the appropriate level. Apply electrical stimulation for 15–30 minutes each time, according to the specific case. It may be necessary to increase the intensity during the course of the session if the patient adapts to the level of stimulation. At the end of each treatment, return the output knobs to '0', turn the stimulator off, remove the electrodes and finally withdraw the needles.

Selection of wave forms

Each wave form has its own characteristics. The appropriate wave form should be selected to give the greatest effect for each particular case.

- Dense wave.
  Decreases the excitability of the nervous system, working first on the sensory nerves and then the motor nerves. It is used to relieve pain, tranquillize the mind and for acupuncture anaesthesia.
- Dispersed wave.
  Increases excitation and tension of the muscles and ligaments. It is used to treat *wei* syndrome and injuries of the muscles, joints, ligaments and tendons.
- Combined dense and dispersed wave.
  Dense and dispersed waves alternate, so there is usually no adaptation to the stimulation by the patient during the session. It is used to treat soft tissue injury, arthritis, sciatica, facial paralysis and localized frostbite.
- Intermittent wave.
  Dense wave occurs at regular intervals. Its function is similar to that of dispersed wave, but there is usually no adaptation to the stimulation by the patient during the session. It is therefore especially suitable for treating *wei* syndrome.

Selection of intensity of stimulation

When the current reaches a certain degree, there will be a sensation of tingling. This is referred to as the sensation threshold. If the current is increased, there will be a twingeing or sensation of stabbing pain. This is the pain threshold. These thresholds vary for each person due to individual differences. The intensity of current for each case is selected according to the nature of the condition and the patient's constitution. Stimulation is started at the lowest degree and gradually increased to the greatest bearable intensity. The current at this point is between the sensation threshold and the pain threshold. Because the range between the two thresholds is narrow, it is essential to regulate the stimulation very carefully in order to achieve the optimum level of stimulation.

Intensity of stimulation is divided clinically into three types, according to the patient's reaction.

- Mild stimulation.
  Marked by localized quivering, but without muscular contraction or pain. The intensity of stimulation is below or near the sensation threshold. Mild stimulation is used for treating neurosism and cardiac diseases, or patients with weak constitutions.
- Moderate stimulation.
  Marked by muscular contraction, but with no severe pain. This level of stimulation falls between the sensation threshold and the pain threshold and is the most commonly used for general cases.
- Strong stimulation.
  Marked by obvious muscular contraction with severe pain. The level of intensity is over the pain threshold. Strong stimulation is usually used for treating schizophrenia, muscular atrophy and paralysis.

Indications

The indications for electroacupuncture are similar to those for body acupuncture. It is especially suitable for treating *wei* syndrome and for pain relief and acupuncture anaesthesia, since the continuous stimulation of the electrical current can increase the needling sensation. Electroacupuncture is also commonly used in scientific research, since parameters such as wave form, frequency and intensity can be controlled and standardized.

Remarks and precautions

- Check that the electrical stimulator is functioning properly before use.
- Determine the positive and negative poles of the circuit before use. Hold the two electrodes, not allowing them to touch. Switch on the stimulator and gradually increase the intensity of the current until a tingling sensation is felt. The electrode with the stronger sensation is negative, the other positive.
- The stimulation provided by electroacupuncture is intense, especially when strong manipulation is applied; it is therefore important to use high quality needles in order to avoid bending or breakage.
- Because the handles of some needles may become oxidized and therefore will not conduct electricity, it is recommended to connect the stimulator directly to the body of the needles.
- It is better to use points on the same side of the body for each pair of electrodes in order to prevent the impulse current from passing through the heart. This is essential in cases with cardiac problems.
- To prevent short circuit, do not allow the outputs of the electrical stimulator to touch each other. This is especially important when the two points being treated are very close together.
- Always increase intensity of current gradually. Abrupt increase may cause severe muscular contraction and pain and lead to bending or breaking of the needles or fainting.
- Intensity of stimulation should be in accordance with the nature of the condition and the patient's personal constitution. Stimulation of the greatest bearable intensity generally achieves the best effects.
- Strong stimulation is forbidden when applying electroacupuncture to points on the face, chest, back and spine.
- Electroacupuncture is contraindicated in cases of severe cardiac disease, for pregnant women and for people prone to fainting or with very weak constitutions.

Appendix 8 Hot salt compress therapy

Hot salt compress therapy, a type of moxibustion, employs the application of hot salt to certain areas of the body, especially Shenque (Ren8), to treat diseases and disorders. Salt is an attribute of the kidneys; Shenque (Ren8), a point on the Ren meridian, is considered to be the centre of life in traditional Chinese medicine. Application of hot salt to Shenque (Ren8) functions to warm the kidney *yang*, strengthen the spleen and restore consciousness. There are also records of early Taoists using this method to preserve health and attain longevity.

Procedure

Heat 500–1000 g of salt in a dry pan over a low fire. Put half of the hot salt in a small bag and apply to Shenque (Ren8). Protect the skin by placing a towel under the bag while it is very hot; when it starts to cool down the towel can be removed. Change to a new hot bag when the first one is no longer hot. Apply for 30–60 minutes, once a day. Ten treatments constitute one course.

Indications

Applying hot salt to Shenque (Ren8) functions to warm the kidney *yang* and strengthen the spleen and stomach, so it is suitable for treating both excessive and deficient cold syndromes such as epigastic pain, abdominal distension, diarrhoea, retention or incontinence of urine and dysmenorrhoea. It is also used as an auxiliary method for treating *jue* syndromes due to deficiency of *qi* or invasion by cold.

Remarks and precautions

● The salt compress should be as hot as can be tolerated to achieve the best results.
● During application of the compress it is essential to check the temperature of the salt and the patient's reactions, especially when treating children or when there is loss of consciousness. Stop treatment if symptoms such as dizziness, headache, palpitation, nausea or vomiting, or profuse sweating occur.
● In addition to Shenque (cRen8), hot salt compresses may also be applied to *ashi* (tender) points when treating pain due to stagnation of *qi* and blood, such as *bi* syndrome and backache.
● It is possible to increase stimulation and improve the effect by adding herbs such as cassia bark and vladimiria root to the salt.
● This method is contraindicated in cases of high fever and heat syndromes and in pregnant women.
● Hot salt compress therapy is ideal for treating cold and deficient conditions and preserving health.

Appendix 9 Point implantation therapy

Point implantation therapy treats diseases and disorders with strong and persistent stimulation by implanting surgical catgut on selected acupuncture points. It is used for treating chronic and refractory problems such as peptic ulcer, epilepsy and asthma.

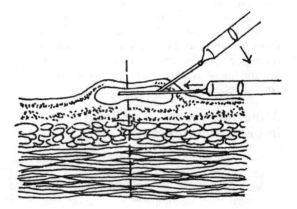

Instruments

Skin disinfectant, towels, syringe, forceps, No. 12 spinal needle with smooth stylet tip, needle holder, No. 0–1 surgical catgut, 0.5–1.0% procaine hydrochloride, scissors, sterile gauze and dressing.

Procedure

1. Implantation with spinal needle.
   Sterilize the local area. Insert a 1–2 cm length of sterilized catgut into the barrel of the spinal needle from the top. Stretching the skin taut, insert the spinal needle until a needling sensation is achieved. Implant the catgut in the point by simultaneously pushing the stylet and withdrawing the syringe. Finally, cover the punctured area with sterile gauze.

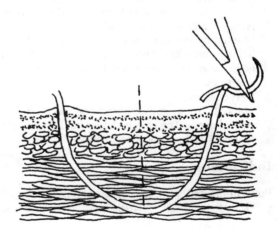

2. Implantation with triangular suture needle.
   Use gentian violet to mark two points 1–2 cm on either side of the point to be treated. Sterilize the local area. Anaesthetize the area between the two marks by infiltrating with 0.5–1.0% procaine hydrochloride. Using a needle holder to grip a triangular suture needle loaded with catgut, insert the needle in through one side, through the subcutaneous tissues and muscle layer and out through the other. Holding the skin between the two puncture sites taut, sever the catgut close to the skin. Release the skin and rub and press until the length of catgut recedes into the subcutaneous tissues and muscle layer (Fig. 32). Finally, cover the punctured area with sterile gauze.

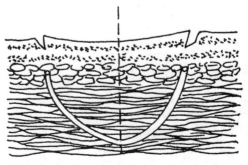

Fig. 32 Point implantation using a triangular suture needle

Normal reactions to point implantation therapy

Localized aseptic inflammation, including mild redness, swelling, heat and pain, commonly occurs for one to five days following implantation due to irritation of the xenogenous protein. More severe reactions may occur in some cases, including exudate or fever to 38°C, with no symptoms of localized infection. These symptoms generally appear within 4–24 hours of implantation and disappear spontaneously within two to four days. No treatment is necessary for any of the above conditions.

Abnormal reactions to point implantation therapy

1. Infection due to incomplete sterilization, or secondary incisional infection.
   Marked by localized redness, swelling and severe pain accompanied by fever occurring within three to four days of implantation. These types of infections should be treated promptly.
2. Allergic reaction to surgical catgut.
   Marked by localized post-implantation redness, itching and fever. Anti-allergy treatment should be given and the catgut immediately removed in severe cases.
3. Nerve injury.
   Marked by aesthesiodermia or paralysis of related nerve. The catgut should be immediately removed and appropriate treatment given.

Indications

Point implantation therapy is used to treat asthma, peptic ulcer, chronic gastritis, nocturnal enuresis, seminal emission, sexual dysfunction, epilepsy, chronic enteritis, dysmenorrhoea, central retinitis, *wei* syndrome and optic atrophy.

Remarks and precautions

- Sterilize strictly to avoid infection.
- When employing a triangular suture needle for implantation, a light and accurate touch should be used to avoid bending the needle.
- The principles used to select points for point implantation therapy are the same as for body acupuncture. However, points rich in muscle, such as those on the back and chest, are most commonly used. Two to four points are selected each time. Treat once every four to five weeks. Five treatments constitute one course.
- The catgut must be implanted between the subcutaneous tissues and muscle layer, or within the muscle layer on points which are rich in muscle. The catgut must not be exposed outside the skin.
- Determine appropriate depth of implantation according to specific points. Take care to avoid injury of the internal organs, large blood vessels, or nerves.
- During repeated treatment of the same point, the location should be changed slightly each time.
- Point implantation is contraindicated in cases of pulmonary tuberculosis during the active stage, in severe heart problems and in pregnant women.
- Check for post-implantation reactions and institute necessary treatment in the event of abnormal reactions.

Appendix 10 Point injection therapy

Point injection therapy utilizes injection of various substances into acupuncture points to treat diseases and disorders. Combining acupuncture and drugs can improve the effectiveness of treatment in some cases.

Instruments

Instruments required are: 1 ml, 2 ml, 5 ml, 10 ml and 20 ml syringes; No. 4–No. 6 syringe needles or No. 5 dental needles.

Commonly used drugs and dosages

Any drug used for intramuscular injection can be used for point injection therapy. Commonly used drugs include vitamins B_1, B_{12} and K_3; 0.25–2.0% procaine hydrochloride solution; atropine, reserpine, antibiotics; normal saline, glucose; and extracts of Chinese herbs such as Chinese angelica root, bupleurum root and red sage root. For example, Chinese angelica root functions to activate the meridians and dredge the collaterals, so it is injected in cases of rheumatic or rheumatoid arthritis. Atropine inhibits the M-cholinergic receptors of the smooth muscles and glands, so it is injected to relieve spasm of the smooth muscles, as in treating gastric spasm.

Dosage depends on location of points to be injected and the characteristics and concentration of the substance being injected. Inject 0.3–0.5 ml for points on the head and face, 0.1 ml for auricular points, 1–2 ml for points on the extremities, 0.5–1 ml for points on the chest and back and 2–5 ml for points on the lumbar and gluteal regions. Dosage should be greater for mildly stimulating substances such as glucose and normal saline; for instance 10–20 ml of glucose is injected for soft tissue injury. Dosage should be correspondingly less for drugs with strongly stimulating properties or for certain drugs such as antibiotics or atropine. In these cases, dosage for each injection is one-tenth to one-third that of routine intramuscular injection. Dosage of extracts of Chinese herbs is generally 1–2 ml per point.

Selection of points

The principles used for selection of points are the same as for body acupuncture, auricular therapy or scalp acupuncture. However, points rich in muscle or *ashi* points are used much more commonly than in other therapies. It is best to treat the minimum number of points; generally two to four points are selected each time.

Procedure

With the patient lying in a comfortable position, sterilize the local area to be treated. Choose syringes of the appropriate size and fill with the substance to be injected. Quickly puncture the point to the subcutaneous tissues, then continue to puncture slowly. Start to inject the drug when a needling sensation is achieved and no blood appears when withdrawing the syringe. If a large amount is to be administered to one point, either inject the solution gradually while slowly withdrawing the syringe, or direct the needle in several different directions while injecting the solution.

Speed of injection depends upon specific conditions. It is usually rapid for excessive and heat syndromes and slow for deficient and cold syndromes.

Indications

Point injection therapy has wide indications. It is especially suitable for soft tissue injury, lumbar muscle strain, cervical spondylopathy, sciatica, rheumatic and rheumatoid arthritis, tennis elbow, scapulohumeral periarthritis, stiff neck, trigeminal neuralgia and intercostal neuralgia.

Remarks and precautions

● Closely monitor pharmacological action, dosage, quality, expiration date, incompatibility, side effects and allergic reactions of each injection. Do skin tests prior to treatment for drugs which may induce allergic reaction, such as penicillin, streptomycin and procaine hydrochloride. Use caution with potentially irritating drugs and do not use drugs with severe side effects.

- Strictly sterilize the local area and use single-use needles to avoid infection.
- Massage the local area for three to five minutes prior to injection to relax the local muscles, improve absorption of drugs and relieve pain.
- The syringe needle may be lifted and thrust to achieve a needling sensation and increase effect, but must not be twirled.
- To prevent injection of drugs into the blood vessels, draw the syringe before starting injection. Inject only if no blood appears in the syringe.
- Do not inject drugs into the articular cavities or the spinal canal. Injection into the articular cavities may result in redness, swelling, heat and pain of the joints. Injection into the spinal canal may result in possibly irreversible spinal cord injury.
- The patient will experience a sensation of electric shock if the needle contacts a nerve trunk. In this case, it is necessary to withdraw the needle slightly before injection in order to avoid nerve injury.
- Points on the chest and back should not be punctured deeply in order to prevent damage to the internal organs or pneumothorax. Points bilateral to the spine should be punctured obliquely toward the spine to prevent pneumothorax. The bladder should be emptied prior to puncturing points on the lower abdomen in order to prevent damage to the bladder.

lower layer of the galea aponeurotica. Resistance will decrease when this depth is reached. Continue to insert the needle horizontally using twirling manipulation, to a depth of 0.5–1.5 *cun* depending on specific conditions.

When the needle has been inserted to the appropriate depth, hold it between the ball of the thumb and the radial side of the index finger and twirl 150–200 times per minute for 2–3 minutes. Repeat two or three times with a 5–10 minute interval between manipulations. Either withdraw the needle at this point, or leave in place for 24 hours to increase stimulation. A helper can withdraw it at the proper time. When treating cases of hemiplegia, instruct the patient to move the affected limbs, or in severe cases provide assistance to move the affected limbs, while the needles are in place.

Electrostimulation is usually applied instead of hand manipulation. For selection of intensity, frequency and wave type, see Appendix 7.

Remarks and precautions

● The stimulation provided by scalp acupuncture is quite strong. Precautions should be taken to prevent fainting, especially when the patient is in a sitting position.
● In cases of cerebral hemorrhage, apply scalp acupuncture only after the patient's blood pressure and general condition have stabilized. In cases of cerebral thrombosis, apply scalp acupuncture as soon as possible after onset in order to improve effect and shorten the course of treatment. Use scalp acupuncture with caution in cases accompanied by high fever, acute infection or heart failure.
● The scalp is rich in blood vessels and bleeds easily, so pressure should be applied to puncture site with sterile cotton immediately after withdrawing the needle.
● Treat once a day or once every other day. Ten treatments constitute one course.

Glossary

Acquired essence: substance derived from food and water and used to maintain the vital activities and mechanisms of the body.

Antipathogenic *qi*: the energy which enables the body to resist pathogens, the opposite of pathogenic *qi*.

***Ashi* points:** 'Oh yes!' points in English. Points with no fixed position or name, determined by positive signs such as tenderness or scleroma.

Back-*shu* points: 12 points on the back, each related physiopathologically to one of the 12 *zangfu* organs. Usually used as main points for treating problems of their corresponding organs.

***Ben*:** the root and trunk of a tree, as opposed to its branches (*biao*). Used in the clinical practice of traditional Chinese medicine to indicate the cause of a disease or disorder as opposed to its manifestations, antipathogenic *qi* as opposed to pathogenic factors, or a primary condition as opposed to its complications.

Biao*:** see ***Ben

Cold: (1) one of the six exogenous pathogens, usually occurring during the winter; (2) deficient cold due to deficiency of the body's *yang qi*, which is insufficient to warm the body. The former is called exogenous cold, the latter endogenous cold.

Congenital essence: original substance essential for building the body and reproduction.

***Cun*:** (1) one of the three portions of the wrist over the radial artery where the pulse is taken: *guan* is located over the eminent head of of the radius at the wrist; *cun* is located adjacent to *guan* on the distal side; and *chi* is located adjacent to *guan* on the proximal side; (2) a relative unit of length used to locate acupuncture points, determined by dividing various parts of the body into segments of equal length. One segment equals one *cun*.

Damp: (1) one of the six exogenous pathogens, usually occurring during the summer; (2) retention of fluid in the body due to reduced function of the spleen and kidneys, which leads to impairment of the water metabolism. The former is called exogenous damp, the latter endogenous damp.

Deficiency: one of the eight principles of traditional Chinese medicine, the opposite of excess.

Its pathogenic change is marked by deficiency of the body's antipathogenic *qi*.

Differentiation of symptoms and signs: one of the most important aspects of traditional Chinese medicine. It allows the cause, nature and location of a disease or disorder to be determined by utilizing the basic theories of TCM to analyse symptoms and signs at various stages of its course.

Dryness: (1) one of the six exogenous pathogens, which usually occurs during autumn and damages the lungs; (2) deficiency of the bodily fluid due to excesssive heat, deficient fire or loss of bodily fluid. The former is called exogenous dryness, the latter endogenous dryness.

Eight confluence points: eight points of the regular meridians located on the extremities and connecting with the eight extraordinary meridians. These points have wide clinical applications.

Eight *hui* (influential) points: eight important points which are closely related to the *zang* and *fu* organs, *qi*, blood, bone, marrow, tendons and blood vessels respectively.

Eight principles: the four pairs of opposite aspects, i.e. *yin* and *yang*, interior and exterior, cold and heat, deficiency and excess. Widely used as guidelines in the differentiation of syndromes.

Even method: a type of puncturing manipulation midway between the reducing and reinforcing methods in which the needle is twirled at a moderate speed or lifted and thrust to a moderate depth. This method is suitable for cases which are neither excessive nor deficient and cases of *yin* deficiency.

Excess: one of the eight principles of traditional Chinese medicine, the opposite of deficiency. It is marked by hyperactivity of pathogens and a strong constitution.

Exterior: one of the eight principles of traditional Chinese medicine, the opposite of interior. Its manifestations are usually superficial and mild.

Extraordinary points: acupuncture points other than those of the twelve regular and Du and Ren meridians, with fixed locations and their own names. They often have special functions.

Fire: (1) one of the five elements; (2) one of the six exogenous pathogens in TCM.

Five elements: also called the five evolutive phases: wood, fire, earth, metal and water. This philosophical theory was integral to medical practice in ancient China. It expounds the unity of matter and the human body, as well as the physiopathological relationship among the five *zang* organs and the other tissues of the body.

Five hearts: the heart, palms of the hands and soles of the feet.

Five orbiculus theory: a theory of ophthalmology which holds that each of the five *zang* organs is physiopathologically related to one of the five orbiculi, i.e. the spleen corresponds to the flesh orbiculus (the eyelid), the heart to the blood orbiculus (the canthus), the lungs to the *qi* orbiculus (the sclera), the liver to the wind orbiculus (the iris) and the kidneys to the water orbiculus (the pupil).

Five *shu* points: five specific points located on each of the twelve regular meridians below the elbows or knees: *jing* 井 (well), *ying* 荥 (spring), *shu* 输 (stream), *jing* 经 (river) and *he* 合 (sea).

Four seas: the Sea of Marrow (the brain), the Sea of Blood (the Chong meridian), the Sea of *qi* (Danzhong (Ren17)) and the Sea of Food (the stomach). Also called the four reservoirs.

Front-*mu* points: twelve points on the chest and abdomen, each related physiopathologically to one of the twelve *zangfu* organs. Usually used as main points for treating problems of their corresponding organs.

***Fu* organs:** the six hollow organs, i.e. the gall-bladder, stomach, large intestine, small intestine, San Jiao and urinary bladder. Related both internally and externally with the six *zang* organs.

Gate of life: the kidney *yang*. It functions to warm the body and promote growth and development, just as the sun illuminates and warms our planet.

Indirect moxibustion: moxibustion performed with an intermediary agent, such as herbal cakes, salt, ginger or garlic, placed between the smoldering moxa cone and the acupuncture point, which increases stimulation and improves effect.

Lower *he* (confluent) points: six specific points of the three Foot Yang meridians, located below the knees. Usually used as main points for treating problems of their corresponding *fu* organs.

***Luo* (collateral) points:** 15 points from which the 15 collaterals stem. Usually used for treating problems of their corresponding internal and external meridians.

Meeting point: the point where two or more meridians cross or converge.

Mental injury: functional derangement of the *qi*, blood and *zangfu* organs, caused by excessive persistent and violent emotions such as joy, anger, melancholy, anxiety, grief, fear and terror.

Meridian theory: one of the most important aspects of traditional Chinese medicine. It describes the physiology and pathology of the meridians and collaterals and their relationship with the *zangfu* organs and serves as a guide for the clinical practice of acupuncture.

Moxa cone: cones made of compressed mugwort herb used in moxibustion. Three sizes are used in clinical practice: large cones are 1 cm high and 1 cm in diameter at the base; medium cones are 0.5 cm high and 0.5 cm in diameter and small cones are the size of a matchhead.

Moxa roll: a cigar-shaped roll of compressed mugwort herb used in moxibustion. The lit end of the roll is held near the skin at a certain acupuncture point or area of the body for therapeutic purposes.

Needling sensation: *deqi* 得气 in Chinese. Includes sensations of soreness, numbness, heaviness, distension, coldness, warmth or even muscular pulsations experienced by the patient during acupuncture. A needling sensation must be felt at the site of the disease or disorder for a cure to be achieved.

Non-scarifying moxibustion: a type of moxa cone moxibustion in which no blisters are raised. Attention must be paid to the patient's level of tolerance and the heat of the burning moxa cone must be kept from burning the skin during treatment. (See **Scarifying moxibustion**)

Pathogenic *qi*: refers to all pathogenic factors in a broad sense, or the six external pathogens in a narrow sense.

Phlegm: a pathogenic substance produced by dysfunction of the *zangfu* organs; usually accumulates in the meridians or internal organs.

Qi: an important concept in TCM, usually translated as vital energy. The original reference is to the air we inhale and exhale; the ancient Chinese used the breath to symbolize life. *Qi* is widely used in TCM to refer to the substance which animates the human body and supports the functioning of its tissues and organs.

Reducing method: a type of puncturing manipulation in which the needle is twirled rapidly or lifted and thrust deeply in order to provide strong stimulation and dissipate pathogenic *qi*. This method is suitable for treating excessive conditions.

Reinforcing method: a type of puncturing manipulation in which the needle is twirled slowly or lifted and thrust shallowly in order to provide moderate stimulation and strengthen antipathogenic *qi*. This method is suitable for treating deficient conditions.

San Jiao: usually translated as Triple Warmer. One of the six *fu* organs, consisting of the Upper Jiao, Middle Jiao and Lower Jiao. The Upper Jiao houses the heart and lungs, the Middle Jiao the spleen and stomach and the Lower Jiao the liver, kidneys, urinary bladder and small and large intestines. The San Jiao synthesizes the functions of the *zangfu* organs, as well as providing passageways for the movement of *qi* and fluids.

Scarifying moxibustion: a type of moxa cone moxibustion in which moxa cones are burned directly on the skin at acupuncture points so small blisters are raised. A scar is left following healing of the lesion. This method provides strong stimulation and is usually used to treat refractory problems such as asthma and chronic gastritis.

Summer heat: one of the six exogenous pathogens, occurring in midsummer.

Syndrome: *zheng* 证 in Chinese. It has a specific meaning in TCM distinct from that in modern medicine. A syndrome is determined by analysing the symptoms and signs of a disease or disorder at various stages of its course in accordance with the theories of TCM. Correct differentiation of syndromes can determine the location, nature, development and prognosis of the condition at each of its stages and is essential for effective treatment.

Wind: (1) one of the six exogenous pathogens, occurring in all seasons; (2) endogenous wind due to deficiency of blood, excessive heat, or hyperactivity of the liver *yang*.

Yin/Yang ☯**:** two of the eight principles of TCM; two opposite yet interrelated aspects of matter or energy. A fundamental theory of traditional Chinese medicine.

Yuan **(primordial)** *qi*: *qi* derived from congenital essence. It provides the primary motive force for life.

Yuan **(source) points:** 12 points located around the wrists and ankles, one on each of the 12 regular meridians. The *yuan* (primordial) *qi* of their corresponding *zangfu* organs originates in these points. Usually used to treat problems of corresponding *zangfu* organs.

Zang **organs:** five solid internal organs, i.e. the heart, liver, spleen, lungs and kidneys. The pericardium is also considered a *zang* organ.

Bibliography

Advances in Treatment of 55 Diseases and Disorders Using Acupuncture and Moxibustion (Zhenjiu zhiliao 55 zhong bingzheng linchuang yan). Wu Xuping *et al.*, Hubei Science and Technology Press, Wuhan. December 1993. (In Chinese)

Chinese Auricular Therapy (Zhongguo erxue liaofa). Bai Xinghua, Scientific and Technical Documents Publishing House, Beijing. October 1994. (Available in English and Chinese)

A Collection of Acupuncture and Moxibustion (Zhenjiu jijin). Zheng Kuishan, Ganshu Science and Technology Press, Lanzhou. December 1988. (In Chinese)

A Collection of Modern Medical Records Concerning Traditional Acupuncture and Moxibustion (Xiandai zhenjiu yi'anxuan). Liu Guanjun, People's Health Press, Beijing. November 1985. (In Chinese)

A Complete Collection of Chinese Moxibustion (Zhongguo jiufa jicui). Tian Chonghuo, *et al.*, Liaoning Science and Technology Press, Shenyang. February 1987. (In Chinese)

Discussion on the Utilization of Commonly Used Acupuncture Points (Changyong shuxu linchuang fahui). Li Shizhen, People's Health Press. Beijing. November 1985. (In Chinese)

The Foundation and Practice of Electroacupuncture (Dianzhen jichu yu linchuang). Zhang Zhaofa *et al.*, China Science and Technology Press, Beijing. January 1993. (In Chinese)

The Journal of Acupuncture and Moxibustion (Zhongguo zhenjiu). Edited by the China Association of Acupuncture and Moxibustion, Beijing. (1981). (In Chinese)

Neijing, The Classic of Medicine. circa 200 B.C. China. Edited by the Shandong College of Traditional Chinese Medicine, People's Health Press, Beijing. 1993. (In Chinese)

Point Injection Therapy (Xuewei yaowu zhushe linfa). Liu Jianhong, *et al.*, Jiangxi Science and Technology Press, Nanchang. April 1989. (In Chinese)

Practical Application of Traditional Chinese Medicine in Internal Medicine (Shiyong zhongyi neike xue). Huang Wendong *et al.*, Shanghai Science and Technology Press, Shanghai. July 1985. (In Chinese)

The Practical Application of Traditional Chinese Medicine in Surgery (Shiyong zhongyi waike xue). Gu Bohua *et al.*, Shanghai Science and Technology Press, Shanghai. November 1985. (In Chinese)

A Record of the Practice of Acupuncture and Moxibustion (Zhenjiu shiyan lu). Shen Zhuobin, Shaanxi Science and Technology Press, Xi'an. April 1983. (In Chinese)

Rehabilitation with Traditional Chinese Medicine (Zhongguo chuantong kangfu yixue). Chen Keji *et al.*, People's Health Press, Beijing. October 1988. (In Chinese)

Useful addresses

All the associations whose contact addresses are listed here are members of the World Federation of Acupuncture and Moxibustion Societies (WFAS).

Australia

Mrs Christine A. Berle
Acupuncture Ethics and Standards
Organization/Australian Acupuncture Association
Federal Office
P.O. Box 84
Merrylands, NSW 2160
Australia

L. J. McMahon, DC, DO, AC, DIP
Australian Acupuncture Federation
23 Beaumont Road
Killara, 2071 NSW
Australia

Canada

Dr Cedric Cheung
The Chinese Medicine and Acupuncture
Association of Canada
154 Wellington Street,
London, Ontario
Canada N6B 2K8
Tel: 519-642-1970

France

Dr Jean Marc Kespi
Confederation Nationale des Associations
Medicales d'Acupuncture
60 boulevard de Latour-Maubourg
750340 Paris Cedex 07
France
Tel: 42 25 84 46

Germany

Dr Gabriel Stux
German Acupuncture Association
Goltsteinstrasse 26. 4000
Dusseldorf
Germany
Tel: 02 11//36 53 83

Hong Kong

Dr Tse Wing-Kwong
Chinese Acupuncture Research Society
(Hong Kong)
P.O. Box 20088
Hennessy Road
Hong Kong
Tel. 566-2293

Ireland

Dr Katherine Chan Mullen
Irish Medical Acupuncture Society
130 Mount Merrion Avenue
Blackrock
Co. Dublin
Ireland

Italy

Dr Aldo Liguori
Italian Association of Acupuncture–Moxibustion
and Traditional Chinese Medicine
via Oreste Reonoli 8. 00152
Rome
Italy
Tel. 06 5897361

Dr Nello Cracolici
Traditional Acupuncture Society of Firenze
via San Vito 7
Firenze
Italy
Tel. 055/704172

Japan

Dr Hideo Yamamura
Japan Society of Acupuncture
44–14 Minamiotsuka 3 Chome Toshima-ku
Tokyo 170
Japan
Tel. Tokyo 985–6188

Netherlands

Dr H. Hummelen
Netherlands Association for Acupuncture
Van Persijnstraat 17
3811 LS Amersfoort
The Netherlands

Dr A. Van der Molen
Association for Traditional Chinese Acupuncture
in the Netherlands
Chopinstraat 33
6561 EM Groesbeek
The Netherlands

Norway

Dr Bernt Rignlien
The Norwegian Association of Classical
Acupuncture
Munchs GT. 7
0165 Oslo 1
Norway
Tel. 02–36 17 74
Fax. 02–36 18 53

People's Republic of China

Dr Hu Ximing
China Association of Acupuncture and
Moxibustion
3 Haiyuncang
Beijing
People's Republic of China
Tel: 401–4411 ext. 3050

Spain

Dr Nogueira Pereza Carlos
Socieoad Espanola de Acupunctores
Profesionales
Plaza Madrid 2
Valladolid 48001
Spain
Tel. 983–397024

Dr Alvine Rose Meunier
Spanish Association for the Study and
Dissemination of Acupuncture and Moxibustion
Zurbano, 74 Madrid
28010 Spain
Tel. 442–26–49

Sweden

Dr Laila Zryd-Carlsson
Swedish Medical Acupuncture Association
K Lostergatan 1
S–211 47 Malmo
Sweden

Dr Jan Lindborg
Swedish Federation of Acupuncture Societies
Cervinsvag 21
S–16358 Spanga
Sweden
Tel. 08–512686

Switzerland

Dr Elisabeth Studer
Swiss Medical Association of Acupuncture and
Moxibustion
Pain Clinic
Hirsch Gaesslein
30 CH–4010 Basel
Switzerland
Tel. 061/237505

United Kingdom

Dr J Goodman
Council for Acupuncture
11 Alderton Crescent
London NW4 3XU
England
Tel. 0171 202 6242

United States of America

Dr Suliang Ku
American Association of Acupuncture and
Oriental Medicine
5473 66th St N.
St Petersburg
FL 33709
USA
Tel. (813) 541–2666

Dr Joseph M. Helms
Liaison Society of United States Medical
Acupuncture Associations
2520 Milvia Street
Berkeley
CA 94704
USA
Tel. (415) 841–3220

Dr Anthony Abbate
Southwest Acupuncture and Moxibustion College
Association
712 W. San Mateo
Sante Fe
NM 87501
USA
Tel. (505) 988–3538

Dr San Hong Hwang
Acupuncture Medicine Association of Southern
California
12751 Brookhurst Way
Garden Grove
CA 92641
USA
Tel. (714) 638–2922

Dr Ching G. Jing
The Federation of Eastern American Acupuncture
Associations
155 W. 68th St, Apt-221 NY 10023
USA
Tel. (212) 787–7959

Dr David P.J. Hung
American Acupuncture Association
42–62 Kissensa Blvd
Flushing
NY 11355
USA
Tel. (718) 886–4431

International

Dr Anita Cignolini
Medical Association for Chinese Medicine in
Europe
Via Santa Sofia 6
20122 Milan
Italy
Tel. 39-2-58 30 32 42

Dr George Serres
Society Internationale d'Acupuncture
3 Rue Rosa Bonheur
75015 Paris
France
Tel. 45 66 40 50

Dr Corral Padilla Jose Luis
Hispanoamerican Association of Acupuncture
C/Antonia Merrce
2 Madrid
28009 Spain
Tel. 2–76–92–89

Index

Abdomen, 230
  acute gastroenteritis, 5
  amenorrhoea, 18
  appendicitis, 21
  bacillary dysentery, 25
  childhood anorexia, 39
  cholecystitis, 44
  cholelithiasis, 44
  chronic diarrhoea, 49
  chronic pelvic inflammatory disease, 51
  competition syndrome, 53
  constipation, 55
  cystitis, 60
  developmental disability, 62
  dysfunctional uterine bleeding, 70
  dysmenorrhoea, 71
  epididymitis, 76
  epilepsy, 79
  gastrointestinal neurosis, 94
  gastroptosis, 96
  jue syndrome, 120
  leukorrhagia, 121
  neurosism, 143
  obesity, 145
  pancreatitis, 149
  Parkinson's disease, 152
  peptic ulcer, 154
  pharyngeal paraesthesia, 158
  premenstrual syndrome, 162
  prostatitis, 165
  urinary retention, 172
  urinary stones, 197
  urticaria, 200
  uterine prolapse, 163
  vomiting, 202
Acne vulgaris, 3–4
Acquired essence, 260
Addresses, 264–6
Adrenal Gland, 231
  acute tonsillitis, 12
  allergic rhinitis, 15
  alopecia areata, 17
  appendicitis, 21
  arrhythmia, 23
  bacillary dysentery, 25
  bi syndrome, 28
  brandy nose, 29
  bronchial asthma, 32
  chloasma, 41
  chronic pelvic inflammatory disease, 51
  chronic pharyngitis, 52
  cystitis, 60
  developmental disability, 62
  diabetes mellitus, 63
  eczema, 74
  epididymitis, 77
  epistaxis, 81

flat wart, 88
furunculosis, 90
haemorrhoids, 101
herpes zoster, 103
jue syndrome, 119
leukorrhagia, 121
mumps, 135
neurodermatitis, 141
otitis media suppurativa, 147
pancreatitis, 149
peripheral facial paralysis, 156
prostatitis, 165
recurrent mouth ulcer, 168
suppurative nasal sinusitis, 186
toothache, 194
urticaria, 200
uterine prolapse, 163
Alcohol withdrawal, 13–14
Allergic rhinitis, 14–15
Alopecia areata, 16–17
Amenorrhoea, 17–19
Anal fissure, 102
Anal fistula, 102
Anal prolapse, 102
Angina pectoris, 19–20
Angioneurotic oedema, 200
Angle of Superior Concha, 232
  prostatitis, 165
Ankle, 229
Anmian (Ex37), 224
Anterior Lobe, 233
  competition syndrome, 53
  menopausal syndrome, 131
  neurosism, 143
  phantom limb pain, 156
  postconcussional syndrome, 159
  prostatitis, 165
  seminal emission, 178
Antihelix, 229–30
Antipathogenic *qi*, 260
Antitragus, 231
Anus, 229
  haemorrhoids, 101
Apex of Antitragus, 231
  bronchial asthma, 32
  epididymitis, 77
  mumps, 135
Apex of Ear, 229
  acne vulgaris, 4
  acute gastroenteritis, 6
  acute mastitis, 10
  acute tonsillitis, 12
  alcohol withdrawal, 14
  allergic rhinitis, 15
  appendicitis, 21
  bacillary dysentery, 25
  bi syndrome, 28
  brandy nose, 29
  cardiac neurosis, 34

central retinitis, 36
cholecystitis, 44
cholelithiasis, 44
chronic pelvic inflammatory disease, 51
competition syndrome, 53
constipation, 55
cutaneous pruritus, 57
cystic hyperplasia of the breast, 58–9
cystitis, 60
dysfunctional uterine bleeding, 70
eczema, 74
epidemic keratoconjunctivitis, 75
epididymitis, 77
epilepsy, 79
erythromelalgia, 83
flat wart, 88
furunculosis, 90
gastritis, 91
haemorrhoids, 102
headache, 100
herpes zoster, 103
hypertension, 108
hysteria, 111
influenza, 115
intercostal neuralgia, 117
jue syndrome, 120
leukorrhagia, 121
Meniere's disease, 129
mumps, 135
myopia, 138
neurodermatitis, 141
neurosism, 143
otitis media suppurativa, 147
phantom limb pain, 156
postconcussional syndrome, 159
prostatitis, 165
Raynaud's disease, 167
recurrent mouth ulcer, 168
simple glaucoma, 183
stye, 185
suppurative nasal sinusitis, 186
toothache, 194
trigeminal neuralgia, 196
urinary retention, 172
urinary stones, 198
urticaria, 200
uterine prolapse, 163
Apex of Tragus, 231
  influenza, 115
Appendicitis, 20–2
Appendix, 233
  appendicitis, 21
Arrhythmia, 22–3
Ashi points, 260
  acute soft tissue injury, 10, 11
  bi syndrome, 28
  calcaneodynia, 32
  cervical spondylopathy, 37

Ashi points (*cont*)
  costal chondritis, 55, 56
  external humeral epicondylitis, 83, 84
  hyperthyroidism, 109
  lumbar muscle strain, 123
  scapulohumeral periarthritis, 173
  thecal cyst, 187
  urinary stones, 197
Auricular massage, 241
Auricular pressure, 241
Auricular taping, 238–9
Auricular therapy, 227–41
  acne vulgaris, 4
  acute gastroenteritis, 5-6
  acute mastitis, 9-10
  acute soft tissue injury, 11
  acute tonsillitis, 12
  alcohol withdrawal, 13–14
  allergic rhinitis, 15
  alopecia areata, 16–17
  amenorrhoea, 18–19
  angina pectoris, 20
  appendicitis, 22
  arrhythmia, 23
  bacillary dysentery, 25
  bi syndrome, 28
  brandy nose, 29
  bronchial asthma, 31–2
  calcaneodynia, 33
  cardiac neurosis, 34
  central retinitis, 35–6
  cervical spondylopathy, 38
  childhood anorexia, 39
  childhood hyperkinetic syndrome,
      40–1
  chloasma, 41
  cholecystitis, 43
  cholelithiasis, 44
  chronic bronchitis, 47
  chronic diarrhoea, 49
  chronic pelvic inflammatory disease,
      51
  chronic pharyngitis, 52
  competition syndrome, 53
  constipation, 55
  costal chondritis, 56
  cutaneous pruritus, 57
  cystic hyperplasia of the breast, 59
  cystitis, 60
  developmental disability, 61–2
  diabetes mellitus, 63
  diagnosis, 235–8
      auricular electrical resistance
          measurement, 237–8
      auricular inspection, 235–6
      auricular palpation, 236–7
  drug withdrawal, 67
  dysfunctional uterine bleeding, 70
  dysmenorrhoea, 72
  eczema, 74
  epidemic keratoconjunctivitis, 75
  epididymitis, 76
  epilepsy, 79
  epistaxis, 81
  erythromelalgia, 82–3
  external humeral epicondylitis, 84

  facial spasm, 85
  flat wart, 88
  furunculosis, 90
  gastritis, 92
  gastrointestinal neurosis, 94
  gastroptosis, 96
  haemorrhoids, 101–2
  headache, 99–100
  herpes zoster, 103
  hiccups, 104–5
  hypertension, 108
  hyperthyroidism, 109
  hysteria, 112
  impotence, 113
  indications, 227–34
  intercostal neuralgia, 117
  jue syndrome, 119–20
  leukorrhagia, 121
  locations of points, 227–34
  lumbar muscle strain, 123–4
  Meniere's disease, 129–30
  menopausal syndrome, 131
  methods, 238–41
  morning sickness, 133
  motion sickness, 134
  mumps, 135
  myocarditis, 136
  myopia, 137–8
  neurodermatitis, 140–1
  neurosism, 143
  nocturnal enuresis, 144
  obesity, 145
  otitis media suppurativa, 146–7
  pancreatitis, 149
  Parkinson's disease, 152
  peptic ulcer, 154
  peripheral facial paralysis, 155–6
  phantom limb pain, 156
  pharyngeal paraesthesia, 158
  points selection, 234–5
  postconcussional syndrome, 159
  premenstrual syndrome, 162
  prostatitis, 165
  Raynaud's disease, 167
  recurrent mouth ulcer, 168–9
  scapulohumeral periarthritis,
      173–4
  sciatica, 175
  seborrhoeic dermatitis, 177
  seminal emission, 178
  simple glaucoma, 182
  sketch map of points, 228
  stiff neck, 184
  stye, 185
  suppurative nasal sinusitis, 186
  temporomandibular joint dysfunction,
      68
  thromboangiitis obliterans, 189
  tobacco withdrawal, 192
  toothache, 194
  trigeminal neuralgia, 196
  urinary retention, 172
  urinary stones, 197–8
  urticaria, 200
  uterine prolapse, 163
  vomiting, 202

Bacillary dysentery, 24–5
Back-*shu* points, 260
Bafeng (Ex23), 222
  bi syndrome, 27
  cerebrovascular accident sequelae,
      180
  eczema, 73
  erythromelalgia, 82
  Raynaud's disease, 166
  thromboangiitis obliterans, 188, 189
Baichongwo (Ex18), 221
Baihuanshu (B30), leukorrhagia, 121
Baihui (Du20)
  acute soft tissue injury, 10
  alcohol withdrawal, 13
  allergic rhinitis, 14, 15
  alopecia areata, 16
  cerebrovascular accident sequelae,
      180
  cervical spondylopathy, 37
  childhood hyperkinetic syndrome, 40
  competition syndrome, 52, 53
  developmental disability, 61
  dian syndrome, 65
  drug withdrawal, 66, 67
  dysmenorrhoea, 71
  epilepsy, 78, 79
  epistaxis, 81
  facial spasm, 85
  gastroptosis, 95
  headache, 98
  hearing loss, 191
  hypertension, 107
  hysteria, 110
  influenza, 114
  jue syndrome, 118, 119
  kuang syndrome, 65
  male infertility, 127
  Meniere's disease, 129
  menopausal syndrome, 131
  neurosism, 142, 143
  nocturnal enuresis, 144
  otitis media suppurativa, 146
  Parkinson's disease, 151
  postconcussional syndrome, 158, 159
  seborrhoeic dermatitis, 176
  seminal emission, 178
  simple glaucoma, 182
  suppurative nasal sinusitis, 187
  tinnitus, 191
  tobacco withdrawal, 192
  uterine prolapse, 163
Bailao (Ex38), 225
  chronic bronchitis, 46
Baliao (B31-B34)
  bi syndrome, 27
  chronic pelvic inflammatory disease,
      50
  haemorrhoids, 101
  impotence, 113
  wei syndrome, 203
Bartholinitis, 51
Baxie (Ex6), 219–20
  bi syndrome, 27
  cerebrovascular accident sequelae,
      179

Baxie (Ex6) (*cont*)
  eczema, 73
  erythromelalgia, 82
  flat wart, 88
  Raynaud's disease, 166
  thromboangiitis obliterans, 188, 189
  wei syndrome, 203, 204
Ben, 260
Bi syndrome, 25–8, 82, 166, 174
Biao see Ben
Biguan (S31), *wei* syndrome, 204
Bitong (Ex32), 223
  suppurative nasal sinusitis, 186
Bizhong (Ex12), 221
Bladder meridian of foot Taiyang, 213
Blepharitis, 185
Blood-letting puncturing, 242–3
  acne vulgaris, 4
  acute mastitis, 9
  acute tonsillitis, 12
  alopecia areata, 17
  auricular therapy technique, 240
  bronchial asthma, 31
  childhood anorexia, 39
  cutaneous pruritus, 57
  eczema, 74
  external humeral epicondylitis, 83–4
  furunculosis, 90
  haemorrhoids, 101
  herpes zoster, 103
  high fever, 106
  hypertension, 107–8
  indications, 242
  neurodermatitis, 140
  precautions, 242–3
  procedure, 242
  seborrhoeic dermatitis, 176
  stye, 185
  urticaria, 200
Body acupuncture
  acne vulgaris, 4
  acute gastroenteritis, 5
  acute intestinal obstruction, 7-8
  acute mastitis, 9
  acute soft tissue injury, 10–11
  acute tonsillitis, 12
  alcohol withdrawal, 13
  allergic rhinitis, 14–15
  alopecia areata, 16
  amenorrhoea, 18
  angina pectoris, 19–20
  appendicitis, 21–2
  arrhythmia, 23
  bacillary dysentery, 24–5
  bi syndrome, 26–8
  brandy nose, 29
  bronchial asthma, 30
  calcaneodynia, 32
  cardiac neurosis, 34
  central retinitis, 35
  cerebrovascular accident sequelae,
    179–81
  cervical spondylopathy, 37
  childhood anorexia, 39
  childhood hyperkinetic syndrome, 40
  cholecystitis, 42

cholelithiasis, 44
chronic bronchitis, 46
chronic diarrhoea, 48–9
chronic pelvic inflammatory disease,
  50
chronic pharyngitis, 51–2
competition syndrome, 52–3
constipation, 54
costal chondritis, 55–6
cutaneous pruritus, 57
cystic hyperplasia of the breast,
  58–9
cystitis, 60
developmental disability, 61
diabetes mellitus, 63
dian syndrome, 64–5
drug withdrawal, 66–7
dysfunctional uterine bleeding,
  69–70
dysmenorrhoea, 71
eczema, 73
epidemic keratoconjunctivitis, 75
epididymitis, 76
epilepsy, 78–9
epistaxis, 81
erythromelalgia, 82
external humeral epicondylitis, 83
facial spasm, 85
female infertility, 87
flat wart, 88
furunculosis, 89–90
gastritis, 91–2
gastrointestinal neurosis, 93–4
gastroptosis, 95–6
haemorrhoids, 101
headache, 98–9
hearing loss, 190–1
herpes zoster, 102–3
hiccups, 104
high fever, 105
hypertension, 107
hyperthyroidism, 109
hysteria, 110–1
impotence, 112
influenza, 114–15
insufficient lactation, 116
intercostal neuralgia, 117
jue syndrome, 118–19
kuang syndrome, 65
leukorrhagia, 121
lochiorrhagia, 122
lumbar muscle strain, 123
malaria, 125
male infertility, 127
Meniere's disease, 129
menopausal syndrome, 131
morning sickness, 132–3
motion sickness, 134
mumps, 134–5
myocarditis, 136
myopia, 137
neurodermatitis, 139–40
neurosism, 142
nocturnal enuresis, 143–4
obesity, 145
otitis media suppurativa, 146

pancreatitis, 148
paralytic strabismus, 149–50
Parkinson's disease, 151
peptic ulcer, 153
peripheral facial paralysis, 155
pharyngeal paraesthesia, 157–8
postconcussional syndrome, 158–9
postpartum uterine contractions, 160
premenstrual syndrome, 161
prostatitis, 164–5
ptosis, 166
Raynaud's disease, 166–7
recurrent mouth ulcer, 168
retention of placenta, 169
scapulohumeral periarthritis, 173
sciatica, 174–5
seborrhoeic dermatitis, 176
seminal emission, 178
simple glaucoma, 182
stiff neck, 183
stye, 184–5
suppurative nasal sinusitis, 186
temporomandibular joint dysfunction,
  68
thecal cyst, 187
thromboangiitis obliterans, 188–9
tinnitus, 190–1
tobacco withdrawal, 192
toothache, 193–4
trigeminal neuralgia, 195
urinary retention, 171
urinary stones, 197
urticaria, 199–200
uterine prolapse, 163
vomiting, 201–2
wei syndrome, 203–4
Brandy nose, 29
Breast cystic hyperplasia, 58–9
Bronchial asthma, 29–32
Bronchitis, chronic, 45–8
Buttock, 230
  sciatica, 175

Calcaneodynia, 32–3
  ashi points, 32
Carbuncle, 90
Cardia, 232
  bacillary dysentery, 25
  competition syndrome, 53
  gastrointestinal neurosis, 94
  gastroptosis, 96
  influenza, 115
  morning sickness, 133
  motion sickness, 134
  postconcussional syndrome, 159
  premenstrual syndrome, 162
  vomiting, 202
Cardiac neurosis, 33–4
Central retinitis, 35–6
Centre of Ear, 229
  acne vulgaris, 4
  cutaneous pruritus, 57
  eczema, 74
  epistaxis, 81
  gastrointestinal neurosis, 94
  hiccups, 104

Cerebrovascular accident sequelae, 179–81
  deviation of mouth, 180
  dysphagia, 180
  dysphasia/aphasia, 180
  incontinence, 180
  lower limbs, 180
  mental disorders, 180–1
Cervical spondylopathy, 36–8
  ashi points, 37
Cervical Vertebrae, 230
  cervical spondylopathy, 38
Cervicitis, 51
Changqiang (Du1)
  cutaneous pruritus, 57
  epilepsy, resting stage, 78
  haemorrhoids, 101
Cheek, 233
  facial spasm, 85
  peripheral facial paralysis, 155
  suppurative nasal sinusitis, 186
  trigeminal neuralgia, 196
Cheilitis, acute/chronic, 169
Chengfu (B36)
  sciatica, 174
Chengjiang (Ren24)
  peripheral facial paralysis, 155
Chengshan (B57)
  cutaneous pruritus, 57
  haemorrhoids, 101
  sciatica, 175
  thromboangiitis obliterans, 188
  wei syndrome, 204
Chest, 230
  acute mastitis, 9
  alcohol withdrawal, 13
  angina pectoris, 20
  arrhythmia, 23
  bronchial asthma, 31
  cardiac neurosis, 34
  chronic bronchitis, 47
  costal chondritis, 56
  cystic hyperplasia of the breast, 58–9
  drug withdrawal, 67
  dysfunctional uterine bleeding, 70
  epilepsy, 79
  hysteria, 111
  intercostal neuralgia, 117
  menopausal syndrome, 131
  myocarditis, 136
  neurosism, 143
  pharyngeal paraesthesia, 158
  premenstrual syndrome, 162
  tobacco withdrawal, 192
  urticaria, 200
Childhood anorexia, 38–9
Childhood hyperkinetic syndrome, 40–1
Chiropractic, 244
Chize (L5)
  acute gastroenteritis, 5
  eczema, 73
  scapulohumeral periarthritis, 173
Chloasma, 41
Cholecystitis, 41–3
Cholelithiasis, 43–5
Chonggu (Ex39), 225

Ciliao (B32)
  female infertility, 87
  leukorrhagia, 121
  male infertility, 127
  uterine prolapse, 163
Ciliaris, 185
Clavicle, 229
  scapulohumeral periarthritis, 173
Cold, 260
Common cold, 115
Competition syndrome, 52–3
Congenital essence, 260
Conjunctivitis, 75
Constipation, 53–5
Contact dermatitis, 74
Costal chondritis, 55–6
Crus of helix, 229
Cun, 260
  acute mastitis, 9
  appliances, 245
  bi syndrome, 28
  cervical spondylopathy, 38
  chronic bronchitis, 47
  external humeral epicondylitis, 83–4
  high fever, 106
  indications, 246
  precautions, 246–7
  procedure, 245–6
  scapulohumeral periarthritis, 173
  urticaria, 200
Cutaneous pruritus, 56–7
Cystitis, 59–60

Dachangshu (B25)
  acne vulgaris, 4
  acute intestinal obstruction, 7, 8
  bacillary dysentery, 25
  constipation, 54
  haemorrhoids, 101
  seborrhoeic dermatitis, 176
  urticaria, 200
Dadun (Liv1)
  epididymitis, 76
  impotence, 112
Dagukong (Ex4), 219
Daheng (Sp15)
  acute intestinal obstruction, 7, 8
  constipation, 54
Daimai (G26)
  leukorrhagia, 121
Daling (P7)
  dian syndrome, 65
  wei syndrome, 204
Damp, 260
Dannangxue (Ex21), 222
  cholecystitis, 44
Danshu (B19)
  cholecystitis, 43
  cholelithiasis, 44, 45
  gastrointestinal neurosis, 93
Danzhong (Ren17)
  acne vulgaris, 4
  acute mastitis, 9
  alcohol withdrawal, 13
  alopecia areata, 16
  amenorrhoea, 18

angina pectoris, 19
arrhythmia, 23
bronchial asthma, 30
cardiac neurosis, 34
cerebrovascular accident sequelae, 181
chronic bronchitis, 46, 47
cystic hyperplasia of the breast, 58
dian syndrome, 64
drug withdrawal, 66, 67
epilepsy, resting stage, 78
gastrointestinal neurosis, 93
hiccups, 104
hyperthyroidism, 109
hysteria, 111
insufficient lactation, 116
jue syndrome, 119
kuang syndrome, 65
menopausal syndrome, 131
morning sickness, 133
myocarditis, 136
Parkinson's disease, 151
pharyngeal paraesthesia, 157
tobacco withdrawal, 192
Dazhui (Du14)
  acne vulgaris, 4
  acute intestinal obstruction, 7
  acute mastitis, 9
  acute tonsillitis, 12
  appendicitis, 21
  bacillary dysentery, 25
  bi syndrome, 27
  bronchial asthma, 30
  cervical spondylopathy, 37, 38
  chronic bronchitis, 46
  cutaneous pruritus, 57
  cystitis, 60
  drug withdrawal, 66, 67
  dysfunctional uterine bleeding, 69
  eczema, 73, 74
  epilepsy, 78, 79, 80
  furunculosis, 89
  headache, 99
  hearing loss, 191
  high fever, 105, 106
  hypertension, 107
  influenza, 114, 115
  kuang syndrome, 65
  malaria, 125
  mumps, 135
  myocarditis, 136
  neck massage, 38
  neurodermatitis, 140
  pancreatitis, 148
  Parkinson's disease, 151
  seborrhoeic dermatitis, 176
  stiff neck, 183
  stye, 185
  thromboangiitis obliterans, 188, 189
  tinnitus, 191
  urticaria, 199, 200
  vomiting, 201
  wei syndrome, 203, 204
Deficiency, 260
Dermatitis medicamentosa, 74
Developmental disability, 61–2
Diabetes mellitus, 62–3

Dian syndrome, 64–6
Diarrhoea, chronic, 48–9
Dichang (S4)
  cerebrovascular accident sequelae,
    180
  Parkinson's disease, 151
  peripheral facial paralysis, 155
  recurrent mouth ulcer, 168
Differentiation of symptoms and signs,
  260
Diji (Sp8)
  amenorrhoea, 18
  chronic diarrhoea, 48
  chronic pelvic inflammatory disease,
    50
  dysmenorrhoea, 71
  lochiorrhagia, 122
  postpartum uterine contractions, 160
Dingchuan (Ex41), 225
  bronchial asthma, 30
  chronic bronchitis, 46, 47
Dingnie Houxiexian (MS7), 257
  phantom limb pain, 156
Dingnie Qianxiexian (MS6), 256–7
  cerebrovascular accident sequelae,
    181
  developmental disability, 61
  Parkinson's disease, 151
Dingpangxian, 1 (MS8), 257
  cerebrovascular accident sequelae,
    181
  developmental disability, 61
  Parkinson's disease, 151
Dingpangxian, 2 (MS9), 257
  cerebrovascular accident sequelae,
    181
  developmental disability, 61
  Parkinson's disease, 151
Dingzhongxian (MS5), 256
  developmental disability, 61
  epilepsy, 79
  Meniere's disease, 129
  Parkinson's disease, 151
Dorsal surface of auricle, 233–4
Drug withdrawal, 66–7
Dry face washing, 138, 139, 191
Dryness, 260
Du (Governor Vessel) meridian, 217
Duodenum, 233
  peptic ulcer, 154
Duyin (Ex24), 222
  retention of placenta, 169
Dysfunctional uterine bleeding, 68–70
Dysmenorrhoea, 70–2

Ear exercises, 191
Ear Shenmen, 230
  acne vulgaris, 4
  acute gastroenteritis, 6
  acute mastitis, 10
  acute soft tissue injury, 11
  alcohol withdrawal, 14
  alopecia areata, 17
  appendicitis, 21
  arrhythmia, 23
  bi syndrome, 28

  bronchial asthma, 32
  cardiac neurosis, 34
  cervical spondylopathy, 38
  childhood hyperkinetic syndrome, 40
  chronic bronchitis, 47
  chronic diarrhoea, 49
  chronic pelvic inflammatory disease,
    51
  chronic pharyngitis, 52
  costal chondritis, 56
  cutaneous pruritus, 57
  cystic hyperplasia of the breast, 58–9
  cystitis, 60
  diabetes mellitus, 63
  drug withdrawal, 67
  dysfunctional uterine bleeding, 70
  dysmenorrhoea, 71
  eczema, 74
  epilepsy, 79
  erythromelalgia, 82
  external humeral epicondylitis, 84
  facial spasm, 85
  furunculosis, 90
  gastrointestinal neurosis, 94
  haemorrhoids, 102
  headache, 99
  herpes zoster, 103
  hiccups, 105
  hypertension, 108
  hysteria, 111
  impotence, 113
  intercostal neuralgia, 117
  lumbar muscle strain, 123
  Meniere's disease, 129
  menopausal syndrome, 131
  morning sickness, 133
  motion sickness, 134
  myocarditis, 136
  neurodermatitis, 141
  neurosism, 143
  pancreatitis, 149
  Parkinson's disease, 152
  peptic ulcer, 154
  phantom limb pain, 156
  pharyngeal paraesthesia, 158
  postconcussional syndrome, 159
  premenstrual syndrome, 162
  prostatitis, 165
  Raynaud's disease, 167
  recurrent mouth ulcer, 168
  scapulohumeral periarthritis, 174
  sciatica, 175
  seminal emission, 178
  simple glaucoma, 183
  stiff neck, 184
  suppurative nasal sinusitis, 186
  temporomandibular joint dysfunction,
    68
  tobacco withdrawal, 192
  toothache, 194
  trigeminal neuralgia, 196
  urinary stones, 198
  urticaria, 200
Eczema, 72–4
  of anus, 102
Effort syndrome *see* Cardiac neurosis

Eight confluent points, 260
Eight *hui* (influential) points, 260
Eight principles, 260
Elbow, 229
  external humeral epicondylitis, 84
Elbow joint *bi* syndrome, 26–7
Electric ophthalmitis, 75
Electroacupuncture, 248–9
  acne vulgaris, 4
  acute intestinal obstruction, 8
  acute soft tissue injury, 11
  alcohol withdrawal, 13
  allergic rhinitis, 15
  amenorrhoea, 18
  angina pectoris, 20
  appendicitis, 22
  appliances, 248
  arrhythmia, 23
  bacillary dysentery, 25
  bi syndrome, 28
  bronchial asthma, 31
  calcaneodynia, 33
  cerebrovascular accident sequelae,
    181
  cervical spondylopathy, 37
  childhood hyperkinetic syndrome, 40
  cholecystitis, 42–3
  cholelithiasis, 44
  chronic bronchitis, 47
  chronic diarrhoea, 49
  chronic pelvic inflammatory disease,
    50
  constipation, 54–5
  cystic hyperplasia of the breast, 59
  cystitis, 60
  developmental disability, 61
  dian and *kuang* syndromes, 65–6
  drug withdrawal, 67
  dysfunctional uterine bleeding, 70
  dysmenorrhoea, 72
  epididymitis, 76
  epilepsy, 79
  external humeral epicondylitis, 83–4
  facial spasm, 85
  female infertility, 87
  flat wart, 88
  gastritis, 92
  gastrointestinal neurosis, 94
  gastroptosis, 96
  haemorrhoids, 101
  headache, 99
  hearing loss, 191
  herpes zoster, 103
  hysteria, 111
  impotence, 113
  indications, 249
  intercostal neuralgia, 117
  jue syndrome, 119
  leukorrhagia, 121
  lumbar muscle strain, 123
  malaria, 125
  male infertility, 128
  Meniere's disease, 129
  menopausal syndrome, 131
  neurodermatitis, 140
  neurosism, 142

Electroacupuncture (*cont*)
  pancreatitis, 148
  paralytic strabismus, 150
  peptic ulcer, 153
  peripheral facial paralysis, 155
  phantom limb pain, 156–7
  postconcussional syndrome, 159
  precautions, 249
  premenstrual syndrome, 161
  procedure, 248
  prostatitis, 165
  ptosis, 166
  Raynaud's disease, 167
  retention of placenta, 171
  scapulohumeral periarthritis, 173
  sciatica, 175
  seminal emission, 178
  stiff neck, 183–4
  stimulation intensity selection, 248–9
  suppurative nasal sinusitis, 186
  thromboangiitis obliterans, 189
  tinnitus, 191
  tobacco withdrawal, 192
  toothache, 194
  trigeminal neuralgia, 196
  urinary retention, 171
  urinary stones, 197
  uterine prolapse, 163
  wave forms selection, 248
  wei syndrome, 204
Endocrine, 232
  acne vulgaris, 4
  acute mastitis, 10
  acute tonsillitis, 12
  alcohol withdrawal, 13
  allergic rhinitis, 15
  alopecia areata, 17
  amenorrhoea, 18
  appendicitis, 21
  bacillary dysentery, 25
  bi syndrome, 28
  brandy nose, 29
  bronchial asthma, 32
  childhood anorexia, 39
  chloasma, 41
  cholecystitis, 44
  cholelithiasis, 44
  chronic bronchitis, 47
  chronic diarrhoea, 49
  chronic pelvic inflammatory disease,
    51
  chronic pharyngitis, 52
  competition syndrome, 53
  cystic hyperplasia of the breast, 58–9
  cystitis, 60
  developmental disability, 62
  diabetes mellitus, 63
  dysfunctional uterine bleeding, 70
  dysmenorrhoea, 71
  eczema, 74
  epididymitis, 77
  flat wart, 88
  furunculosis, 90
  gastritis, 91
  gastrointestinal neurosis, 94
  haemorrhoids, 101

  herpes zoster, 103
  hyperthyroidism, 109
  impotence, 113
  jue syndrome, 119
  leukorrhagia, 121
  menopausal syndrome, 131
  morning sickness, 133
  mumps, 135
  neurodermatitis, 141
  obesity, 145
  otitis media suppurativa, 147
  pancreatitis, 149
  peripheral facial paralysis, 156
  premenstrual syndrome, 162
  prostatitis, 165
  recurrent mouth ulcer, 168
  seborrhoeic dermatitis, 177
  suppurative nasal sinusitis, 186
  toothache, 194
  urticaria, 200
  uterine prolapse, 163
Enteroparalysis, 55
Epangxian 1 (MS2), 255
Epangxian 2 (MS3), 255–6
Epangxian 3 (MS4), 256
Epididymitis, 75–7
Epilepsy, 77–80
Epistaxis, 80–2
Erbai (Ex11), 220
  haemorrhoids, 101
Ermen (SJ21)
  hearing loss, 190
  kuang syndrome, 65
  Meniere's disease, 129
  otitis media suppurativa, 146
  tinnitus, 190
Erysipelas, 90
Erythromelalgia, 82–3
Even method, 260
Excess, 260
Exterior, 260
External ear, 231
  Meniere's disease, 129
  motion sickness, 134
  otitis media suppurativa, 146
  trigeminal neuralgia, 196
External Genitals, 229
  epididymitis, 76
  impotence, 113
  leukorrhagia, 121
  prostatitis, 165
External humeral epicondylitis, 83–4
External nose, 231
  influenza, 115
  trigeminal neuralgia, 196
Extraordinary acupuncture points,
    219–26, 260
Eye 1, 233
Eye 2, 233
  epidemic keratoconjunctivitis, 75
  myopia, 137
  simple glaucoma, 182
  stye, 185
Eye, 233
  central retinitis, 35
  epidemic keratoconjunctivitis, 75

  facial spasm, 85
  hyperthyroidism, 109
  myopia, 137
  peripheral facial paralysis, 155
  simple glaucoma, 182
  stye, 185
Ezhongxian (MS1), 255
  epilepsy, 79
  Meniere's disease, 129

Facial spasm, 84–5
Feishu (B13)
  acne vulgaris, 4
  allergic rhinitis, 15
  bronchial asthma, 30
  chronic bronchitis, 46, 47
  cutaneous pruritus, 57
  eczema, 73, 74
  furunculosis, 89
  high fever, 106
  influenza, 114, 115
  neurodermatitis, 140
  seborrhoeic dermatitis, 176
  tobacco withdrawal, 192
  urticaria, 199, 200
  wei syndrome, 204
Female infertility, 86–7
Fengchi (G20)
  acne vulgaris, 4
  acute tonsillitis, 12
  allergic rhinitis, 14, 15
  alopecia areata, 16
  bi syndrome, 27
  central retinitis, 35
  cerebrovascular accident sequelae,
    180, 181
  cervical spondylopathy, 37
  childhood hyperkinetic syndrome, 40
  competition syndrome, 52, 53
  cutaneous pruritus, 57
  developmental disability, 61
  dian syndrome, 65
  drug withdrawal, 66, 67
  eczema, 73
  epidemic keratoconjunctivitis, 75
  epilepsy, resting stage, 78
  epistaxis, 81
  facial spasm, 85
  furunculosis, 89
  headache, 98
  hearing loss, 190
  high fever, 105
  hypertension, 107
  hyperthyroidism, 109
  hysteria, 110, 111
  influenza, 114
  kuang syndrome, 65
  Meniere's disease, 129
  menopausal syndrome, 131
  mumps, 134, 135
  myopia, 137, 138, 139
  neck massage, 38
  neurodermatitis, 140
  neurosism, 142, 143
  otitis media suppurativa, 146
  paralytic strabismus, 149

Fengchi (G20) (*cont*)
Parkinson's disease, 151
peripheral facial paralysis, 155
postconcussional syndrome, 158, 159
ptosis, 166
recurrent mouth ulcer, 168
seborrhoeic dermatitis, 176
simple glaucoma, 182
stiff neck, 183
stye, 184, 185
suppurative nasal sinusitis, 186
tinnitus, 190
toothache, 193
trigeminal neuralgia, 195
urticaria, 199
vomiting, 201
wei syndrome, 203
Fengfu (Du16)
cerebrovascular accident sequelae, 180
epilepsy, resting stage, 78, 80
epistaxis, 81
kuang syndrome, 65
Fenglong (S40)
amenorrhoea, 18
angina pectoris, 20
arrhythmia, 23
bronchial asthma, 30
cerebrovascular accident sequelae, 181
chronic bronchitis, 46
dian syndrome, 64
epilepsy, resting stage, 78
gastrointestinal neurosis, 94
headache, 99
hearing loss, 191
hypertension, 107
hyperthyroidism, 109
hysteria, 111
jue syndrome, 119
kuang syndrome, 65
Meniere's disease, 129
menopausal syndrome, 131
neurosism, 142
Parkinson's disease, 151
peripheral facial paralysis, 155
pharyngeal paraesthesia, 157
tinnitus, 191
Fengmen (B12)
acne vulgaris, 4
Fengshi (G31)
bi syndrome, 27
eczema, 73
hearing loss, 191
hysteria, 111
tinnitus, 191
wei syndrome, 204
Fetal position abnormality, 3
Fever, 105–6
Fingers, 229
Fire, 260
Five elements, 261
Five hearts, 261
Five orbiculus theory, 261
Five *shu* points, 261
Flat wart, 88
Folliculitis, chronic, 90

Forehead, 231
childhood hyperkinetic syndrome, 40
developmental disability, 62
drug withdrawal, 67
epilepsy, 79
frontal headache, 100
impotence, 113
influenza, 115
mumps, 135
nocturnal enuresis, 144
obesity, 145
Parkinson's disease, 152
suppurative nasal sinusitis, 186
Four seas, 261
Front-*mu* points, 261
Frontal Surface of Earlobe, 233
Fu organs, 261
Fuliu (K7)
hyperthyroidism, 109
Parkinson's disease, 151
Furunculosis, 89–90
Futu (LI18)
hyperthyroidism, 109
wei syndrome, 204

Gallbladder meridian of foot Shaoyang, 216
Gallstones *see* Cholelithiasis
Ganshu (B18)
amenorrhoea, 18
central retinitis, 35
gastrointestinal neurosis, 93
hypertension, 107
myopia, 137
Parkinson's disease, 151
wei syndrome, 204
Gaohuang (B43)
chronic bronchitis, 46, 47
Gastritis, 90–2
Gastroenteritis, acute, 5-6
Gastrointestinal neurosis, 93–4
Gastroptosis, 95–6
Gate of life, 261
Geshu (B17)
acne vulgaris, 4
alopecia areata, 16
angina pectoris, 20
arrhythmia, 23
cutaneous pruritus, 57
eczema, 73, 74
gastrointestinal neurosis, 93
hiccups, 104
neurodermatitis, 140
peptic ulcer, 153
seborrhoeic dermatitis, 176
urticaria, 199, 200
Glaucoma, simple, 182–3
Globus hystericus, 93, 94
Gongsun (Sp4)
acute gastroenteritis, 5
hiccups, 104
morning sickness, 133
pancreatitis, 148
vomiting, 201
Gongzhong (Ex14), 221
Groove of Dorsal Surface, 234

hypertension, 108
Guanchong (SJ1)
epidemic keratoconjunctivitis, 75
mumps, 134, 135
Guangming (G37)
central retinitis, 35
hysteria, 111
myopia, 137
simple glaucoma, 182
Guanmen (S22)
gastroptosis, 95
Guanyuan (Ren4)
acute intestinal obstruction, 7, 8
amenorrhoea, 18
angina pectoris, 20
arrhythmia, 23
bi syndrome, 27
bronchial asthma, 30
cerebrovascular accident sequelae, 180, 181
childhood anorexia, 39
chronic bronchitis, 46
chronic diarrhoea, 48, 49
chronic pelvic inflammatory disease, 50
constipation, 54
diabetes mellitus, 63
drug withdrawal, 66, 67
dysfunctional uterine bleeding, 69
dysmenorrhoea, 71, 72
epididymitis, 76
epilepsy, 78, 79
female infertility, 87
gastritis, 91
gastroptosis, 95
habitual miscarriage, 97
hearing loss, 191
impotence, 112, 113
jue syndrome, 119
lochiorrhagia, 122
male infertility, 127, 128
neurosism, 142
nocturnal enuresis, 143, 144
obesity, 145
Parkinson's disease, 151
postpartum uterine contractions, 160
prostatitis, 165
retention of placenta, 169
seminal emission, 178
thromboangiitis obliterans, 188, 189
tinnitus, 191
urinary retention, 171
urinary stones, 197
uterine prolapse, 163
wei syndrome, 204
Guilai (S29)
amenorrhoea, 18
chronic pelvic inflammatory disease, 50
dysmenorrhoea, 71, 72
epididymitis, 76
female infertility, 87
male infertility, 127
postpartum uterine contractions, 160

Haemorrhoids, 100–2
Hanyan (G4)
headache, 99

Headache, 97–100
Hearing loss, 190–1
Heart
  acne vulgaris, 4
  acute soft tissue injury, 11
  angina pectoris, 20
  arrhythmia, 23
  cardiac neurosis, 34
  childhood hyperkinetic syndrome, 40
  competition syndrome, 53
  cutaneous pruritus, 57
  eczema, 74
  epilepsy, 79
  erythromelalgia, 82
  facial spasm, 85
  furunculosis, 90
  hypertension, 108
  hyperthyroidism, 109
  hysteria, 111
  impotence, 113
  jue syndrome, 119
  menopausal syndrome, 131
  myocarditis, 136
  neurodermatitis, 141
  neurosism, 143
  Parkinson's disease, 152
  premenstrual syndrome, 162
  Raynaud's disease, 167
  recurrent mouth ulcer, 168
  seminal emission, 178
  thromboangiitis obliterans, 188, 189
  urticaria, 200
Heart of Dorsal Surface, 234
Heart meridian of hand Shaoyin, 211
Heding (Ex19), 221–2
  bi syndrome, 27
Heel, 229
  calcaneodynia, 32
Hegu (LI4)
  acne vulgaris, 4
  acute intestinal obstruction, 7
  acute tonsillitis, 12
  alcohol withdrawal with convulsions, 13
  allergic rhinitis, 14
  appendicitis, 21
  bacillary dysentery, 24
  bi syndrome, 26, 27
  brandy nose, 29
  cerebrovascular accident sequelae, 179, 180
  childhood hyperkinetic syndrome, 40
  cholecystitis, 43
  cholelithiasis, 44
  chronic pelvic inflammatory disease, 50
  chronic pharyngitis, 51, 52
  cutaneous pruritus, 57
  cystitis, 60
  drug withdrawal, 67
  dysmenorrhoea, 71
  eczema, 73
  epidemic keratoconjunctivitis, 75
  epileptic attack, 78
  epistaxis, 81
  erythromelalgia, 82

  external humeral epicondylitis, 83
  facial spasm, 85
  flat wart, 88
  furunculosis, 89
  headache, 99
  hearing loss, 191
  herpes zoster, 102
  high fever, 105
  hyperthyroidism, 109
  hysteria, 110
  influenza, 114
  jue syndrome, 119
  malaria, 125
  neurodermatitis, 139
  pancreatitis, 148
  paralytic strabismus, 149
  Parkinson's disease, 151
  peptic ulcer, 153, 154
  peripheral facial paralysis, 155
  postconcussional syndrome, 159
  premenstrual syndrome, 161
  ptosis, 166
  Raynaud's disease, 166
  recurrent mouth ulcer, 168
  retention of placenta, 169
  scapulohumeral periarthritis, 173
  seborrhoeic dermatitis, 176
  stye, 185
  suppurative nasal sinusitis, 186
  temporomandibular joint dysfunction, 68
  thecal cyst, 187
  thromboangiitis obliterans, 188
  tinnitus, 191
  toothache, 193
  trigeminal neuralgia, 195
  urticaria, 199
  vomiting, 201
  wei syndrome, 203, 204
Helix 1-Helix 6, 229
Helix, 229
Herpes zoster, 102–3
Hiccups, 103–5
Hip, 229
Hot salt compress therapy, 250
  chronic diarrhoea, 49
  gastrointestinal neurosis, 94
  impotence, 112–13
  indications, 250
  peptic ulcer, 154
  postpartum uterine contractions, 160
  precautions, 250
  procedure, 250
  urinary retention, 171
Houxi (SI3)
  acute soft tissue injury, 10
  bi syndrome, 26, 27
  cerebrovascular accident sequelae, 179
  cervical spondylopathy, 37
  eczema, 73
  headache, 99
  hysteria, 110
  malaria, 125
  Parkinson's disease, 151
  scapulohumeral periarthritis, 173

  stiff neck, 183
  wei syndrome, 203, 204
Huantiao (G30)
  bi syndrome, 27
  cerebrovascular accident sequelae, 180
  cervical spondylopathy, 37
  hysteria, 110
  sciatica, 175
  wei syndrome, 203, 204
Huanzhong (Ex16), 221
Huaroumen (S24)
  dian syndrome, 64
  kuang syndrome, 65
Huatuojiaji (Ex46), 225–6
  acute mastitis, 9
  bi syndrome, 27
  cerebrovascular accident sequelae, 179, 180
  diabetes mellitus, 63
  gastroptosis, 95
  herpes zoster, 102
  intercostal neuralgia, 117
  peptic ulcer, 153
  phantom limb pain, 156, 157
  sciatica, 175
  wei syndrome, 203, 204
Hydrocele of tunica vaginalis, 77
Hypertension, 106–8
Hyperthyroidism, 108–10
Hysteria, 110–11

Ileus, acute *see* Intestinal obstruction, acute
Impetigo herpetiformis, 90
Impotence, 112–13
Indirect moxibustion, 261
Inferior concha, 231–2
Influenza, 114–15
Intercostal neuralgia, 116–17
Internal Ear, 233
  Meniere's disease, 129
  motion sickness, 134
  otitis media suppurativa, 146
  postconcussional syndrome, 159
Internal Genitals, 230
  amenorrhoea, 18
  chronic pelvic inflammatory disease, 51
  competition syndrome, 53
  cystic hyperplasia of the breast, 58–9
  dysfunctional uterine bleeding, 70
  dysmenorrhoea, 71
  epididymitis, 76
  hyperthyroidism, 109
  impotence, 113
  leukorrhagia, 121
  menopausal syndrome, 131
  mumps, 135
  premenstrual syndrome, 162
  prostatitis, 165
  uterine prolapse, 163
Internal nose, 231
  epistaxis, 81
  influenza, 115
  suppurative nasal sinusitis, 186
Intestinal obstruction, acute, 6-8

Jaw, 233
  mumps, 135
  temporomandibular joint dysfunction, 68
  toothache, 194
  trigeminal neuralgia, 196
Jiache (S6)
  acne vulgaris, 4
  cerebrovascular accident sequelae, 180
  flat wart, 88
  mumps, 134, 135
  Parkinson's disease, 151
  peripheral facial paralysis, 155
  recurrent mouth ulcer, 168
  temporomandibular joint dysfunction, 68
  toothache, 193, 194
  trigeminal neuralgia, 195
Jiachengjiang (Ex34), 224
  trigeminal neuralgia, 195
Jianjing (G21)
  acne vulgaris, 4
  acute mastitis, 9
  cervical spondylopathy, 37
  cystic hyperplasia of the breast, 58
  furunculosis, 89
  scapulohumeral periarthritis, 173
Jianliao (SJ14)
  bi syndrome, 26
  scapulohumeral periarthritis, 173
Jianqian (Ex15), 221
  scapulohumeral periarthritis, 173
Jianshi (P5)
  dian syndrome, 65
  kuang syndrome, 65
  malaria, 125
  wei syndrome, 204
Jianyu (LI15)
  bi syndrome, 26
  cerebrovascular accident sequelae, 179
  cervical spondylopathy, 37
  scapulohumeral periarthritis, 173
  wei syndrome, 203
Jianzhen (S19)
  scapulohumeral periarthritis, 173
Jiaosun (SJ20)
  headache, 99
Jiehexue (Ex42), 225
Jiuwei (Ren15)
  dian syndrome, 64
  epilepsy, resting stage, 78
  kuang syndrome, 65
Jiexi (S41)
  bi syndrome, 27
  cerebrovascular accident sequelae, 180
  eczema, 73
  erythromelalgia, 82
  Raynaud's disease, 166
  thecal cyst, 187
  thromboangiitis obliterans, 188
  wei syndrome, 203
Jimen (Sp11)
  wei syndrome, 204

Jingbi (Ex40), 225
Jingming (B1)
  myopia self massage exercise, 138, 139
  paralytic strabismus, 150
Jinjin and Yuye (Ex33), 223–4
  cerebrovascular accident sequelae, 180
Jinsuo (Du8)
  epilepsy, resting stage, 78
Jue syndrome, 117–120
Jueyinshu (B14)
  angina pectoris, 19
  arrhythmia, 23
  cardiac neurosis, 34
  dian syndrome, 65
  myocarditis, 136
Juque (Ren14)
  kuang syndrome, 65
  peptic ulcer, 153

Keratitis, 75
Keratoconjunctivitis, epidemic, 74–5
Kidney, 232
  allergic rhinitis, 15
  alopecia areata, 16–17
  amenorrhoea, 18
  bi syndrome, 28
  bronchial asthma, 31
  calcaneodynia, 32
  cardiac neurosis, 34
  central retinitis, 35
  cervical spondylopathy, 38
  childhood hyperkinetic syndrome, 40
  chloasma, 41
  chronic bronchitis, 47
  chronic diarrhoea, 49
  chronic pharyngitis, 52
  costal chondritis, 56
  cystitis, 60
  developmental disability, 61
  diabetes mellitus, 63
  drug withdrawal, 67
  eczema, 74
  epididymitis, 76
  epilepsy, 79
  facial spasm, 85
  hypertension, 108
  hyperthyroidism, 109
  impotence, 113
  leukorrhagia, 121
  lumbar muscle strain, 123
  menopausal syndrome, 131
  myopia, 138
  neurosism, 143
  nocturnal enuresis, 144
  obesity, 145
  otitis media suppurativa, 147
  Parkinson's disease, 152
  postconcussional syndrome, 159
  prostatitis, 165
  recurrent mouth ulcer, 169
  scapulohumeral periarthritis, 174
  sciatica, 175
  seminal emission, 178
  simple glaucoma, 182

  thromboangiitis obliterans, 188, 189
  toothache, 194
  urinary retention, 172
  urinary stones, 197
  uterine prolapse, 163
Kidney of Dorsal Surface, 234
Kidney meridian of foot Shaoyin, 214
Knee, 229
Kongzhui (L6)
  bronchial asthma, 30
  wei syndrome, 204
Kouheliao (LI19), trigeminal neuralgia, 195
Kuang syndrome, 64–6
Kunlun (B60)
  acute soft tissue injury, 10
  bi syndrome, 27
  calcaneodynia, 32
  furunculosis, 89
  lumbar muscle strain, 123
  sciatica, 175
  stiff neck, 183
  thromboangiitis obliterans, 188
  trigeminal neuralgia, 195
  wei syndrome, 204

Lactation, insufficient, 115–16
Lanweixue (Ex22), 222
Laogong (P8)
  competition syndrome, 53
  kuang syndrome, 65
  recurrent mouth ulcer, 168
  wei syndrome, 204
Large Intestine, 233
  acute gastroenteritis, 5
  acute tonsillitis, 12
  bacillary dysentery, 25
  brandy nose, 29
  bronchial asthma, 31
  chronic bronchitis, 47
  chronic diarrhoea, 49
  competition syndrome, 53
  constipation, 55
  drug withdrawal, 67
  eczema, 74
  external humeral epicondylitis, 84
  facial spasm, 85
  flat wart, 88
  furunculosis, 90
  gastrointestinal neurosis, 94
  gastroptosis, 96
  haemorrhoids, 101
  herpes zoster, 103
  obesity, 145
  peripheral facial paralysis, 155
  scapulohumeral periarthritis, 174
  seborrhoeic dermatitis, 177
  temporomandibular joint dysfunction, 68
  toothache, 194
  trigeminal neuralgia, 196
  uterine prolapse, 163
Large Intestine meridian of hand Yangming, 209
Laryngitis, 52
Leukorrhagia, 120–1

Liangmen (S21)
  gastroptosis, 95
  peptic ulcer, 153, 154
Liangqiu (S34)
  appendicitis, 21
  gastritis, 91
  gastroptosis, 96
  hysteria, 111
  pancreatitis, 148
  peptic ulcer, 153
  wei syndrome, 204
Lianquan (Ren23)
  cerebrovascular accident sequelae,
    180
  chronic pharyngitis, 51, 52
  deafness with muteness, 191
  hysteria, 111
  kuang syndrome, 65
Lidui (S45)
  acute tonsillitis, 12
  epistaxis, 81
  recurrent mouth ulcer, 168
  toothache, 193
Lieque (L7)
  chronic pharyngitis, 51
Ligou (Liv5)
  chronic pelvic inflammatory disease,
    50
  cutaneous pruritus, 57
  eczema, 73
  epididymitis, 76
  impotence, 112
  leukorrhagia, 121
  male infertility, 127
  mumps, 135
  urinary retention, 171
  urinary stones, 197
  uterine prolapse, 163
Lineiting (Ex25), 222
Lingtai (Du10)
  furunculosis, 89
Liver, 232
  acute mastitis, 9
  acute soft tissue injury, 11
  alcohol withdrawal, 13
  alopecia areata, 17
  amenorrhoea, 18
  angina pectoris, 20
  appendicitis, 21
  arrhythmia, 23
  bi syndrome, 28
  calcaneodynia, 32
  cardiac neurosis, 34
  central retinitis, 35
  cervical spondylopathy, 38
  childhood anorexia, 39
  childhood hyperkinetic syndrome, 40
  chloasma, 41
  cholecystitis, 44
  cholelithiasis, 44
  chronic pelvic inflammatory disease,
    51
  competition syndrome, 53
  costal chondritis, 56
  cutaneous pruritus, 57
  cystic hyperplasia of the breast, 58–9

developmental disability, 62
drug withdrawal, 67
dysfunctional uterine bleeding, 70
dysmenorrhoea, 71
eczema, 74
epidemic keratoconjunctivitis, 75
epididymitis, 76
epilepsy, 79
erythromelalgia, 82
external humeral epicondylitis, 84
facial spasm, 85
flat wart, 88
gastritis, 91
gastrointestinal neurosis, 94
haemorrhoids, 101
herpes zoster, 103
hiccups, 104
hypertension, 108
hyperthyroidism, 109
hysteria, 111
impotence, 113
intercostal neuralgia, 117
jue syndrome, 119
leukorrhagia, 121
lumbar muscle strain, 123
menopausal syndrome, 131
morning sickness, 133
motion sickness, 134
mumps, 135
myopia, 138
neurodermatitis, 141
neurosism, 143
occipital headache, 100
Parkinson's disease, 152
peptic ulcer, 154
pharyngeal paraesthesia, 158
postconcussional syndrome, 159
premenstrual syndrome, 162
prostatitis, 165
Raynaud's disease, 167
recurrent mouth ulcer, 168
scapulohumeral periarthritis, 174
seborrhoeic dermatitis, 177
seminal emission, 178
simple glaucoma, 182
stiff neck, 184
stye, 185
thromboangiitis obliterans, 188, 189
tobacco withdrawal, 192
uterine prolapse, 163
vomiting, 202
Liver of Dorsal Surface, 234
Liver meridian of foot Juэyin, 217
Liver Yang, 229
  simple glaucoma, 182
Lochiorrhagia, 122
Lochiostasis, 160
Lower ear root, 234
Lower *he* (confluent) points, 261
Lumbar muscle strain, 123–4
Lumbosacral Vertebrae, 230
  lumbar muscle strain, 123
  nocturnal enuresis, 144
  prostatitis, 165
  sciatica, 175
  urinary retention, 172

urinary stones, 197
Lung, 231
  acne vulgaris, 4
  acute tonsillitis, 12
  allergic rhinitis, 15
  alopecia areata, 16–17
  brandy nose, 29
  bronchial asthma, 31
  chronic bronchitis, 47
  chronic pharyngitis, 52
  constipation, 55
  cutaneous pruritus, 57
  drug withdrawal, 67
  eczema, 74
  epidemic keratoconjunctivitis, 75
  epistaxis, 81
  erythromelalgia, 82
  flat wart, 88
  furunculosis, 90
  influenza, 115
  neurodermatitis, 141
  obesity, 145
  Raynaud's disease, 167
  scapulohumeral periarthritis, 174
  seborrhoeic dermatitis, 177
  suppurative nasal sinusitis, 186
  thromboangiitis obliterans, 188, 189
  tobacco withdrawal, 192
  urticaria, 200
  uterine prolapse, 163
Lung of Dorsal Surface, 234
Lung meridian of hand Taiyin, 209
Luo (collateral) points, 261
Luozhen (Ex8), 220

Malaria, 124–6
Male infertility, 126–8
Mastitis, acute, 8-10
Meeting point, 261
Meniere's disease, 128–30
Menopausal syndrome, 130–2
Mental injury, 261
Meridians, 209–18, 261
Middle of Superior Concha, 232
  appendicitis, 21
  bacillary dysentery, 25
  constipation, 55
  gastritis, 91
  gastrointestinal neurosis, 94
  gastroptosis, 96
  menopausal syndrome, 131
  obesity, 145
  pancreatitis, 149
  vomiting, 202
Middle Triangular Fossa, 230
Midpoint of Rim, 231
  amenorrhoea, 18
  chloasma, 41
  cystic hyperplasia of the breast, 58–9
  diabetes mellitus, 63
  dysfunctional uterine bleeding, 70
  dysmenorrhoea, 71
  hyperthyroidism, 109
  impotence, 113
  leukorrhagia, 121
  menopausal syndrome, 131

Midpoint of Rim (*cont*)
  nocturnal enuresis, 144
  obesity, 145
  Parkinson's disease, 152
  premenstrual syndrome, 162
Mingmen (Du4)
  bi syndrome, 27
  cerebrovascular accident sequelae, 181
  chronic bronchitis, 46
  chronic diarrhoea, 48
  constipation, 54
  diabetes mellitus, 63
  dysfunctional uterine bleeding, 70
  dysmenorrhoea, 71, 72
  epilepsy, 79
  female infertility, 87
  headache, 99
  impotence, 112
  lumbar muscle strain, 123
  male infertility, 127, 128
  myocarditis, 136
  neurosism, 142
  sciatica, 175
Minimal brain dysfunction *see*
    Childhood hyperkinetic syndrome
Miscarriage, habitual, 96–7
Morning sickness, 132–3
Motion sickness, 133–4
Mouth, 232
  alcohol withdrawal, 13
  chronic pharyngitis, 52
  facial spasm, 85
  influenza, 115
  recurrent mouth ulcer, 168
  temporomandibular joint dysfunction,
    68
  tobacco withdrawal, 192
  toothache, 194
Mouth ulcer, recurrent, 167–9
Moxa cone, 140, 261
Moxa roll, 31, 261
Moxibustion
  abnormal fetal position, 3
  acute gastroenteritis, 5
  acute intestinal obstruction, 7, 8
  allergic rhinitis, 15
  alopecia areata, 16
  amenorrhoea, 18
  bi syndrome, 28
  bronchial asthma, 30–1
  calcaneodynia, 33
  cervical spondylopathy, 38
  childhood anorexia, 39
  chronic bronchitis, 46–7
  chronic pelvic inflammatory disease, 50
  crude herb (medicinal vesculation), 31
  drug withdrawal, 67
  dysfunctional uterine bleeding, 70
  dysmenorrhoea, 72
  eczema, 73
  epididymitis, 76
  epistaxis, 81
  external humeral epicondylitis, 83
  female infertility, 87
  ginger, 46–7
  habitual miscarriage, 97

herbal moxibustion/medicinal
    vesiculation, 140
  impotence, 112–13
  insufficient lactation, 116
  jue syndrome, 119
  leukorrhagia, 121
  lochiorrhagia, 122
  malaria, 125–6
  male infertility, 128
  morning sickness, 133
  moxa cone, 140, 261
  moxa roll, 31, 46, 261
  neurodermatitis, 140
  nocturnal enuresis, 144
  non-scarifying, 261
  otitis media suppurativa, 146
  peptic ulcer, 154
  peripheral facial paralysis, 155
  postpartum uterine contractions, 160
  Raynaud's disease, 167
  retention of placenta, 170
  scapulohumeral periarthritis, 173
  scarifying, 31, 47, 48, 262
  sciatica, 175
  seminal emission, 178
  suppurative nasal sinusitis, 187
  thecal cyst, 187
  thromboangiitis obliterans, 189
  urinary retention, 171
  uterine prolapse, 163
Muchuang (G16)
  myopia, 137
Mumps, 134–5
Myocarditis, 135–6
Myopia, 137–9

Naohu (Du17)
  headache, 99
Naoshu (SI10)
  bi syndrome, 26
Nasal self-massage
  allergic rhinitis, 15
Neck, 230
  hyperthyroidism, 109
  mumps, 135
  stiff neck, 184
Neck massage, 38
Neck stretching exercises, 38
Needling sensation, 261
Neiguan (CP6)
  impotence, 112
Neiguan (P6)
  acute gastroenteritis, 5
  acute intestinal obstruction, 7
  acute mastitis, 9
  alcohol withdrawal, 13
  alopecia areata, 16
  amenorrhoea, 18
  angina pectoris, 19
  appendicitis, 21
  arrhythmia, 23
  bacillary dysentery, 25
  cardiac neurosis, 34
  central retinitis, 35
  cerebrovascular accident sequelae, 180
  childhood hyperkinetic syndrome, 40

cholecystitis, 43
  cholelithiasis, 44
  competition syndrome, 53
  constipation, 54
  cystic hyperplasia of the breast, 58
  cystitis, 60
  developmental disability, 61
  drug withdrawal, 66, 67
  dysmenorrhoea, 71
  epilepsy, resting stage, 78
  facial spasm, 85
  female infertility, 87
  gastritis, 91
  gastrointestinal neurosis, 93
  gastroptosis, 95, 96
  headache, 99
  hiccups, 104
  hypertension, 107
  hyperthyroidism, 109
  hysteria, 110, 111
  influenza, 114, 115
  insufficient lactation, 116
  jue syndrome, 119
  kuang syndrome, 65
  malaria, 125
  male infertility, 127
  Meniere's disease, 129
  menopausal syndrome, 131
  morning sickness, 132, 133
  motion sickness, 134
  mumps, 135
  myocarditis, 136
  neurosism, 142
  pancreatitis, 148
  Parkinson's disease, 151
  peptic ulcer, 153, 154
  pharyngeal paraesthesia, 157
  premenstrual syndrome, 161
  seminal emission, 178
  tobacco withdrawal, 192
  vomiting, 201
  wei syndrome, 204
Neiting (S44)
  acute mastitis, 9
  acute tonsillitis, 12
  allergic rhinitis, 15
  bacillary dysentery, 25
  constipation, 54
  diabetes mellitus, 63
  furunculosis, 89
  headache, 99
  herpes zoster, 102
  malaria, 125
  obesity, 145
  stye, 185
  suppurative nasal sinusitis, 186
  thecal cyst, 187
  trigeminal neuralgia, 195
Neurocirculatory asthenia *see* Cardiac
    neurosis
Neurodermatitis, 139–41
Neurosism, 141–3
Niehouxian (MS11), 258
  hearing loss, 191
  Meniere's disease, 129
  tinnitus, 191

Nieqianxian (MS10), 258
Nocturnal enuresis, 143–4
Non-scarifying moxibustion, 261

Obesity, 144–5
Occiput, 231
    alcohol withdrawal, 14
    arrhythmia, 23
    bronchial asthma, 32
    cardiac neurosis, 34
    central retinitis, 35
    cervical spondylopathy, 38
    childhood hyperkinetic syndrome, 40
    chronic bronchitis, 47
    chronic diarrhoea, 49
    competition syndrome, 53
    cutaneous pruritus, 57
    cystic hyperplasia of the breast, 58–9
    developmental disability, 62
    drug withdrawal, 67
    dysfunctional uterine bleeding, 70
    eczema, 74
    epilepsy, 79
    erythromelalgia, 82
    facial spasm, 85
    herpes zoster, 103
    hypertension, 108
    impotence, 113
    influenza, 115
    Meniere's disease, 129
    menopausal syndrome, 131
    motion sickness, 134
    mumps, 135
    myocarditis, 136
    myopia, 138
    neurodermatitis, 141
    neurosism, 143
    occipital headache, 100
    Parkinson's disease, 152
    peptic ulcer, 154
    phantom limb pain, 156
    recurrent mouth ulcer, 168
    seminal emission, 178
    simple glaucoma, 182
    temporomandibular joint dysfunction, 68
    tobacco withdrawal, 192
    toothache, 194
    trigeminal neuralgia, 196
    urticaria, 200
Oesophagus, 232
    gastrointestinal neurosis, 94
    pharyngeal paraesthesia, 158
Optic atrophy, 36
Oral contraceptives, 19
Otitis media catarrhalis, 147
Otitis media suppurativa, 146–7

Pancreas & Gallbladder, 232
    cholecystitis, 44
    cholelithiasis, 44
    costal chondritis, 56
    diabetes mellitus, 63
    facial spasm, 85
    furunculosis, 90
    headache, 100

herpes zoster, 103
    intercostal neuralgia, 117
    Meniere's disease, 129
    mumps, 135
    myopia, 138
    otitis media suppurativa, 147
    pancreatitis, 149
    peripheral facial paralysis, 155–6
    sciatica, 175
    stiff neck, 184
    suppurative nasal sinusitis, 186
Pancreatitis, 147–9
Pangguangshu (B28)
    cystitis, 60
    nocturnal enuresis, 144
    prostatitis, 164
    urinary stones, 197
Paralytic strabismus, 149–50
Parkinson's disease, 150–2
Pathogenic *qi*, 261
Pelvic inflammation, acute, 51
Pelvic inflammatory disease, chronic, 49–51
Pelvis, 230
    amenorrhoea, 18
    chronic pelvic inflammatory disease, 51
    cystitis, 60
    dysfunctional uterine bleeding, 70
    dysmenorrhoea, 71
    epididymitis, 76
    leukorrhagia, 121
    premenstrual syndrome, 162
    prostatitis, 165
    uterine prolapse, 163
Peptic ulcer, 152–4
Pericardium meridian of hand Jueyin, 214
Peripheral Crus of Helix, 232–3
Peripheral facial paralysis, 154–6
Phantom limb pain, 156–7
Pharyngeal paraesthesia, 157–8
Pharyngitis, chronic, 51–52
Phlegm, 261
Pigen (Ex48), 226
Pishu (B20)
    allergic rhinitis, 15
    amenorrhoea, 18
    bronchial asthma, 30, 31
    cardiac neurosis, 34
    cerebrovascular accident sequelae, 181
    childhood anorexia, 39
    chronic bronchitis, 46, 47
    chronic diarrhoea, 48
    developmental disability, 61
    diabetes mellitus, 63
    dian syndrome, 65
    epilepsy, 79
    gastritis, 91
    gastrointestinal neurosis, 93
    haemorrhoids, 101
    hiccups, 104
    malaria, 125
    neurosism, 142
    pancreatitis, 148

peptic ulcer, 153
    pharyngeal paraesthesia, 157
    premenstrual syndrome, 161
    urticaria, 199
    vomiting, 201
Point implantation therapy, 251–2
    abnormal reactions, 252
    bronchial asthma, 31
    chronic bronchitis, 47
    diabetes mellitus, 63
    epilepsy, 79
    gastritis, 92
    gastroptosis, 96
    indications, 252
    instruments, 251
    nocturnal enuresis, 144
    normal reactions, 252
    peptic ulcer, 154
    precautions, 252
    procedure, 251
    scapulohumeral periarthritis, 173
    wei syndrome, 204–5
Point injection therapy, 253–4
    acute soft tissue injury, 11
    bi syndrome, 28
    cervical spondylopathy, 37
    costal chondritis, 56
    developmental disability, 61
    drugs/drug dosages, 253
    external humeral epicondylitis, 83
    hiccups, 104
    impotence, 113
    indications, 253
    instruments, 253
    lumbar muscle strain, 123
    points selection, 253
    precautions, 253–4
    procedure, 253
    scapulohumeral periarthritis, 173
    urinary retention, 171
Postconcussional syndrome, 158–9
Postpartum uterine contractions, 159–60
Premature ejaculation, 113, 178
Premature labour, 3
Premenstrual syndrome, 160–2
Prostate hyperplasia, 165
Prostatitis, 164–5
Ptosis, 165–6

Qi, 261
Qianzheng (Ex35), 224
Qihai (Ren4)
    dysmenorrhoea, 71
    seminal emission, 178
Qihai (Ren6)
    acute intestinal obstruction, 7, 8
    acute mastitis, 9
    amenorrhoea, 18
    bacillary dysentery, 25
    bronchial asthma, 30
    cerebrovascular accident sequelae, 180, 181
    chronic bronchitis, 46
    constipation, 54
    diabetes mellitus, 63
    dysfunctional uterine bleeding, 70

Qihai (Ren6) (*cont*)
  epileptic attack, 78
  female infertility, 87
  gastroptosis, 95
  habitual miscarriage, 97
  haemorrhoids, 101
  headache, 99
  insufficient lactation, 116
  jue syndrome, 119
  lochiorrhagia, 122
  male infertility, 127, 128
  menopausal syndrome, 131
  neurodermatitis, 140
  obesity, 145
  Parkinson's disease, 151
  peptic ulcer, 153
  postpartum uterine contractions, 160
  thromboangiitis obliterans, 188, 189
  urticaria, 199
  uterine prolapse, 163
  wei syndrome, 204
Qimen (Liv14)
  insufficient lactation, 116
Qiuhou (Ex31), 223
  central retinitis, 35
  paralytic strabismus, 150
  simple glaucoma, 182
Qiuxu (G40)
  bi syndrome, 27
  costal chondritis, 55
  wei syndrome, 204
Qixue (K13)
  female infertility, 87
Quanliao (SI18)
  flat wart, 88
  trigeminal neuralgia, 195
Quchi (LI11)
  acne vulgaris, 4
  acute tonsillitis, 12
  appendicitis, 21
  bacillary dysentery, 24, 25
  bi syndrome, 26, 27
  brandy nose, 29
  cerebrovascular accident sequelae, 179
  constipation, 54
  cutaneous pruritus, 57
  diabetes mellitus, 63
  dysfunctional uterine bleeding, 69
  eczema, 73, 74
  erythromelalgia, 82
  external humeral epicondylitis, 83
  furunculosis, 89
  high fever, 105
  hypertension, 107
  hysteria, 110, 111
  neurodermatitis, 139
  obesity, 145
  Raynaud's disease, 166
  seborrhoeic dermatitis, 176
  thromboangiitis obliterans, 188
  urticaria, 199
  wei syndrome, 203, 204
Qugu (Ren2)
  chronic pelvic inflammatory disease, 50

  cutaneous pruritus, 57
  female infertility, 87
  impotence, 113
  leukorrhagia, 121
  male infertility, 127
  mumps, 135
  retention of placenta, 169
  uterine prolapse, 163
Ququan (Liv8)
  uterine prolapse, 163
Quze (P3)
  kuang syndrome, 65
  malaria, 125
  vomiting, 201
  wei syndrome, 204

Raynaud's disease, 166–7
Rectum, 229
  bacillary dysentery, 25
  chronic diarrhoea, 49
  constipation, 55
  gastrointestinal neurosis, 94
  gastroptosis, 96
  haemorrhoids, 101
  Parkinson's disease, 152
Recurrent mouth ulcer, 168–9
Reducing method, 261–2
Reinforcing method, 262
Ren (Conception Vessel) meridian, 218
Renying (S9)
  hypertension, 107
  hyperthyroidism, 109
Renzhong (Du26)
  epileptic attack, 78
Retention of placenta, 169–70
Rhinitis, chronic, 15
Riyue (G24)
  cholecystitis, 43
  cholelithiasis, 44, 45
  pancreatitis, 148
Root of Ear Vagus, 233
  arrhythmia, 23
  cholecystitis, 44
  cholelithiasis, 44
Rugen (S18)
  acute mastitis, 9
  cystic hyperplasia of the breast, 58
  insufficient lactation, 116
  wei syndrome, 204

San Jiao, 232, 262
  appendicitis, 21
  arrhythmia, 23
  bacillary dysentery, 25
  brandy nose, 29
  cholecystitis, 44
  cholelithiasis, 44
  chronic pelvic inflammatory disease, 51
  chronic pharyngitis, 52
  constipation, 55
  cystitis, 60
  diabetes mellitus, 63
  eczema, 74
  epididymitis, 76
  external humeral epicondylitis, 84
  facial spasm, 85

gastritis, 91
gastroptosis, 96
herpes zoster, 103
leukorrhagia, 121
Meniere's disease, 129
mumps, 135
obesity, 145
otitis media suppurativa, 147
pancreatitis, 149
peripheral facial paralysis, 155
pharyngeal paraesthesia, 158
prostatitis, 165
recurrent mouth ulcer, 168
scapulohumeral periarthritis, 174
seborrhoeic dermatitis, 177
temporomandibular joint dysfunction, 68
toothache, 194
trigeminal neuralgia, 196
urinary retention, 172
urinary stones, 197
San Jiao (Triple Energizer) meridian of hand Shaoyang, 215
Sanjiaojiu (Ex43), 225
Sanyinjiao (Sp6)
  acne vulgaris, 4
  acute intestinal obstruction, 7, 8
  acute mastitis, 9
  alcohol withdrawal, 13
  alopecia areata, 16
  amenorrhoea, 18
  angina pectoris, 20
  arrhythmia, 23
  bacillary dysentery, 24
  bi syndrome, 27, 28
  cardiac neurosis, 34
  cerebrovascular accident sequelae, 180, 181
  childhood anorexia, 39
  childhood hyperkinetic syndrome, 40
  cholecystitis, 43
  cholelithiasis, 44
  chronic bronchitis, 46
  chronic diarrhoea, 48
  chronic pelvic inflammatory disease, 50
  competition syndrome, 53
  constipation, 54
  cutaneous pruritus, 57
  cystic hyperplasia of the breast, 58
  cystitis, 60
  developmental disability, 61
  diabetes mellitus, 63
  dian syndrome, 65
  drug withdrawal, 66, 67
  dysfunctional uterine bleeding, 69
  dysmenorrhoea, 71, 72
  epididymitis, 76
  epilepsy, 78, 79
  epistaxis, 81
  facial spasm, 85
  female infertility, 87
  gastritis, 91, 92
  gastrointestinal neurosis, 93
  gastroptosis, 95
  habitual miscarriage, 97

Sanyinjiao (Sp6) *(cont)*
  haemorrhoids, 101
  headache, 99
  herpes zoster, 103
  hiccups, 104
  hypertension, 107
  hyperthyroidism, 109
  hysteria, 111
  impotence, 112, 113
  insufficient lactation, 116
  jue syndrome, 119
  kuang syndrome, 65
  leukorrhagia, 121
  lochiorrhagia, 122
  malaria, 125
  male infertility, 127, 128
  Meniere's disease, 129
  menopausal syndrome, 131
  myocarditis, 136
  myopia, 137
  neurodermatitis, 139
  neurosism, 142
  nocturnal enuresis, 143
  obesity, 145
  otitis media suppurativa, 146
  Parkinson's disease, 151
  peptic ulcer, 153
  postconcussional syndrome, 159
  postpartum uterine contractions, 160
  premenstrual syndrome, 161
  prostatitis, 164
  Raynaud's disease, 167
  recurrent mouth ulcer, 168
  retention of placenta, 169
  seborrhoeic dermatitis, 176
  seminal emission, 178
  simple glaucoma, 182
  thromboangiitis obliterans, 188, 189
  tobacco withdrawal, 192
  urinary stones, 197
  urticaria, 199
  uterine prolapse, 163
  vomiting, 202
  wei syndrome, 204
Sanyinjiao (Sp6) eczema, 73
Scalp acupuncture, 255–9
  central retinitis, 36
  cerebrovascular accident sequelae, 181
  developmental disability, 61
  epilepsy, 79
  hearing loss, 191
  indications, 255–8
  Meniere's disease, 129
  Parkinson's disease, 151
  phantom limb pain, 156
  precautions, 259
  procedure, 258–9
  scalp line locations, 255–8
Scaphoid fossa, 229
Scapulohumeral periarthritis, 172–4
Scarifying moxibustion, 31, 47, 48, 262
Sciatic nerve, 230
  sciatica, 175
Sciatica, 174–5
Seborrhoeic dermatitis, 176–7

Seminal emission, 177–8
Shangjuxu (S37)
  acute gastroenteritis, 5
  acute intestinal obstruction, 7
  appendicitis, 21
  bacillary dysentery, 24
  chronic diarrhoea, 48
  constipation, 54
  gastrointestinal neurosis, 93
  headache, 99
  Parkinson's disease, 151
Shangming (Ex29), 223
Shangwan (Ren13)
  morning sickness, 133
  peptic ulcer, 153
Shangxing (Du23)
  allergic rhinitis, 15
  developmental disability, 61
  epistaxis, 81
  kuang syndrome, 65
  suppurative nasal sinusitis, 187
Shangyang (LI1)
  acute tonsillitis, 12
  brandy nose, 29
  epistaxis, 81
  recurrent mouth ulcer, 168
  urticaria, 199
Shaofu (H8)
  wei syndrome, 204
Shaohai (H3)
  wei syndrome, 204
Shaoshang (L11)
  acute tonsillitis, 12
  epistaxis, 81
  influenza, 114
  mumps, 134, 135
  recurrent mouth ulcer, 168
  urticaria, 199
Shaoze (SI1)
  acute mastitis, 9
  insufficient lactation, 116
Shenmai (B62)
  bi syndrome, 27
  headache, 99
  scapulohumeral periarthritis, 173
Shenmen (H7)
  arrhythmia, 23
  cardiac neurosis, 34
  developmental disability, 61
  dian syndrome, 65
  facial spasm, 85
  hyperthyroidism, 109
  impotence, 112
  male infertility, 127
  menopausal syndrome, 131
  myocarditis, 136
  neurosism, 142
  seminal emission, 178
  wei syndrome, 204
Shenque (Ren8)
  acute gastroenteritis, 5
  acute intestinal obstruction, 7, 8
  childhood anorexia, 39
  chronic diarrhoea, 48, 49
  constipation, 54
  drug withdrawal, 67

  female infertility, 87
  gastritis, 91
  gastrointestinal neurosis, 94
  gastroptosis, 95
  habitual miscarriage, 97
  impotence, 112
  jue syndrome, 119
  lochiorrhagia, 122
  malaria, 125
  male infertility, 128
  nocturnal enuresis, 144
  peptic ulcer, 154
  retention of placenta, 169, 170
  seminal emission, 178
  urinary retention, 171
  urticaria, 200
Shenshu (B23)
  amenorrhoea, 18
  bi syndrome, 27
  bronchial asthma, 30, 31
  central retinitis, 35
  cerebrovascular accident sequelae, 181
  chronic bronchitis, 46, 47
  developmental disability, 61
  diabetes mellitus, 63
  dysmenorrhoea, 71
  epilepsy, 79
  facial spasm, 85
  female infertility, 87
  headache, 99
  hearing loss, 191
  hiccups, 104
  hypertension, 107
  impotence, 112
  lumbar muscle strain, 123
  male infertility, 127, 128
  myopia, 137
  neurosism, 142
  nocturnal enuresis, 144
  obesity, 145
  Parkinson's disease, 151
  postconcussional syndrome, 159
  prostatitis, 165
  sciatica, 175
  seminal emission, 178
  tinnitus, 191
  urinary retention, 171
  urinary stones, 197
  uterine prolapse, 163
  wei syndrome, 204
Shenting (Du24)
  headache, 99
Shenzhu (Du12)
  chronic bronchitis, 46
  furunculosis, 89
Shiqizhui (Ex50), 226
  dysmenorrhoea, 71
Shixuan (Ex1), 219
  acute tonsillitis, 12
  epileptic attack, 78
  erythromelalgia, 82
  high fever, 105, 106
  influenza, 114, 115
  jue syndrome, 118, 119
  malaria, 125

Shixuan (Ex1) (*cont*)
  mumps, 135
  wei syndrome, 204
Shoubei Yaotongdian (Ex9), 220
Shoulder, 229
  scapulohumeral periarthritis, 173
Shoulder joint *bi* syndrome, 26
Shousanli (LI10)
  appendicitis, 21
  bi syndrome, 26
  external humeral epicondylitis, 83
  Parkinson's disease, 151
  scapulohumeral periarthritis, 173
  wei syndrome, 204
Shouxiaojie (Ex53), 226
  acute soft tissue injury, 10
Shuaigu (G8)
  headache, 99
Shugu (B65)
  sciatica, 175
Shuifen (Ren9)
  bi syndrome, 27
Shuigou (Du26)
  acute soft tissue injury, 10
  alcohol withdrawal with convulsions,
    13
  competition syndrome, 53
  hysteria, 110
  jue syndrome, 118, 120
  kuang syndrome, 65
  mumps, 135
Shuitu (S10)
  hyperthyroidism, 109
Sibai (S2)
  acne vulgaris, 4
  flat wart, 88
  myopia, 137, 138, 139
  peripheral facial paralysis, 155
  trigeminal neuralgia, 195
Sifeng (Ex2), 219
  bronchial asthma, 31
  childhood anorexia, 39
Sinusitis, suppurative nasal, 185-7
Siqiang (Ex17), 221
Sishencong (Ex26), 222-3
  cerebrovascular accident sequelae,
    180, 181
  headache, 99
  impotence, 112
  Parkinson's disease, 151
  postconcussional syndrome, 159
  tobacco withdrawal, 192
Sizhukong (SJ23)
  paralytic strabismus, 150
  ptosis, 166
Small intestine, 233
  angina pectoris, 20
  childhood anorexia, 39
  chronic diarrhoea, 49
  gastrointestinal neurosis, 94
  scapulohumeral periarthritis, 174
  stiff neck, 184
Small intestine meridian of hand
  Taiyang, 212
Soft tissue injury, acute, 10-11
  ashi points, 10

Spermatitis, 77
Spermatopathy, 113
Spermophlebectasia, 77
Spinal joint *bi* syndrome, 27
Spleen, 231
  acute gastroenteritis, 6
  acute soft tissue injury, 11
  alcohol withdrawal, 13
  allergic rhinitis, 15
  alopecia areata, 16-17
  amenorrhoea, 18
  angina pectoris, 20
  appendicitis, 21
  bacillary dysentery, 25
  bi syndrome, 28
  brandy nose, 29
  bronchial asthma, 31
  cardiac neurosis, 34
  central retinitis, 35
  childhood anorexia, 39
  childhood hyperkinetic syndrome, 40
  chloasma, 41
  cholecystitis, 44
  cholelithiasis, 44
  chronic bronchitis, 47
  chronic diarrhoea, 49
  chronic pelvic inflammatory disease,
    51
  competition syndrome, 53
  constipation, 55
  cutaneous pruritus, 57
  cystitis, 60
  developmental disability, 62
  diabetes mellitus, 63
  drug withdrawal, 67
  dysfunctional uterine bleeding, 70
  eczema, 74
  epilepsy, 79
  epistaxis, 81
  facial spasm, 85
  gastritis, 91
  gastrointestinal neurosis, 94
  gastroptosis, 96
  haemorrhoids, 101
  hiccups, 104
  hypertension, 108
  hyperthyroidism, 109
  hysteria, 111
  impotence, 113
  leukorrhagia, 121
  lumbar muscle strain, 123
  menopausal syndrome, 131
  morning sickness, 133
  myocarditis, 136
  myopia, 138
  neurosism, 143
  obesity, 145
  pancreatitis, 149
  Parkinson's disease, 152
  peptic ulcer, 154
  pharyngeal paraesthesia, 158
  Raynaud's disease, 167
  recurrent mouth ulcer, 169
  scapulohumeral periarthritis, 174
  seborrhoeic dermatitis, 177
  seminal emission, 178

stiff neck, 184
stye, 185
suppurative nasal sinusitis, 186
thromboangiitis obliterans, 188, 189
urticaria, 200
uterine prolapse, 163
vomiting, 202
Spleen of Dorsal Surface, 234
Spleen meridian of foot Taiyin, 211
Stiff neck, 183-4
  stimulation intensity selection, 183-4
Stomach, 232
  acne vulgaris, 4
  acute gastroenteritis, 5
  acute mastitis, 9
  acute tonsillitis, 12
  alcohol withdrawal, 13
  angina pectoris, 20
  appendicitis, 21
  bacillary dysentery, 25
  brandy nose, 29
  cardiac neurosis, 34
  childhood anorexia, 39
  childhood hyperkinetic syndrome, 40
  chloasma, 41
  cholecystitis, 44
  cholelithiasis, 44
  competition syndrome, 53
  constipation, 55
  cystic hyperplasia of the breast, 58-9
  developmental disability, 62
  drug withdrawal, 67
  facial spasm, 85
  frontal headache, 100
  furunculosis, 90
  gastritis, 91
  gastrointestinal neurosis, 94
  gastroptosis, 96
  herpes zoster, 103
  hiccups, 104
  hypertension, 108
  influenza, 115
  jue syndrome, 120
  morning sickness, 133
  myocarditis, 136
  neurosism, 143
  pancreatitis, 149
  peptic ulcer, 154
  peripheral facial paralysis, 155
  postconcussional syndrome, 159
  premenstrual syndrome, 162
  seminal emission, 178
  suppurative nasal sinusitis, 186
  temporomandibular joint dysfunction,
    68
  toothache, 194
  trigeminal neuralgia, 196
  urticaria, 200
  vomiting, 202
Stomach meridian of foot Yangming,
  210
Stump neuralgia, 157
Stye, 184-5
Subcortex, 231
  acute mastitis, 10
  alcohol withdrawal, 14

Subcortex (*cont*)
  alopecia areata, 17
  amenorrhoea, 18
  angina pectoris, 20
  arrhythmia, 23
  bacillary dysentery, 25
  calcaneodynia, 32
  cardiac neurosis, 34
  central retinitis, 35
  childhood hyperkinetic syndrome, 40
  chronic diarrhoea, 49
  competition syndrome, 53
  cutaneous pruritus, 57
  cystic hyperplasia of the breast, 58–9
  developmental disability, 62
  diabetes mellitus, 63
  drug withdrawal, 67
  dysfunctional uterine bleeding, 70
  dysmenorrhoea, 71
  epilepsy, 79
  facial spasm, 85
  gastritis, 91
  gastrointestinal neurosis, 94
  gastroptosis, 96
  haemorrhoids, 102
  headache, 99
  hiccups, 105
  hypertension, 108
  hyperthyroidism, 109
  hysteria, 111
  impotence, 113
  intercostal neuralgia, 117
  jue syndrome, 119
  Meniere's disease, 129
  menopausal syndrome, 131
  morning sickness, 133
  mumps, 135
  myocarditis, 136
  myopia, 138
  neurodermatitis, 141
  neurosism, 143
  nocturnal enuresis, 144
  obesity, 145
  otitis media suppurativa, 147
  Parkinson's disease, 152
  peptic ulcer, 154
  peripheral facial paralysis, 156
  phantom limb pain, 156
  pharyngeal paraesthesia, 158
  postconcussional syndrome, 159
  premenstrual syndrome, 162
  Raynaud's disease, 167
  seborrhoeic dermatitis, 177
  seminal emission, 178
  simple glaucoma, 183
  stiff neck, 184
  thromboangiitis obliterans, 188, 189
  tobacco withdrawal, 192
  trigeminal neuralgia, 196
  urinary retention, 172
  vomiting, 202
Suliao (Du25)
  brandy nose, 29
Summer heat, 262
Superior concha, 232
Superior Triangular Fossa, 230

  hypertension, 108
Sympathesis
  acute gastroenteritis, 6
  appendicitis, 21
  arrhythmia, 23
  bacillary dysentery, 25
  bronchial asthma, 32
  central retinitis, 35
  erythromelaegia, 82
  gastrointestinal neurosis, 94
  hiccups, 104
  hypertension, 108
  hyperthyroidism, 109
  jue syndrome, 119
  menopausal syndrome, 131
  pancreatitis, 149
  Parkinson's disease, 152
  peptic ulcer, 154
  Raynaud's disease, 167
  seborrhoeic dermatitis, 177
  thromboangiitis obliterans, 188, 189
  urinary retention, 172
  urinary stones, 198
  vomiting, 202
Syndrome, 262

Taibai (Sp3)
  bi syndrome, 27
Taichong (Liv3)
  acute intestinal obstruction, 7
  acute mastitis, 9
  acute soft tissue injury, 10
  alcohol withdrawal with convulsions, 13
  alopecia areata, 16
  amenorrhoea, 18
  cardiac neurosis, 34
  central retinitis, 35
  cerebrovascular accident sequelae, 180, 181
  cervical spondylopathy, 37
  childhood hyperkinetic syndrome, 40
  cholecystitis, 43
  cholelithiasis, 44
  chronic pelvic inflammatory disease, 50
  constipation, 54
  cystic hyperplasia of the breast, 58
  diabetes mellitus, 63
  dysmenorrhoea, 71
  epididymitis, 76
  epilepsy, 78, 79
  erythromelalgia, 82
  facial spasm, 85
  female infertility, 87
  gastritis, 91, 92
  gastrointestinal neurosis, 93
  headache, 99
  hearing loss, 191
  herpes zoster, 103
  hiccups, 104
  hypertension, 107
  hyperthyroidism, 109
  hysteria, 110
  impotence, 112
  insufficient lactation, 116

  jue syndrome, 119
  kuang syndrome, 65
  male infertility, 127
  Meniere's disease, 129
  menopausal syndrome, 131
  morning sickness, 133
  mumps, 135
  myopia, 137
  neurosism, 142
  pancreatitis, 148
  paralytic strabismus, 149
  Parkinson's disease, 151
  peptic ulcer, 153, 154
  pharyngeal paraesthesia, 157
  postconcussional syndrome, 159
  premenstrual syndrome, 161
  Raynaud's disease, 167
  recurrent mouth ulcer, 168
  seminal emission, 178
  simple glaucoma, 182
  thecal cyst, 187
  thromboangiitis obliterans, 188, 189
  tinnitus, 191
  urinary retention, 171
  vomiting, 201
Taixi (K3)
  acute intestinal obstruction, 7
  amenorrhoea, 18
  bi syndrome, 28
  calcaneodynia, 32
  cardiac neurosis, 34
  central retinitis, 35
  cerebrovascular accident sequelae, 181
  cervical spondylopathy, 37
  childhood hyperkinetic syndrome, 40
  chronic bronchitis, 46
  chronic pharyngitis, 51
  constipation, 54
  cutaneous pruritus, 57
  developmental disability, 61
  diabetes mellitus, 63
  dysmenorrhoea, 71
  epilepsy, 79
  epileptic attack, 78
  facial spasm, 85
  female infertility, 87
  gastritis, 91
  gastrointestinal neurosis, 94
  gastroptosis, 95
  headache, 99
  hearing loss, 191
  hypertension, 107
  hyperthyroidism, 109
  impotence, 112
  kuang syndrome, 65
  lumbar muscle strain, 123
  malaria, 125
  male infertility, 127
  Meniere's disease, 129
  menopausal syndrome, 131
  myopia, 137
  neurosism, 142
  Parkinson's disease, 151
  peptic ulcer, 153
  postconcussional syndrome, 159

Taixi (K3) (*cont*)
  prostatitis, 165
  recurrent mouth ulcer, 168
  sciatica, 175
  seminal emission, 178
  simple glaucoma, 182
  thromboangiitis obliterans, 188, 189
  tinnitus, 191
  toothache, 194
  wei syndrome, 204
Taiyang (Ex30), 223
  allergic rhinitis, 15
  central retinitis, 35
  cerebrovascular accident sequelae,
    180
  cervical spondylopathy, 37
  childhood hyperkinetic syndrome, 40
  competition syndrome, 53
  epidemic keratoconjunctivitis, 75
  headache, 98, 99
  hypertension, 107
  hyperthyroidism, 109
  hysteria, 111
  influenza, 114
  kuang syndrome, 65
  Meniere's disease, 129
  menopausal syndrome, 131
  myopia, 137, 138, 139
  neurosism, 143
  paralytic strabismus, 149
  Parkinson's disease, 151
  peripheral facial paralysis, 155
  postconcussional syndrome, 158, 159
  simple glaucoma, 182
  stye, 185
  trigeminal neuralgia, 195
  wei syndrome, 203
Taiyuan (L9)
  thromboangiitis obliterans, 188
Taodao (Du13)
  malaria, 125
Tarsal cyst, 185
Teeth, 233
  jue syndrome, 119
  temporomandibular joint dysfunction,
    68
  toothache, 194
  trigeminal neuralgia, 196
Temple, 231
  developmental disability, 62
  epilepsy, 79
  headache, 100
  influenza, 115
  mumps, 135
  otitis media suppurativa, 146
Temporomandibular joint dysfunction,
  68
Thecal cyst, 187
Thoracic Vertebrae, 230
  acute mastitis, 9
  cholecystitis, 44
  cholelithiasis, 44
  costal chondritis, 56
  cystic hyperplasia of the breast,
    58–9
  intercostal neuralgia, 117

Throat, 231
  acute tonsillitis, 12
  chronic pharyngitis, 52
  gastrointestinal neurosis, 94
  influenza, 115
  pharyngeal paraesthesia, 158
Thromboangiitis obliterans, 188–90
Thrombotic phlebitis, 190
Tianding (LI17)
  hyperthyroidism, 109
Tianjing (SJ10)
  bi syndrome, 26
Tianshu (S25)
  acute gastroenteritis, 5
  acute intestinal obstruction, 7, 8
  alcohol withdrawal, 13
  appendicitis, 21
  bacillary dysentery, 24
  childhood anorexia, 39
  cholecystitis, 43
  cholelithiasis, 44
  chronic diarrhoea, 48, 49
  competition syndrome, 53
  constipation, 54
  diabetes mellitus, 63
  dian syndrome, 64
  gastritis, 91
  gastrointestinal neurosis, 93
  gastroptosis, 95
  headache, 99
  hysteria, 111
  malaria, 125
  obesity, 145
  Parkinson's disease, 151
  peptic ulcer, 153
  seborrhoeic dermatitis, 176
  urticaria, 199
Tiantu (Ren22)
  bronchial asthma, 30, 32
  cerebrovascular accident sequelae,
    180
  chronic bronchitis, 46
  chronic pharyngitis, 51, 52
  deafness with muteness, 191
  hysteria, 111
  pharyngeal paraesthesia, 157, 158
Tianzhu (B10)
  headache, 99
  stiff neck, 183
  wei syndrome, 203
Tianzong (SI11)
  bi syndrome, 26
  cervical spondylopathy, 37
  scapulohumeral periarthritis, 173
Tiaokou (S38)
  scapulohumeral periarthritis, 173
Tinggong (SI19)
  hearing loss, 190
  Meniere's disease, 129
  otitis media suppurativa, 146
  temporomandibular joint dysfunction,
    68
  tinnitus, 190
Tinghui (G2)
  hearing loss, 191
  hysteria, 111

Meniere's disease, 129
  otitis media suppurativa, 146
  tinnitus, 191
Tinnitus, 190–1
Tituo (Ex44), 225
  uterine prolapse, 163
Tobacco withdrawal, 192–3
Toes, 229
Tongli (H5)
  cerebrovascular accident sequelae, 180
  deafness with muteness, 191
  hysteria, 111
  kuang syndrome, 65
  myocarditis, 136
Tongtian (B7)
  allergic rhinitis, 15
Tongue, 233
  recurrent mouth ulcer, 168
  tobacco withdrawal, 192
Tongziliao (G1)
  hyperthyroidism, 109
  paralytic strabismus, 150
Tonsil, 233
  acute tonsillitis, 12
Tonsillitis, acute, 11–12
Tonsillitis, chronic, 52
Toothache, 193–4
Touwei (S8)
  headache, 98
Toxaemia of pregnancy, 3
Trachea, 231
  bronchial asthma, 31
  chronic bronchitis, 47
  influenza, 115
  tobacco withdrawal, 192
  urticaria, 200
Tragus, 231
Triangular fossa, 230
Trigeminal neuralgia, 194–6

Upper Ear Root, 233
  epistaxis, 81
Ureter, 232
  urinary stones, 197
Urethra, 229
  cystitis, 60
  prostatitis, 165
  urinary retention, 172
  urinary stones, 197
Urinary Bladder, 232
  cystitis, 60
  furunculosis, 90
  haemorrhoids, 101
  lumbar muscle strain, 123
  occipital headache, 100
  sciatica, 175
  stiff neck, 184
  urinary retention, 172
  urinary stones, 197
  uterine prolapse, 163
Urinary incontinence, 144, 180
Urinary retention, 170–2
Urinary stones, 196–8
Urticaria, 199–200
Uterine atony, 170
Uterine prolapse, 162–4

Vomiting, 200–2
Vulvitis, 51

Waiguan (SJ5)
  bi syndrome, 26, 27
  cerebrovascular accident sequelae,
    179
  cervical spondylopathy, 37
  erythromelalgia, 82
  hearing loss, 191
  hysteria, 110, 111
  mumps, 134, 135
  Parkinson's disease, 151
  Raynaud's disease, 166
  scapulohumeral periarthritis, 173
  thecal cyst, 187
  thromboangiitis obliterans, 188
  tinnitus, 191
  wei syndrome, 203, 204
Waiguan (SJ5)
Wailing (S26)
  gastroptosis, 95
Wangu (G12)
  bi syndrome, 27
  hearing loss, 191
  neurosism, 143
  tinnitus, 191
  wave forms selection, 248
Wei syndrome, 202–5
Weiguanxiashu (Ex47), 226
Weishang (Ex52), 226
  gastroptosis, 95
Weishu (B21)
  amenorrhoea, 18
  childhood anorexia, 39
  gastritis, 91, 92
  gastrointestinal neurosis, 93
  hiccups, 104
  pancreatitis, 148
  peptic ulcer, 153, 154
  vomiting, 201, 202
Weizhong (B40)
  acne vulgaris, 4
  acute gastroenteritis, 5
  acute soft tissue injury, 10
  bi syndrome, 27
  cutaneous pruritus, 57
  eczema, 73, 74
  furunculosis, 89
  herpes zoster, 103
  kuang syndrome, 65
  lumbar muscle strain, 123
  malaria, 125
  neurodermatitis, 140
  sciatica, 174
  seborrhoeic dermatitis, 176
  thromboangiitis obliterans, 188, 189
  urticaria, 200
  wei syndrome, 204
Wind, 262
Wind Stream, 229
  allergic rhinitis, 15
  bi syndrome, 28
  bronchial asthma, 32
  diabetes mellitus, 63
  eczema, 74

flat wart, 88
furunculosis, 90
leukorrhagia, 121
motion sickness, 134
mumps, 135
neurodermatitis, 141
recurrent mouth ulcer, 168
suppurative nasal sinusitis, 186
urticaria, 200
Wrist joint *bi* syndrome, 27

Xiaguan (S7)
  acne vulgaris, 4
  cerebrovascular accident sequelae,
    180
  peripheral facial paralysis, 155
  recurrent mouth ulcer, 168
  temporomandibular joint dysfunction,
    68
  toothache, 193
  trigeminal neuralgia, 195
Xiajuxu (S39)
  pancreatitis, 148
  peptic ulcer, 153
Xialiao (B34)
  haemorrhoids, 101
  leukorrhagia, 121
Xiaogukong (Ex5), 219
Xiaohai (SI8)
  bi syndrome, 26
Xiawan (Ren10)
  gastritis, 91
  gastroptosis, 95
  peptic ulcer, 153
Xiaxi (G43)
  bi syndrome, 27
  epidemic keratoconjunctivitis, 75
  headache, 99
  hearing loss, 191
  premenstrual syndrome, 161
  suppurative nasal sinusitis, 186
  tinnitus, 191
  trigeminal neuralgia, 195
Xingjian (Liv2)
  cholecystitis, 43
  cholelithiasis, 44
  cystic hyperplasia of the breast, 58
  dysfunctional uterine bleeding, 69
  epidemic keratoconjunctivitis, 75
  epilepsy, 79
  gastritis, 91
  headache, 99
  hypertension, 107
  hyperthyroidism, 109
  jue syndrome, 119
  lochiorrhagia, 122
  neurosism, 142
  peptic ulcer, 153
  premenstrual syndrome, 161
  suppurative nasal sinusitis, 186
  trigeminal neuralgia, 195
Xinhui (Du22)
  epistaxis, 81
Xinshu (B15)
  arrhythmia, 23
  cardiac neurosis, 34

dian syndrome, 65
furunculosis, 89
male infertility, 127
myocarditis, 136
neurosism, 142
seminal emission, 178
Xiyan (Ex20), 222
  bi syndrome, 27
Xuanzhong (G39)
  bi syndrome, 27
  cerebrovascular accident sequelae,
    180, 181
  cervical spondylopathy, 37
  hysteria, 111
  stiff neck, 183
  thromboangiitis obliterans, 188
  wei syndrome, 203, 204
Xuehai (Sp10)
  amenorrhoea, 18
  bacillary dysentery, 24
  chronic diarrhoea, 48
  cutaneous pruritus, 57
  cystitis, 60
  diabetes mellitus, 63
  dysfunctional uterine bleeding, 69
  dysmenorrhoea, 71
  eczema, 73, 74
  epididymitis, 76
  female infertility, 87
  lochiorrhagia, 122
  neurodermatitis, 139
  postpartum uterine contractions, 160
  retention of placenta, 169
  seborrhoeic dermatitis, 176
  thromboangiitis obliterans, 188, 189
  urinary retention, 171
  urticaria, 199
  wei syndrome, 204

Yamen (Du15)
  deafness with muteness, 191
Yangbai (G14)
  peripheral facial paralysis, 155
  ptosis, 166
  trigeminal neuralgia, 195
Yangchi (SJ4)
  bi syndrome, 27
  eczema, 73
  wei syndrome, 204
Yanglao (SI6)
  bi syndrome, 27
Yanglingquan (G34)
  acute soft tissue injury, 10
  cardiac neurosis, 34
  cerebrovascular accident sequelae, 180
  cervical spondylopathy, 37
  cholecystitis, 43, 44
  cholelithiasis, 44, 45
  constipation, 54
  costal chondritis, 55
  dysfunctional uterine bleeding, 69
  dysmenorrhoea, 71
  gastritis, 91, 92
  headache, 99
  herpes zoster, 102
  hiccups, 104

Yanglingquan (G34) (*cont*)
  hypertension, 107
  hysteria, 110, 111
  intercostal neuralgia, 117
  male infertility, 127
  morning sickness, 133
  neurosism, 142
  pancreatitis, 148
  Parkinson's disease, 151
  peptic ulcer, 153
  premenstrual syndrome, 161
  scapulohumeral periarthritis, 173
  sciatica, 175
  vomiting, 201
  wei syndrome, 203, 204
Yangxi (LI5)
  bi syndrome, 27
Yaoqi (Ex51), 226
  epilepsy, resting stage, 78
Yaoshu (Du2)
  cerebrovascular accident sequelae,
    180
  leukorrhagia, 121
Yaoyan (Ex49), 226
Yaoyangguan (Du3)
  bi syndrome, 27
  male infertility, 128
  sciatica, 175
  seminal emission, 178
Yatong (Ex7), 220
Yifeng (SJ17)
  acute tonsillitis, 12
  cerebrovascular accident sequelae,
    180
  eczema, 73
  facial spasm, 85
  hearing loss, 191
  hysteria, 111
  kuang syndrome, 65
  Meniere's disease, 129
  mumps, 134
  otitis media suppurativa, 146
  peripheral facial paralysis, 155
  stiff neck, 183
  tinnitus, 191
  toothache, 193
Yiming (Ex36), 224
Yin/Yang, 262
Yinbai (Sp1)
  dysfunctional uterine bleeding, 69
  retention of placenta, 169
Yingchuang (S16)
  cystic hyperplasia of the breast, 58
  insufficient lactation, 116
Yingxiang (LI20)
  allergic rhinitis, 14, 15
  brandy nose, 29
  epistaxis, 81
  influenza, 114
  suppurative nasal sinusitis, 186, 187
Yinjiao (Du28)
  haemorrhoids, 101
Yinjiao (Ren7)
  bi syndrome, 27
  female infertility, 87
  premenstrual syndrome, 161

Yinlingquan (Sp9)
  alcohol withdrawal, 13
  bacillary dysentery, 24
  cholecystitis, 43
  cholelithiasis, 44
  chronic pelvic inflammatory disease,
    50
  cystitis, 60
  impotence, 112
  leukorrhagia, 121
  malaria, 125
  male infertility, 127
  morning sickness, 133
  obesity, 145
  scapulohumeral periarthritis, 173
  urinary retention, 171
  urinary stones, 197
  uterine prolapse, 163
  wei syndrome, 204
Yinshi (S33)
  wei syndrome, 204
Yintang (Ex27), 223
  allergic rhinitis, 14, 15
  headache, 98
  suppurative nasal sinusitis, 186,
    187
Yinxi (H6)
  angina pectoris, 20
  arrhythmia, 23
  hyperthyroidism, 109
  myocarditis, 136
Yongquan (K1)
  epistaxis, 81
  hypertension, 107
  hysteria, 110, 111
  jue syndrome, 119
  kuang syndrome, 65
Yuan (primordial) *qi*, 262
Yuan (source) points, 262
Yuji (L10)
  bronchial asthma, 30
  chronic bronchitis, 46
  diabetes mellitus, 63
  scapulohumeral periarthritis, 173
  wei syndrome, 204
Yuyao (Ex28), 223
  myopia, 137
  paralytic strabismus, 150
  trigeminal neuralgia, 195
  wei syndrome, 203

Zang organs, 262
Zanzhu (B2)
  acne vulgaris, 4
  epidemic keratoconjunctivitis, 75
  headache, 98
  hyperthyroidism, 109
  myopia, 137
  paralytic strabismus, 150
  ptosis, 166
  trigeminal neuralgia, 195
  wei syndrome, 203
Zhangmen (Liv13)
  pharyngeal paraesthesia, 157
Zhaohai (K6)
  bi syndrome, 27

chronic pharyngitis, 51
  constipation, 54
  recurrent mouth ulcer, 168
  trigeminal neuralgia, 195
  wei syndrome, 204
Zhenshang Pangxian (MS13), 258
  central retinitis, 36
Zhenshang Zhengzhongxian (MS12),
  258
Zhenxia Pangxian (MS14), 258
Zhibian (B54)
  bi syndrome, 27
  cerebrovascular accident sequelae,
    180
  sciatica, 174
  wei syndrome, 203
Zhigou (SJ6)
  acute intestinal obstruction, 7
  acute soft tissue injury, 10
  cholecystitis, 43
  cholelithiasis, 44
  constipation, 54
  costal chondritis, 55, 56
  herpes zoster, 102
  intercostal neuralgia, 117
  obesity, 145
Zhishi (B52)
  male infertility, 127
  seminal emission, 178
Zhiyin (B67)
  abnormal fetal position, 3
  cystitis, 60
  dysmenorrhoea, 71
  furunculosis, 89
  haemorrhoids, 101
  prostatitis, 165
  urinary stones, 197
Zhizheng (SI7)
  flat wart, 88
Zhongchong (P9)
  jue syndrome, 118, 120
Zhongfu (L1)
  bronchial asthma, 30
  chronic bronchitis, 46
Zhongji (Ren3)
  alcohol withdrawal, 13
  amenorrhoea, 18
  cholecystitis, 43
  cholelithiasis, 44
  chronic pelvic inflammatory disease,
    50
  cutaneous pruritus, 57
  cystitis, 60
  eczema, 73
  female infertility, 87
  hysteria, 111
  impotence, 112
  leukorrhagia, 121
  male infertility, 127
  obesity, 145
  prostatitis, 164
  urinary retention, 171, 172
  urinary stones, 197
  wei syndrome, 204
Zhongkui (Ex3), 219
Zhongquan (Ex10), 220

Zhongwan (Ren12)
  acute intestinal obstruction, 7, 8
  alcohol withdrawal, 13
  amenorrhoea, 18
  angina pectoris, 20
  appendicitis, 21
  arrhythmia, 23
  bacillary dysentery, 24
  bi syndrome, 27
  bronchial asthma, 30
  cerebrovascular accident sequelae,
    181
  childhood anorexia, 39
  cholecystitis, 43
  cholelithiasis, 44
  chronic bronchitis, 46, 47
  chronic diarrhoea, 48
  cystic hyperplasia of the breast,
    58–9
  cystitis, 60
  diabetes mellitus, 63
  dian syndrome, 64, 65
  drug withdrawal, 66, 67
  epilepsy, 78, 79
  gastritis, 91, 92
  gastrointestinal neurosis, 93
  gastroptosis, 95
  headache, 99
  hearing loss, 191
  hiccups, 104
  hypertension, 107
  hyperthyroidism, 109
  hysteria, 111
  impotence, 112
  influenza, 114
  insufficient lactation, 116
  jue syndrome, 119
  kuang syndrome, 65
  malaria, 125
  Meniere's disease, 129
  menopausal syndrome, 131
  morning sickness, 132, 133
  myocarditis, 136
  neurosism, 142
  obesity, 145
  otitis media suppurativa, 146
  pancreatitis, 148
  Parkinson's disease, 151
  peptic ulcer, 153, 154
  pharyngeal paraesthesia, 157
  premenstrual syndrome, 161
  tinnitus, 191
  tobacco withdrawal, 192
  urticaria, 199
  vomiting, 201
  wei syndrome, 204
Zhongzhu (SJ3)
  acute soft tissue injury, 10
  flat wart, 88
  hearing loss, 190
  kuang syndrome, 65

  otitis media suppurativa, 146
  peripheral facial paralysis, 155
  scapulohumeral periarthritis, 173
  stiff neck, 183
  thecal cyst, 187
  tinnitus, 190
Zhoujian (Ex13), 221
Zhouliao (LI12)
  external humeral epicondylitis, 83
Zigongxue (Ex45), 225
  dysfunctional uterine bleeding, 70
  female infertility, 87
  habitual miscarriage, 97
  uterine prolapse, 163
Zulinqi (G41)
  cystic hyperplasia of the breast, 58
  headache, 99
  hypertension, 107
  hyperthyroidism, 109
  Meniere's disease, 129
  neurosism, 142
  otitis media suppurativa, 146
Zusanli (S36)
  acne vulgaris, 4
  acute gastroenteritis, 5
  acute intestinal obstruction, 7
  acute mastitis, 9
  alcohol withdrawal, 13
  allergic rhinitis, 14, 15
  alopecia areata, 16
  amenorrhoea, 18
  angina pectoris, 20
  appendicitis, 21
  arrhythmia, 23
  bacillary dysentery, 25
  bi syndrome, 27
  brandy nose, 29
  bronchial asthma, 30, 32
  cardiac neurosis, 34
  central retinitis, 35
  cerebrovascular accident sequelae,
    180, 181
  cervical spondylopathy, 37
  childhood anorexia, 39
  childhood hyperkinetic syndrome,
    40
  cholecystitis, 43
  cholelithiasis, 44, 45
  chronic bronchitis, 46
  chronic diarrhoea, 48
  chronic pharyngitis, 51, 52
  competition syndrome, 52
  constipation, 54
  cutaneous pruritus, 57
  cystic hyperplasia of the breast, 58
  developmental disability, 61
  diabetes mellitus, 63
  dian syndrome, 64
  drug withdrawal, 66, 67
  dysfunctional uterine bleeding, 70
  eczema, 73

  epilepsy, 78, 79
  erythromelalgia, 82
  facial spasm, 85
  female infertility, 87
  gastritis, 91
  gastrointestinal neurosis, 93
  gastroptosis, 95
  habitual miscarriage, 97
  haemorrhoids, 101
  headache, 99
  hearing loss, 191
  herpes zoster, 103
  hiccups, 104
  hypertension, 107
  hyperthyroidism, 109
  hysteria, 110, 111
  impotence, 112
  influenza, 114
  insufficient lactation, 116
  jue syndrome, 119
  leukorrhagia, 121
  lochiorrhagia, 122
  malaria, 125
  male infertility, 127
  Meniere's disease, 129
  menopausal syndrome, 131
  morning sickness, 132, 133
  myocarditis, 136
  myopia, 137
  neurodermatitis, 140
  neurosism, 142
  nocturnal enuresis, 144
  obesity, 145
  otitis media suppurativa, 146
  pancreatitis, 148
  Parkinson's disease, 151
  peptic ulcer, 153, 154
  pharyngeal paraesthesia, 157
  postpartum uterine contractions, 160
  premenstrual syndrome, 161
  prostatitis, 165
  ptosis, 166
  Raynaud's disease, 166
  sciatica, 175
  seborrhoeic dermatitis, 176
  temporomandibular joint dysfunction,
    68
  thecal cyst, 187
  thromboangiitis obliterans, 188
  tinnitus, 191
  tobacco withdrawal, 192
  trigeminal neuralgia, 195
  urinary stones, 197
  urticaria, 199
  uterine prolapse, 163
  vomiting, 201, 202
  wei syndrome, 203, 204
Zutonggu (B66)
  bi syndrome, 27
Zuxiaojie (Ex54), 226
  acute soft tissue injury, 10